Emergence and Control of Zoonotic Ortho- and Paramyxovirus Diseases

John Libbey Eurotext
127, avenue de la République
92120 Montrouge
Tél.: 33 (0) 1 46 73 06 60
e-mail: contact@john-libbey-eurotext.fr
http://www.john-libbey-eurotext.fr

John Libbey and Company Ltd
Collier House,
163-169 Brompton Road, Knightsbridge
London SW3 1 PY, England
Tel.: 44 (0) 20 75 81 24 49

CIC Edizioni Internazionali
Corso Trieste 42
00198 Roma, Italia
Tel.: 39 06 841 26 73

ISBN: 2-7420-0408-4

Emergence and Control of Zoonotic Ortho- and Paramyxovirus Diseases

Symposium Proceedings
13-15 December 2000

Editors:
Betty Dodet,
Marissa Vicari

John Libbey EUROTEXT

Contents

Paramyxoviruses

Emergence and Control of Zoonotic Ortho- and Paramyxovirus Diseases
B. Dodet, M. Vicari, eds.

Foreword

Researchers continue to identify micro-organisms that provoke new diseases in humans. In the emergence of these diseases an essential factor is the role played by animals, which act as a reservoir for certain viruses, capable, under favourable conditions, of infecting humans or crossing the species barrier.

The third symposium on emerging diseases organised by the Mérieux Foundation in December, 2000, was devoted to two families of viruses, *Orthomyxoviridae* and *Paramyxoviridae* which infect numerous species of vertebrates and are responsible for various zoonoses:

Orthomyxoviruses are mostly known as influenza, or flu, viruses. Their global impact on public health is considerable. Influenza has been known since antiquity but it continues to re-emerge as a result of genetic mutations or reorganisations, and is at the origin of seasonal epidemics and pandemics which can be very deadly.

Paramyxoviruses infect numerous animal species. In humans, they are responsible for several flu-like respiratory syndromes. However, new paramyxoviruses of the *Henipavirus* genus emerged in the 1990's with the appearance of severe encephalitis and raised mortality rates in humans.

Opening the symposium, Peter Daszak spoke of phases of emergence of diseases throughout the history of mankind, underlining the role of environmental disruptions, especially those due to the intervention of man. His presentation is reported on page 1.

The first part of this work is devoted to influenza: the ecology of influenza viruses, wild, aquatic birds as the principal reservoir, the role of domestic aquatic birds and farm animals; epidemiology of the flu in various animals species and genetic evolution of the virus. Methods of fighting the risk of pandemics are also discussed, focusing on the example of recent alerts; updating and production of vaccines in urgent situations, and the utilisation of antivirals.

The second part is dedicated to *Paramyxoviridae*. It begins with an overview of the evolution of the epidemiology of paramyxovirus diseases in various animal species (terrestrial carnivores and aquatic mammals). A large section is reserved for emerging henipaviruses and their etiology, showing that bats play an important role in the natural cycle of these viruses: Hendra virus, responsible for encephalitis in horses and humans in Australia since 1994, and Nipah virus, responsible for the encephalitis epidemic that hit the pork farmers of Malaysia in 1998. Nipah virus is currently under study, notably at the BSL4 Jean Mérieux Laboratory in Lyon. This was one of the last projects of Dr. Charles Mérieux, who dedicated his life to the fight against infectious diseases and to their prevention, and who died in January 2001. We would like to express our sincere appreciation in dedicating this work to him.

Betty Dodet
Scientific Director
Fondation Mérieux

Emergence and Control of Zoonotic Ortho- and Paramyxovirus Diseases
B. Dodet, M. Vicari, eds.

Viral emergence in the human-wildlife continuum

Peter Daszak[1, 2], Andrew A. Cunningham[2], Alex D. Hyatt[3]
[1] *Consortium for Conservation Medicine, LDEO, New York, USA*
[2] *Institute of Zoology, Zoological Society of London, London, UK*
[3] *Australian Animal Health Laboratory, CSIRO, Victoria 3220, Australia*

Ecology, evolution and the five phases of disease emergence

The emergence of a number of key infectious diseases over the past two decades has fostered a quiet revolution in our approach to infectious disease research, surveillance and control. This revolution began in the 1980s, partly in response to decreased funding for surveillance programs [1, 2], but largely following the emergence of antibiotic resistant microbes, AIDS and a number of other novel diseases [3, 4]. Now, almost ten years after the publication of the Institute of Medicines report on emerging infections [5], we understand a great deal about the demographic factors that drive this phenomenon and have become proficient in rapidly responding to emergence events [6-8]. However, diseases continue to emerge: pandemic influenza remains a key threat to developed countries [9]; urbanization in the tropics continues to throw up outbreaks of dengue hemorrhagic fever and a host of other emerging infectious diseases (EIDs) [8]; an Old World pathogen, West Nile virus, recently emerged in the New World, amid great public concern [10]; and the latter half of the 1990s has seen the emergence of three new paramyxovirus diseases in Australia and South-East Asia [11, 12].

Emergence is a complex process that essentially involves interactions between host, pathogen and environment. Ultimately, disease emergence is driven by ecological changes that are almost entirely a product of human alteration of the environment [13-15]. These act within a background of pathogen biodiversity, to favor the transmission of (or, in evolutionary terms, select for) those pathogens most suited to the altered environmental conditions. Thus, in simple terms, the emergence of Lyme disease in the USA was driven by a shift in agriculture (an anthropogenic environmental change) and reforestation of the North-Eastern USA, increased deer and white-footed mouse populations and increased transmission of *Borrelia burgdorferi* to humans living in close proximity to this changed habitat [16]. The complexity of disease emergence arises from interaction between an array of ecological changes, a diverse assemblage of microbes and complex interrelations between host populations. For Lyme disease, this complexity means that population cycles of the introduced gypsy moth (the larvae of which browse on oak foliage) are predictors for disease risk in humans [17], since defoliation causes cycles in the abundance of oak mast and the white-footed deermouse on which *Ixodes* ticks feed.

The environmental changes that drive emergence include global changes in demography, technology and behaviour (*e.g.* urbanization, air travel, agricultural intensification) that have been discussed previously [4, 5, 18]. In addition, a number of less well-understood anthropogenic impacts such as global climate change, biodiversity loss, fragmentation of wildlife habitat, pollution and, in some cases, natural (or non-human mediated) environmental oscillations such as El Nino Southern Oscillation confound this process. Microbial diversity is enhanced by the unique mutation rates of some microbes (*e.g.* RNA virus "quasispecies"), the ability of others to reassort genetic elements of different strains to produce new levels of virulence (*e.g.* influenza virus) and the sheer magnitude of a pool of known and unknown zoonotic agents, some of which may have the potential to jump into new host species [19]. Zoonotic disease emergence is, in turn, influenced by interactions between three key populations: humans, their domesticated animals and wildlife. These populations exist within a host-pathogen ecological continuum; sharing pathogens, habitats, ecology and environment, and ultimately sharing the environmental changes that drive disease emergence [20].

The importance of anthropogenic environmental change in the emergence of EIDs can be traced back through human history to reveal five phases of disease emergence (here we define "emergence" according to the IOM and other key references – see [20]). Each phase involves a shift of ecology and environment that changes host-pathogen dynamics or allows clashes between previously isolated host populations and their pathogens. Three phases are well-known. In the first, the emergence of a range of pathogenic diseases coincided with the development of increasingly close relationships with domestic animals [21]. Some human pathogens, *e.g.* measles virus, likely evolved from ancestral domestic animal pathogens (rinderpest, or a rinderpest-like ancestor) [22]. Second, the aggregation of humans into large, dense city populations was a key ecological event, producing the conditions required for outbreaks of diseases such as cholera, typhoid and plague, and allowing human populations to rise above threshold densities for pathogen endemicity, resulting in the persistence of newly emerged diseases such as measles and smallpox [21].

The third phase of human-mediated infectious disease emergence began in the late 15th century as Europeans colonized the globe. Here, diseases such as measles increased the competitive edge of invading Europeans over the immunologically naive endemic peoples, leading to extreme depopulation rates, and the virtual extinction of some New World tribes [23]. These events were essentially the origins of globalization, and have been followed by continual expansion of global trade and human, domestic animal and wildlife populations. This phase mirrors an hypothesized natural, prehistoric, phase of disease emergence in animals (and, presumably, plants). As land bridges formed throughout prehistory, previously isolated populations of animals (and their pathogens) must have made contact for the first time, and emergence followed. Such a scenario has been proposed to explain a number of extinction events following land-bridge formation, culminating in a series of Pleistocene megafaunal extinctions. These Pleistocene extinctions coincided with the expansion of human populations across the Beringean land bridge into North America, and in other parts of the globe. Introduction of a pathogenic agent into these naive populations by either humans or associated animals has been hypothesized as a cause of these extinctions [24]. Current research is using new "ancient DNA" technology to identify viral elements in well-preserved carcasses from these extinction events.

The most recent, fourth, phase of anthropogenic disease emergence encompasses the events of the last few decades; the emergence of new diseases such as post-antibiotic multi-drug resistant tuberculosis, hantavirus pulmonary syndrome and variant Creutzfeldt-Jakob disease (CJD). These are driven by unparalleled changes in technology, agriculture, and demography that allow rapid dissemination of new viral strains, increased opportunity for transmission of foodborne illnesses, and selection of antibiotic resistant microbes [5].

We can hypothesize a further phase of anthropogenic disease emergence which threatens to become significant in the future. As human populations expand and increasing pressure is placed on the last remaining areas of wilderness, we predict the increasing importance of emergence due to encroachment. Encroachment exposes a now "globalized" population of humans and domestic animals to the zoonotic pool of known and unknown pathogens. Such encroachment has driven emergence of classical zoonoses (*e.g.* Nipah virus disease), or zoonoses defined in a broader sense to include agents that have recently evolved from wildlife pathogens following host jumps (*e.g.* HIV).

The aim of the current paper is to discuss recent advances in our understanding of the roles wildlife populations and ecological changes play in disease emergence. We propose that understanding disease emergence, particularly in the current phase, requires an holistic, interdisciplinary approach that fuses medical, microbiological and veterinary research with recent advances in theoretical and experimental ecology, conservation biology and wildlife biology. This may be particularly applicable to ortho- and paramyxovirus emergence, which are intrinsically bound within the human-wildlife continuum.

Wildlife EIDs and pathogen pollution

Over the past few years a growing number of infectious disease outbreaks have been reported from wildlife populations. By following the same criteria that define EIDs in human populations many of these can be classed as emerging [20]. These wildlife EIDs have resulted in a series of mass mortalities, population declines and even extinctions in the last two decades. Wildlife EIDs include diseases caused by domestic animal pathogens such as canine distemper virus, responsible for mass mortality of African wild dogs and the near-extinction of the North American black-footed ferret. Plague, a disease that still remains enzootic in North America following the last great pandemic in the 1860s, causes mortality rates as high as 98% in prairie dogs during cyclical outbreaks, and was a significant factor in the initial demise of the last wild black-footed ferret population [25]. A group of newly described morbilliviruses have emerged as significant causes of mortality in marine mammals, along with a range of marine EIDs, including diseases of hard and soft corals, fibropapillomatosis of sea turtles and others [26]. New infections of garden birds such as mycoplasmal conjunctivitis in house finches in the USA and salmonellosis in passerines in the UK have emerged apparently as a product of the artificially high density and rate of interspecies contact that backyard feeders foster [27, 28]. Less well-known diseases such as kangaroo blindness (caused by an orbivirus), or pilchard herpesvirus disease, have emerged over large areas, causing extensive wildlife mortality [29, 30]. Endangered species in captive breeding programs can be particularly hard hit by wildlife EIDs, especially where allopatric, closely related hosts are mixed [31]. Such interspecies transmission has led to the death of Asian elephants in captivity following infection by a herpesvirus originating as a non-pathogenic infection of African elephants [32]. Of particular interest is a recently discovered fungal disease of amphibians, cutaneous chytridiomycosis, that has been implicated in a global series of multi-species population declines and extinctions previously hypothesized to be a symptom of global climate change or ozone depletion [33, 34]. Wildlife EIDs are expanding in impact, geographic range or moving into new host populations on a global scale, causing mass mortality events and population declines that appear to be unsustainable in the long term. What are the factors driving these events, and why are they emerging now?

Firstly, we must ascertain if these events are a byproduct of increased surveillance. There has undoubtedly been a growing interest in wildlife disease following advances in our understanding of the role parasites and pathogens play in the population biology of wild animals [35]. However, there is little doubt that such noticeable mass mortalities as recent die-offs of seals, porpoises and dolphins are a novel phenomenon. Similarly, even though disease was not thought to be a cause of amphibian population declines until recently, these declines were noticed by ecologists simultaneously in Australia and the New World, suggesting a recent phenomenon. Finally, a number of wildlife diseases have clinical signs that are noticeable by the public, such as the haemorrhaging and ulcers associated with a new ranavirus disease of European amphibians [36] and the swollen eyelids associated with songbird mycoplasmal conjunctivitis [28]. The obvious clinical signs and unsustainability of these events support a recent emergence hypothesis, since if they had been longterm phenomena, diseased animals and mass mortalities would likely have been reported earlier.

Our recent analysis of the underlying causes of wildlife EIDs suggests two interrelated factors that appear to have driven emergence in the majority of cases: spill-over from domestic animal hosts and "pathogen pollution". Spill-over is responsible for a number of wildlife EIDs. Canine parvovirus, reported from wolves in America; sarcoptic mange, which has spread throughout fox populations in Europe and wombats in Australia; canine distemper, which has emerged in the endangered black-footed ferret, African wild dogs and lions. Spill-over of pathogens from large domestic animal reservoir populations is a particular threat to small or fragmented populations of wild animals. For example, the large reservoir of domesticated dogs in the Serengeti, Africa, is thought to have led to repeated outbreaks of canine distemper and rabies in African wild dogs. The continued presence of domestic dogs raises the overall population above the threshold density for enzootic transmission. The result is continual transmission to small, fragmented wild dog populations, and local extinctions of this species, as recently occurred in the Serengeti [37]. Spill-over events are a subset of a much more significant cause of disease emergence – the anthropogenic introduction of pathogens (often with their introduced hosts) into new geographic regions, termed pathogen pollution [20]. Pathogen pollution is thought to have driven the emergence of red squirrel poxvirus disease and crayfish plague in the UK, diseases which may have been introduced with their respective North American host species [38, 39]. Introduction of salmonid fish infected with whirling disease has devastated populations of farmed and wild salmonid fish throughout Europe and now North America [40]. Mycoplasmal infections in North American tortoises are thought to have originated from infected captive individuals released into the environment without disease screening [41].

Pathogen pollution has a particularly high impact on immunologically naive populations. Thus, the introduction of exotic birds infected by avian pox and avian malaria into Hawaii during early European colonization, along with the *Culex* mosquito vector for these diseases in 1826, is thought to have led to extinction of a third of the endemic bird fauna [42]. These threats continue. Toxoplasmosis, a disease that requires cats for completion of its life cycle, has been introduced onto Hawaii and threatens the remnant populations of a number of endemic birds [43]. In some cases of host-pathogen co-introduction, the higher impact of the introduced pathogen on endemic populations increases the competitive advantage of the invader in a process known as apparent competition [44]. Thus, the parapox virus currently emerging in UK red squirrels appears to be a co-evolved pathogen of introduced grey squirrels, which have expanded throughout the UK, usurping the native species [39].

Pathogen pollution is a form of global anthropogenic environmental change that may rival chemical pollution in its insidious effects on ecosystems, its rapid dissemination and its global nature. Its roots lie in the globalization of trade and transport of wild animals and their products (for pets, hunting, food or conservation). For example, translocation of rabies-infected raccoons by hunters in the late 1970s led to re-emergence of this disease as a threat to human health in the USA [45]. Outbreaks of pilchard herpesvirus disease off the coast of Australia cost the economy over A$12 million. The source of infection is thought to be importation of frozen mixed by-catch (bait fish that includes pilchards) to feed farmed tuna or discharge of pathogen-contaminated ballast water [30]. Because of the hidden nature of pathogen pollution, introduced diseases occur in remote regions thought to be beyond human influence. For example, *Salmonella* of potentially human origin and antibodies to infectious bursal disease virus (a poultry pathogen) have been reported in Antarctic penguins [46, 47]. The presumed source is inadequately disposed food waste from previous Antarctic expeditions and subsequent transmission throughout the native avian population. Outbreaks of canine distemper, a disease of domestic dogs, have been reported in crabeater seals and a Siberian seal, possibly due to contact with sledge dogs on previous expeditions [48, 49]. More recently, canine distemper has been identified as the cause of mass mortalities of Caspian seals [50]. The exponential growth in international trade, development of new technologies and opening of new markets continue to bring exotic pathogens into contact with new host populations. Such events, when viewed individually, appear of moderate impact, such as the recent discovery of influenza A in farmed ostriches, a relatively new livestock industry that has recently expanded worldwide [51]. However, when viewed together, these new forms of pathogen pollution represent serious risks to human and wildlife health. For example, dumping of ballast water from ocean-going ships in foreign harbours is a well-recognized source of invasive species. Recently, pathogenic strains of *Vibrio cholerae* were detected in ballast water from an ocean-going vessel [52]. Pathogen movement from humans to wildlife represents another form of public health threat. Influenza B virus has recently been isolated from naturally-infected Dutch harbour seals [53]. Sequence analyses and serology suggest that this is a strain that circulated in humans 4 to 5 years earlier, and therefore is a direct health threat to humans. Pathogen pollution *via* deposition of runoff and sewage effluent may be increasing threats to marine wildlife. Toxoplasmosis and soil-borne pathogens such as *Coccidioides immitis* have been described from marine mammals and the impact of *Aspergillus sydowii* on sea fans has been particularly high [54]. International air travel continues to grow, bringing with it new disease risks, such as the recent outbreak of West Nile virus disease in New York [10]. Global air travel volume doubled between 1985 and 1996 and the number of new routes offered has increased in direct proportion to this growth [55]. Projections suggest this trend will continue as countries put an annually higher share of their gross domestic product into international air travel, both for human transport and movement of produce.

Our understanding of disease introduction events may benefit from recent advances in ecology. The past decade has seen a boost in research into the ecology and impact on ecosystems of invasive species, a group that is gaining recognition as serious threat to ecosystem stability [56, 57]. These have focused on a series of devastating events such as the introduction of the brown tree snake to Guam that has resulted in the almost complete extinction of its avian fauna. Pathogen pollution is the disease equivalent of biological invasions. It follows that the impact of wildlife infectious disease emergence on populations may also be greater than previously recognized. Wildlife EIDs have led to mass mortality, population declines, local and species extinctions [15, 20, 58]. Data on the size of epizootic mass mortalities in wildlife populations are rare, but often significant. For example, in 1988, an outbreak of phocid distemper virus in seals led to over 17,000 deaths. Epizootic amphibian chytridiomycosis has led to complete removal of multi-species amphibian assemblages (local extinction) throughout Central and North America and Australia. In Australia, the disease probably caused the global extinction of at least one species and possibly of at least two others. Wildlife infectious disease emergence, in particular that caused by pathogen pollution, is an especially important consideration for animals translocated for captive breeding and reintroduction programs [31]. A growing number of species maintained solely in captivity (*e.g.* the Guam rail, a number of *Partula* spp. snails and Rothschilds mynah) are at particular risk from disease emergence. These animals are usually maintained in close proximity to allopatric species and their pathogens. The only definitively proven example of extinction of a species by an infectious agent was a species of Polynesian tree snail, *Partula turgida*, kept solely in captivity that died out in 1996, following an outbreak of microsporidiosis [59].

Zoonoses and new threats to wildlife populations: conservation biology meets public health?

There is a distinct zoonotic skew in the diseases that have recently emerged in humans. Analysis suggests that of 1,709 infectious organisms pathogenic to humans, 49% are zoonotic (*i.e.* can be transmitted from animals to humans), whereas of the 156 considered "emerging", 73% are zoonotic [60]. Thus, zoonotic pathogens are over three times more likely to be emerging than non-zoonotic microbes. If we take a less strict view of the definition of zoonosis and include microbes that have recently shifted hosts from wildlife to humans (*e.g.* HIV-1 and HIV-2, [61]), or microbes that have been demonstrated transmissible to animals in captivity or under other unusual conditions (*e.g. M. tuberculosis*, identified in captive elephants, [62]) the zoonotic skew is even more dramatic. In classical zoonoses, wildlife populations act as pathogen reservoirs, but are themselves largely unaffected. There are some obvious exceptions to this rule. The recent outbreak of West Nile virus in New York resulted in the mortality of many thousands of wild birds and of a range of captive exotic species at the zoological gardens in New York [63]. This link has proved useful for surveillance because the outbreak in humans (a dead-end host) usually follows avian die-offs.

The emergence of pathogens that cause no or few clinical signs in their wildlife reservoirs may be more difficult to detect, or predict. Murphy [8] commented on this problem, suggesting that the solution is rapid response to emergence events, followed up by detailed, collaborative investigations. It appears that this unpredictability arises in part due to the range of anthropogenic factors that act in synchrony with encroachment to drive emergence. This situation has occurred three times recently with the emergence of Hendra virus and Menangle virus in Australia and Nipah virus in Malaysia and Singapore [12, 64-66]. These viruses belonging to the family *Paramyxoviridae* share a common biological characteristic in that they all emerged from fruitbat reservoirs belonging to the family Pteropodidae (also known as flying foxes) and are amplified in domestic animal hosts such as horses (for Hendra virus – suggested genus *Henipavirus*, subfamily *Paramyxovirus*) and pigs (for Menangle virus – genus *Rubulavirus*, subfamily *Paramyxovirus*; and for Nipah virus – suggested genus *Henipavirus*, subfamily *Paramyxovirus*). The emergence of Hendra virus and Nipah virus in particular is of great concern to public health. They are lethal to humans, and the isolation of a further virus, Tioman virus (genus *Rubulavirus* within the subfamily *Paramyxovirus*), in a fruitbat reservoir suggests that related viruses await discovery. Predicting emergence is difficult due to limited data on the mode of transmission between bats and domestic animals. Evidence to date indicates a close relationship between fruitbats and piggeries where diseases associated with Nipah and Menangle viruses occur. For Nipah virus, it appears that emergence is a product of encroachment of both humans and intensively farmed pigs into wildlife (fruitbat) habitat. The isolation of Nipah virus from bat urine (Chua, personnal communication) suggests that co-habitation between bats and pigs could be the key to emergence. Infection within high density pig populations generates high viral loads (including those of respiratory origin), resulting in rapid dissemination of the virus between pigs and human "handlers". Movement of pigs to other geographic regions may have increased the efficiency of the spread. The mode of transmission of Hendra virus between fruitbats and horses is more obscure as Hendra virus appears not to be highly contagious and has only been isolated from the uterine fluids of bats [67] and the urine of experimentally infected horses [68]. There are a number of considerations that increase the complexity of predicting future emergence of either these, or other unknown viruses (*e.g.* Tioman and others) within fruit bat reservoirs. First, the presence of antibodies to Nipah virus in five bat species suggests that modeling emergence may be difficult since each reservoir host is likely to have different ecological and behavioural patterns. Secondly, the finding of another novel paramyxovirus (Tioman virus) in a relatively small survey of a fruit bat population suggests that many more viruses exist that have the potential to emerge. Third, encroachment, habitat destruction (*e.g.* deforestation) and exploitation for food add unpredictable dimensions to fruitbat ecology, and therefore the ecology of their viruses. Finally, extending the hypothesis that fruitbats harbour a high diversity of known viruses (*e.g.* Hendra, Menangle, Nipah and Australian bat lyssavirus) and probably unknown viruses suggests they may represent a more widespread threat to human and veterinary health than previously thought. Fruitbats are key colonizers of oceanic islands in the Pacific and Indian Oceans. In many cases, they are the only mammals to have naturally colonized islands. Even the youngest archipelagos are many millions of years old, and earlier colonization by fruitbats has led the evolution of a diverse group of fruitbat species, each localized to single oceanic islands or small groups of islands (*i.e.* island endemics). If the initial colonizers of these islands were infected by viruses, it is possible that extended periods of co-evolution in isolation has led to a greater increase in virus diversity within the families *Paramyxoviridae* and *Rhabdoviridae* to name but two. If emergence of these putative island viruses requires intensively-farmed domesticated animal amplifier hosts, then island emergence may occur as island economies expand. Clearly, a focused biodiversity survey of fruitbat viruses will be a key step forward. Unraveling the complexity of emergence of these viruses may have greater lessons since chain events leading to emergence are not unique to the paramyxoviruses. Ebola virus has also been hypothesized to emerge *via* a chain event [69]. The reservoir is still unknown, but chimpanzees could be viewed as amplifiers, or intermediates, between the wildlife reservoir and the human population. Finally, chain events are thought to be crucial to the emergence of pandemic influenza which follows reassortment of avian and human virus gene segments in a pig host [9].

Anthropogenic factors such as habitat loss, pollution, habitat fragmentation, loss of biodiversity, overexploitation, encroachment, climate change and introduction of invasive species directly affect wildlife populations, significantly altering the species complement, often removing some species entirely (*e.g.* niche specialists, those with small populations, low fecundity species or top predators) and forcing communities so that they resemble those in early stages of succession [35]. These population changes are likely to affect parasite ecology and in some cases drive disease emergence. The impact of these "new" environmental changes on wildlife populations has been the subject of a great deal of research in ecology and conservation biology fields (*e.g.* theoretical and experimental studies of biological invasions) that may be directly applicable to understanding disease emergence. There is growing evidence that these new anthropogenic factors play a significant role in emergence. For example, an outbreak of phocine distemper in European harbour seals may have resulted from forced migration of enzootically-infected harp seals from Greenland, following overfishing by humans in those waters [70]. Deforestation led to the emergence of Mayaro and Oropouche viruses in Brazilian woodcutters as a result of expansion into isolated ecosystems [8]. In a more subtle way, anthropogenic fragmentation of wildlife habitat may lead to disease emergence by reducing patch size. Patch size is directly related to species diversity, and if habitat fragmentation favours the emergence of key reservoir species over other less-efficient reservoirs, emergence may follow. Recent work by Ostfeld and Keesing [71] has provided initial data that suggest reservoir biodiversity is related to Lyme disease risk. In the case of Lyme disease, they demonstrate a "dilution effect", whereby increasing diversity of reservoir species with low competence lowers the influence of competent reservoirs on disease transmission [72]. Extrapolation from these studies supports a prediction that anthropogenic fragmentation or biodiversity loss may influence emergence of a wide range of vector-borne diseases [73]. The role of chemical pollution in disease emergence is also in the early stages of investigation. A current debate concerning the potential role of PCB residues in marine mammal morbillivirus emergence remains unresolved, but preliminary experimental data suggest a link [74]. Similar debates underlie increasing awareness of the potential role of global anthropogenic climate change in driving disease emergence, particularly those transmitted by vectors whose life cycles are greatly influenced by climate [75, 76].

The zoonotic potential of human interactions with wildlife has led to conflict between public health concerns and conservation strategies. For example, brucellosis was introduced into North America with infected domestic cattle during early colonization and, in an early example of pathogen pollution, infected native bison. The disease has now been eradicated from ranched cattle, but persists in bison where it threatens to spill back into domestic herds [77]. The clash between conservationists and ranchers is highly politicized with bison that leave national park boundaries for ranchland being shot on a regular basis. Zoonotic reservoirs of disease are selectively exterminated in the UK (*e.g.* badgers, which are thought to be reservoirs of tuberculosis) and the USA (*e.g.* prairie dogs, which can harbour *Yersinia pestis*). As human and domestic animal populations continue to expand and encroach into natural habitats, these problems are likely to become more numerous and complex. For example, the Southern elephant seal was once hunted to near extinction in the Eastern seaboard of the USA. Its legal protection as an endangered species has allowed its population to expand back into its former range. Brownell *et al.* [78] recently suggested that recent eradication of natural predators in California will lead to further, artificial range expansion, close contact with domestic animals and the risk of disease emergence. The conservationists dilemma is whether to prevent future beaching to reduce the risk of disease emergence, or remove the contact with domestic animals [79]. Ecotourism has become an increasingly important form of conservation. This pragmatic approach of raising tourist revenue while, at the same time, increasing public awareness of wildlife conservation, has been so successful that the United Nations has designated 2002 as the Year of Ecotourism [80]. However, ecotourism raises a novel EID problem: the transmission of pathogens of humans to endangered wildlife. Repeated outbreaks of respiratory infections in habituated chimps in the Gombe National Park, Tanzania [81], and of intestinal parasites of probable human origin in habituated mountain gorillas [82] have led to an interventionist approach. An epizootic of respiratory disease with six deaths in habituated mountain gorillas in Rwanda, and serological and pathological evidence of measles virus led to mass vaccination of gorillas against measles virus [83]. A series of outbreaks of a paralytic disease in habituated chimpanzees at Gombe led to mass vaccination of chimpanzees against poliovirus [81]. Contact between ecotourists and endangered species is likely to increase in the future, bringing a real possibility of introduction of virulent pathogens into naive wildlife populations and potentially devastating depopulation. The threats are significant: in a survey of 43 tourists viewing apes in Uganda, evidence of active herpesvirus infection, influenza, tuberculosis and chicken pox were detected [84].

Conservation biologists have recently begun to discuss the concept of parasite conservation [*e.g.* 85]. Extinction of species with host-specific parasites is likely to lead to the loss of parasite biodiversity ("co-extinction", [86]) and parasite conservation measures have been proposed [87]. This raises interesting ethical issues, since parasites are the only group containing species for which internationally co-ordinated, global eradication programmes exist (*e.g.* the WHO programmes for eradication of smallpox, polio and riverblindness). Agents of these diseases may become the first living organisms wilfully forced into extinction by humans. Ethical arguments for the conservation of smallpox are unlikely to guide policy. However, conservation of parasites of endangered species may have practical advantages for the maintenance of host immunity in captive-bred animals destined for release into the wild [88].

New initiatives, new challenges: conservation medicine and a broader view of disease emergence

We have outlined some of the ecological aspects of disease emergence that demonstrate commonalities underlying this complex process. Humans, wildlife and domestic animals exist within a continuum of habitat, environment and pathogens. Disease emergence across these populations is essentially driven by different forms of the same anthropogenic environmental changes that act within a background of microbial diversity. The complexity of this process and of the resulting threats to public health and conservation suggests that integration across disciplines will become increasingly important in understanding EIDs. In many ways, this is a return to an earlier approach described by Murphy [8], whereby disease emergence is investigated by a large research community skilled in diverse fields (*e.g.* entomology, ecology, mammalogy and virology) and adopting a holistic perspective to understanding emergence. The time appears to be ripe for a fusion of diverse disciplines and a new approach to emergence. There is increasing interest in the impact on disease dynamics of less well-understood environmental changes such as biodiversity loss, habitat fragmentation, climate change and others. This approach has begun, and will continue, to integrate ecology and conservation biology into the microbiological sciences. Theoretical advances in wildlife diseases (*e.g.* Modeling) have led to important experimental demonstrations of the role of infections in population biology. Advances in our understanding of biological invasions can be directly applied to disease emergence [56, 57]. For example, it has been demonstrated that biodiverse environments are more able to resist invasion [89]. Can this be extrapolated to disease introduction events? Are populations with more biodiverse pathogen assemblages more resistant to invasion? While this may seem a difficult connection, a recent hypothesis on the origin of *Salmonella enteritidis* as an EID suggests that emergence was a cross-species invasion event [90]. The key to emergence is suggested to be antibiotic prophylaxis in the poultry industry that led to removal of *S. gallinarum* and *S. pullorum* during the 1960s and the exposure of a vacant niche in the gut, which was subsequently filled by *S. enteritidis*. These three pathogens share a common immunodominant surface antigen, therefore herd immunity prior to removal of the former two species would have prevented the latter from becoming established. Ecological research has demonstrated that habitat fragmentation leads to "edge effects" – the increased susceptibility of habitats to degredation as the proportion of habitat size that is unbuffered from outside influences increases. This may also be directly applicable to disease emergence since an increased proportion of edge exposure may increase contact with exotic pathogens.

Integrating diverse fields of biology may require new approaches and the development of new fields. One such approach is the developing field of "Conservation Medicine". The principal goals of conservation medicine are to investigate the relationship between environmental changes (such as habitat loss, pollution, fragmentation, encroachment) and both human and nonhuman animal health and to develop solutions to problems at the interface between environmental and health sciences [91]. This approach encompasses ecosystem health, human health as it relates to the global environment, and emerging diseases. In fact, the field of conservation medicine originated as a direct response to the complexity that underlies disease emergence [88]. This new field may not represent completely new concepts, but rather a fusion of disciplines under one umbrella that will act to promote a holistic view of disease emergence and to promote collaboration at the ground level by bringing medical and veterinary students into contact with ecologists, zoologists and conservation biologists.

Acknowledgements

P.D. is supported by a National Science Foundation IRCEB Grant (IBN#9977063) and Consortium for Conservation Medicine core funding from the V. Kann Rasmussen Foundation.

References

1. Krause RM. *The restless tide: the persistent challenge of the microbial world.* Washington DC: National foundation for infectious diseases; 1981.
2. Berkelman RL, Bryan RT, Osterholm, MT, LeDuc JW, Hughes JM. Infectious disease surveillance: a crumbling foundation. *Science* 1994; 264: 368-70.
3. Cohen ML. Epidemiology of drug resistance: implications for a post-antimicrobial era. *Science* 1992; 257: 1050-5.
4. Krause RM. The origins of plagues: old and new. *Science* 1992; 257: 1073-8.
5. Lederberg J, Shope RE, Oakes SC Jr. Emerging infections: microbial threats to health in the United States. Washington DC: Institute of Medicine, National Academy Press; 1992.
6. Mahy BWJ, Murphy FA. Emergence and re-emergence of viral infections. In: Mahy BWJ, Collier L, eds. *Topley & Wilson's Microbiology and Microbial Infections, Vol. 1: Virology.* London: Edward Arnold, 1997: 1011-25.
7. Binder S, Levitt AM, Sacks JJ, Hughes JM. Emerging infectious diseases: public health issues for the 21st century. *Science* 1999; 284: 1311-3.
8. Murphy FA. Emerging zoonoses. *Emerg Infect Dis* 1998; 4: 429-35.
9. Webster RG. Influenza: An emerging disease. *Emerg Infect Dis* 1998; 4: 436-41.
10. Lanciotti RS, Roehrig JT, Deubel V, Smith J, Parker M, Steele K, *et al.* Origin of the West Nile virus responsible for an outbreak of encephalitis in the northeastern United States. *Science* 1999; 286: 2333-7.
11. Mackenzie JS. Emerging viral diseases: an Australian perspective. *Emerg Infect Dis* 1999; 5: 1-8.
12. Chua KB, Bellini WJ, Rota PA, Harcourt BH, Tamin A, Lam SK, *et al.* Nipah virus: a recently emergent deadly paramyxovirus. *Science* 2000; 288: 1432-5.
13. Schrag SJ, Wiener P Emerging infectious diseases: what are the relative roles of ecology and evolution? *Trends Ecol Evol* 1995; 10: 319-24.
14. Garnett GP, Holmes EC The ecology of emergent infectious disease. *Biosci* 1996; 46: 127-35.
15. Daszak P, Cunningham AA, Hyatt AD. Anthropogenic environmental change and the emergence of infectious diseases in wildlife. *Acta Tropica* 2001; 78: 103-16.
16. Barbour AG, Fish D. The Biological and social phenomenon of Lyme disease. *Science* 1993; 260: 1610-6.
17. Jones CG, Ostfield RS, Richard MP, Schauber EM, Wolff JO. Chain reactions linking acorns to gypsy moth outbreaks and Lyme disease risk. *Science* 1998; 279: 1023-6.
18. Morse SS. Examining the origins of emerging viruses. In: Morse SS, ed. *Emerging Viruses.* New York: Oxford University Press, 1993: 10-28.
19. Morse SS. *Emerging Viruses.* New York: Oxford University Press, 1993.

20. Daszak P, Cunningham AA, Hyatt AD. Emerging infectious diseases of wildlife – threats to biodiversity and human health. *Science* 2000; 287: 443-9.
21. Dobson AP, Carper ER. Infectious diseases and human population history. *Bioscience* 1996; 46: 115-26.
22. Norrby E, Sheshbaeradaran H, McCullough, KC, Carpenter WC, Orvell C. Is rinderpest virus the archevirus of the Morbillivirus genus? *Intervirol* 1985; 23: 228-32.
23. Crosby AW. Ecological imperialism. The biological expansion of Europe, 900-1900. New York: Cambridge University Press, 1986.
24. MacPhee RDE, Marx PA. The 40,000 year plague: humans, hyperdisease, and first-contact extinctions. In: Goodman SM, Patterson BD, eds. *Natural change and human impact in Madagascar*. Washington DC: Smithsonian Institution Press, 1997: 169-217.
25. Thorne ET, Williams ES. Disease and endangered species: the black-footed ferret as a recent example. *Conserv Biol* 1988; 2: 66-74.
26. Harvell CD, Kim K, Burkholder JM, Colwell RR, Epstein PR, Grimes DJ, *et al.* Emerging marine diseases – climate links and anthropogenic factors. *Science* 1999; 285: 1505-10.
27. Kirkwood JK. Population density and infectious disease at bird tables. *Vet Rec* 1998; 142: 468.
28. Fischer JR, Stallknecht DE, Luttrell MP, Dhondt AA, Converse KA. Mycoplasmal conjunctivitis in wild songbirds: the spread of a new contagious disease in a mobile host population. *Emerg Infect Dis* 1997; 3: 69-72.
29. Hooper PT, Lunt RA, Gould AR, Hyatt AD, Russell GM, Kattenbelt JA, *et al.* Epidemic of blindness in kangaroos – evidence of a viral aetiology. *Austr Vet J* 1999; 77: 529-36.
30. Whittington RJ, Jones JB, Hine PM, Hyatt AD. Epizootic mortality in the pilchard Sardinops sagax neopilchardus in Australia and New Zealand in 1995. I. Pathology and epizootiology. *Dis Aquat Org* 1997; 28: 1-16.
31. Cunningham AA. Disease risks of wildlife translocations. *Conserv Biol* 1996; 10: 349-53.
32. Richman LK, Montali RJ, Garber RL, Kennedy MA, Lehnhardt J, Hildebrandt T, *et al.* Novel endotheliotropic herpesviruses fatal for Asian and African elephants. *Science* 1999; 283: 1171-6.
33. Berger L, Speare R, Daszak P, Green DE, Cunningham AA, Goggin CL, *et al.* Chytridiomycosis causes amphibian mortality associated with population declines in the rainforests of Australia and Central America. *Proc Natl Acad Sci USA* 1998; 95: 9031-6.
34. Daszak P, Berger L, Cunningham AA, Hyatt AD, Green DE, Speare R. Emerging infectious diseases and amphibian population declines. *Emerg Infect Dis* 1999; 5: 735-48.
35. Dobson AP, May RM. Disease and conservation. In: Soule M, ed. *Conservation biology: the science of scarcity and diversity*. Massachusetts: Sinauer Associates Inc, 1986: 345-65.
36. Cunningham AA, Langton TES, Bennett PM, Lewin JF, Drury SEN, Gough RE, *et al.* Pathological and microbiological findings from incidents of unusual mortality of the common frog Rana temporaria. *Phil Trans R Soc Lond B* 1996; 351: 1529-57.
37. Cleaveland S, Dye C. Maintenance of a microparasite infecting several host species: rabies in the Serengeti. *Parasitology* 1995; 111: S33-S47.
38. Alderman DJ. Geographical spread of bacterial and fungal diseases of crustaceans. *Rev Sci Tech Office Int Epizooties* 1996; 15: 603-32.
39. Sainsbury AW, Nettleton P, Gilray J, Gurnell J. Grey squirrels have high seroprevalence to a parapoxvirus associated with deaths in red squirrels. *Anim Conserv* 2000; 3: 229-33.
40. Hoffman GL. Intercontinental and transcontinental dissemination and transfaunation of fish parasites with emphasis on whirling disease *Myxosoma cerebralis*. In: Snieszko SF, ed. *Symposium on the diseases of fishes and shellfishes*. Washington DC: American Fisheries Society, 1970: 69-81.
41. Jacobson ER. Implications of infectious diseases for captive propagation and introduction programs of threatened/endangered reptiles. *J Zoo Wildl Med* 1993; 24: 245-55.
42. Warner RE. The role of introduced diseases in the extinction of the endemic Hawaiian avifauna. *Condor* 1968; 70: 101-20.
43. Work TM, Massey GM, Rideout BA, Gardiner CH, Ledig DB, Kwok OCH, *et al.* Fatal toxoplasmosis in free-ranging endangered'Alala from Hawaii. *J Widl Dis* 2000; 36: 205-12.
44. Hudson P, Greenman J. Competition mediated by parasites: biological and theoretical progress. *Trends Ecol Evol* 1998; 1310: 387-90.
45. Rupprecht CE, Smith JS, Fekadu M, Childs JE. The ascension of wildlife rabies: a cause for public health concern or intervention? *Emerg Infect Dis* 1995; 1: 107-14.
46. Gardner H, Kerry K, Riddle M, Brouwer S, Gleeson L. Poultry virus infection in Antarctic penguins. *Nature* 1997; 387: 245.

47. Olsen B, Bergstrom S, McCafferty DJ, Sellin M, Wistrom J. *Salmonella enteritidis* in Antarctica: zoonosis in man or humanosis in penguins? *Lancet* 1996; 348: 1319-20.
48. Mamaev LV, Denikina NN, Belikov SI, Volchkov VE, Visser IKG, Fleming M, *et al.* Characterization of morbilliviruses isolated from Lake Baikal seals *(Phoca sibirica)*. *Vet Microbiol* 1995; 44: 251-9.
49. Bengston JL, Boveng P, Franzen U, Have P, Heide-Jorgensen MP, Harkionen TJ. Antibodies to canine distemper virus in antarctic seals. *Mar Mamm Sci* 1991; 7: 85-7.
50. Kennedy S, Kuiken T, Jepson PD, Deaville R, Forsyth M, Barrett T, *et al.* Canine distemper virus identified as cause of recent mass mortality in Caspian seals *(Phoca caspica)*. *Emerg Infect Dis* 2000; 6: 637-9.
51. Alexander DJ, Brown IH. Recent zoonoses caused by influenza A viruses. *Rev Sci Tech OIE* 2000; 19: 197-225.
52. Ruiz GM, Rawlings TK, Dobbs FC, Drake LA, Mullady T, Huq A, *et al.* Global spread of microorganisms by ships. *Nature* 2000; 408: 49-50.
53. Osterhaus ADME, Rimmelzwaan GF, Martina BEE, Bestebroer TM, Fouchier RAM. Influenza B virus in seals. *Science* 2000; 288: 1051-3.
54. Smith GW, Ives LD, Nagelkerken IA, Ritchie KB. Aspergillosis associated with Caribbean sea fan mortalities. *Nature* 1996; 382: 487.
55. Boeing. Current Market Outlook 2000: Into the Next Century. Demand for Air Travel. Http://www.boeing.com/commercial/cmo/3at00.htm Published 2000.
56. Vitousek PM, D'Antonio CM, Loope LL, Wesbrooks R. Biological invasions as global environmental change. *Am Sci* 1996; 84: 468-78.
57. Vitousek PM, Mooney HA, Lubchenco J, Melillo JM. Human domination of Earth's ecosystems. *Science* 1997; 277: 494-9.
58. Daszak P, Cunningham AA. Extinction by infection. *Trends Ecol Evol* 1999; 14: 279.
59. Cunningham AA, Daszak P. Extinction of a species of land snail due to infection with a microsporidian parasite. *Conserv Biol* 1998; 12: 1139-41.
60. Taylor LH, Woolhouse MEJ. Zoonoses and the risk of disease emergence. *Proc Int Conf Emerg Infect Dis* Atlanta, USA, 2000: Board 122.
61. Hahn BH, Shaw GM, de Cock KM, Sharp PM. AIDS as a zoonosis: scientific and public health implications. *Science* 2000; 287: 607-14.
62. Michalak K, Austin C, Diesel S, Maichle B, Zimmerman P, Maslow JN. *Mycobacterium tuberculosis* infection as a zoonotic disease: transmission between humans and elephants. *Emerg Infect Dis* 1998; 4: 283-7.
63. Steele KE, Linn MJ, Schoepp RJ, Komar N, Geisbert TW, Manduca RM, *et al.* Pathology of fatal West Nile virus infections in native and exotic birds during the 1999 outbreak in New York City, New York. *Vet Pathol* 2000; 37: 208-24.
64. Murray K, Selleck P, Hooper P, Hyatt A, Gould A, Gleeson L. A morbillivirus that caused fatal disease in horses and humans. *Science* 1995; 268: 94-7.
65. Philbey AW, Kirkland PD, Ross AD, Davis RJ, Gleeson AB, Love RJ, *et al.* An apparently new virus family Paramyxoviridae infectious for pigs, humans, and fruit bats. *Emerg Infect Dis* 1998; 4: 269-71.
66. Goh KJ, Tan CT, Chew NK, Tan PSK, Kamarulzaman A, Sarji SA, *et al.* Clinical features of Nipah virus encephalitis among pig farmers in Malaysia. *N Engl J Med* 2000; 342: 1229-35.
67. Haplin K, Yonung PL, Field H, Mackenzie JS. Newly discovered viruses of flying foxes. *Vet Microbiol* 1999; 68: 83-7.
68. Williamson MM, Hooper PT, Selleck PW, Gleeson LJ, Daniels PW, *et al.* Transmission studies of Hendra virus (equine morbillivirus) in fruit bats, horses and cats. *Austr Vet J* 1998; 76: 813-8.
69. Monath TP. Ecology of Marburg and Ebola viruses: speculations and directions for future research. *J Infect Dis* 1999; 179: S127-S38.
70. Heidejorgensen MP, Harkonen T, Dietz R, Thompson PM. Retrospective of the 1988 european seal epizootic. *Dis Aquat Org* 1992; 13: 37-62.
71. Ostfeld RS, Keesing F. Biodiversity and disease risk: the case of Lyme disease. *Conserv Biol* 2000; 14: 722-8.
72. Schmidt JA, Ostfeld RS. Biodiversity and the dilution effect in disease ecology. *Ecology* 2001 (in press).
73. Ostfeld RS, Keesing F. The function of biodiversity in the ecology of vector-borne zoonotic diseases. *Can J Zool* 2000; 57: 1-18.
74. Ross PS, Vos JG, Birnbaum LS, Osterhaus ADME. PCBs are a health risk for humans and wildlife. *Science* 2000; 289: 1878-9.

75. Colwell RR. Global climate and infectious disease: the cholera paradigm. *Science* 1996; 274: 2025-31.
76. Epstein PR. Climate and health. *Science* 1999; 285: 347-8.
77. Dobson A, Meagher M. The population dynamics of brucellosis in the Yellowstone National Park. *Ecology* 1996; 774: 1026-36.
78. Brownell RL, Curry BE, Van Bonn W, Ridgway SH. Conservation conundrum. *Science* 2000; 288: 2319.
79. Daszak P, Cunningham AA, Hyatt AD. Conservation conundrum, response. *Science* 2000b; 288: 2320.
80. WTO World Tourism Organization. International year of ecotourism IYE. Http://www.world-tourism.org/omt/ecotourism2002.htm Published 2000.
81. Goodall J. *In the shadow of man*. Revised edition. London: Weidenfeld & Nicholson, 1988.
82. Weber W. Primate Conservation and ecotourism in Africa. In: Potter CC, Cohen JJ, Janczewski D, eds. *Perspectives on biodiversity: case studies of genetic resource conservation and development*. Washington DC: American Association for the Advancement of Science Press, 1993: 129-50.
83. Hastings BE, Gibbons LM, Williams JE. Parasites of free-ranging mountain gorillas: Survey and epidemiological factors. *Proc Joint Meeting AAZV and AAWV*, Oakland, California; 1992: 301-2.
84. Adams HR, Sleeman J, New JC. A medical survey of tourists visiting Kibale National Park, Uganda, to determine the potential risk for disease transmission to chimpanzees Pan troglodytes from ecotourism. *Proc AAZV*; 1999: 270-1.
85. Windsor DA. Heavenly hosts. *Nature* 1990; 348: 104.
86. Stork NE, Lyall CHC. Extinction or "co-extinction" rates? *Nature* 1993; 366: 307.
87. Gompper ME, Williams ES. Parasite conservation and the black-footed ferret recovery program. *Conserv Biol* 1998; 123: 730-2.
88. Daszak P, Cunningham AA. Emerging diseases: a key role for Conservation Medicine. In: Aguirre AA, Ostfeld RS, House CA, Tabor GM, Pearl MC, eds. *Conservation Medicine: ecological health in practice*. New York: Oxford University Press, 2001 (in press).
89. Stachowicz JJ, Whitlatch RB, Osman RW. Species diversity and invasion resistance in a marine ecosystem. *Science* 1999; 5444: 1577-9.
90. Bäumler, AJ, Hargis, BM, Tsolis RM. Tracing the origins of Salmonella outbreaks. *Science* 2000; 287: 50-2.
91. Ostfield RS, Pearl MC, Meffe G. Conservation medicine: the birth of another crisis discipline. In: *Conservation Medicine*. New York: Oxford University Press, 2001 (in press).

Orthomyxoviruses: influenza

Emergence and Control of Zoonotic Ortho- and Paramyxovirus Diseases
B. Dodet, M. Vicari, eds.

Role of aquatic birds migration in influenza transmission

François Moutou
Laboratoire d'études et de recherches en pathologie animale et zoonoses, Agence française de sécurité sanitaire des aliments, Maisons-Alfort, France

It has been known for some time that birds represent the gene reservoir for type A influenza viruses. All 15 known subtypes have been found in this Vertebrate class [1]. Within the 10,000 or so recognized living species of birds [2, 3], some orders and families do play a special role in influenza virus epidemiology, as virus strains have already been reported in 12 different orders of birds [4]. However, aquatic birds are considered of really special importance within the class [4, 5]. Altogether, there are a little over 1,000 different species, including fresh, brackish and sea aquatic birds, representing some 10% of the whole class biodiversity. It must be realized that even these 10% are far from being all well known.

More precisely, aquatic birds include a number of different families and orders, mainly ducks (family Anatidae, order Anseriformes) and waders (families Charadriidae and Scolopacidae, order Charadriiformes). Even if some seven or eight other orders (out of 30) do include aquatic birds and may play a role in influenza epidemiology, these two groups are the most important, as ducks and waders can be numerous, are often gregarious, at least during certain periods of time, are hunted and so get into contact with human beings and human activities, and are migratory, so cross many countries, even continents, and theoretically, could carry viruses over oceans from one land to another. This is why they are closely monitored, as they could be seen as the origin of any new influenza epidemics, within domestic stock or in human populations. However, their own ecology, their special habits and physiological or behavioural adaptations to migration, making them able to face very different natural conditions, from Arctic breeding grounds to tropical wintering wetlands, could suggest a certain kind of relationship between these birds and their viruses.

This presentation will start by a short recall on bird migration, and then will present some evidence of the importance of the biology of aquatic birds in influenza epidemiology. In the discussion, some ideas aimed at preventing virus transmission between wild birds and other species, man included, will be proposed.

Bird migration

Migration presentation

Aquatic birds migration is just one example of migration within the world of birds. Most of the material for this section comes from [2] and [6].

It is not because it is easy to see a flock of snow geese *(Anser caerulescens)* or of common cranes *(Grus grus)* flying South, high above our heads in a "V" shape, that migrations are easy to understand. The real origin of migrations is still the object of debate. It may be linked to climate modification at the end of ice age. Different species were able, then, to expand their range to the North and to find new feeding grounds. Theoretical ecologists are still working on this subject, as some speciation processes may be linked to migration [7]. It must be noticed that migration can also exist under tropical conditions, with the balance between dry and rainy seasons. In Africa, the dry season corresponds to our European summer time, so that only African residents are left, then, in Africa. During our winter time, in the same way, only our European residents are sharing the limited food left or accessible in Europe. This may decrease competition in a time of food shortage.

It must also be realized that, from fully migratory species to fully resident species, many in between situations do exist, and that, with time, populations within the same species, areas within larger regions, and climatic conditions, movements may be quite different. Some birds breeding in the Arctic will winter in temperate Europe, whereas birds breeding around the 45 °N latitude may spend winter on the Mediterranean shores or even in sub-Saharan countries. The same figures can be seen in the New World, between the high Arctic and tropical South America, or between Eastern Siberia and South-East Asia.

A peculiar species may seem to be present all year long in the same place, when in fact different individuals from different populations will replace each other, following seasons.

Some populations will fly according to a quite precise schedule, from one year to the other, following the same route, when others will wait until water freezes and food becomes out of reach to move away in any favourable direction. Some will fly non-stop from Europe to tropical Africa, or from mid-Atlantic USA states to Brazil over the golf of Mexico, others will stop many times all along the way. It must also be understood that, in Eurasia, the global direction of bird migration is NE/SW, so that many aquatic birds arriving along our Atlantic shores are coming from Arctic Siberia. This is for instance the case of the brant *(Branta bernicla)*, also present, but with other populations, in North America.

Migration flyways and numbers

As aquatic birds are linked to water, be it fresh, brackish or sea water, their migration flyways have been well known for years and years, by ornithologists and by hunters, as some of their favourite resting places are a real "tradition". In France for instance, some wetlands are very famous for their high numbers of ducks and waders during the fall and winter seasons. The Baie de Somme, the Rhine river valley, the Der lake, the Dombes, or the Camargue, not forgetting some others, like the lake of Annecy, are just a few among them. As most of these species were, are, or could be game species, they are monitored by agencies like *Office National de la Chasse et de la Faune Sauvage* (National Hunting and Wildlife Agency). Surveys are performed to get an idea of the numbers of species, and of individuals within species, travelling across a country like France, which is only part of their home range, year after year, to see if hunting bags are adapted to the known dynamics of the populations. These estimations are performed from Siberia to Africa, the real area of concern, with the help of similar national agencies, when present, or with NGOs, and with international teams and networks, as birds ignore political borders. For instance, in France, between November 1997 and March 1998, monthly reports gave figures, for ducks and coots, 30 species altogether, numbering from 268,315 to 629,772 birds. Two species represented nearly 45% of the whole community, the mallard *(Anas platyrhynchos)* and the Eurasian coot *(Fulica atra)*. In January 1997, one year earlier, the figure raised up to 837,000 birds. These surveys concern 1352 wetlands all over the country [8]. In Western Europe, the commonest species is the mallard with an estimated population of 15 to 20 million individuals, whereas one of the rarest aquatic birds is the Eurasian avocet *(Recurvirostra avosetta)* with only 60,000 birds for the same region.

The map of the flyways of the white stork *(Ciconia ciconia)*, a very popular species here, even if it numbers are now decreasing, highlights some useful information *(Figure 1)*. This bird, like many large species, will glide or soar, using ascending air currents, also called thermal columns or bubbles, present over land, and will not cross easily a large piece of water. Active flapping flight will exhaust the storks quite rapidly, so they need these "thermal pathways", overland. Between Europe and Africa, the Mediterranean sea will be crossed either over the Gibraltar strait, to the West, or over the Near East shores, to the East. Using ringed individuals, it has been possible to determine that two sub-populations exist, in Europe as in Africa, with few genetic exchanges.

Another situation may be seen in *Figure 2*, where common cranes *(Grus grus)* are wintering in discrete distant tropical areas, whereas they spend the summer time spread over a large and unique area of the sub-Arctic.

A third example comes from the migration scheme of the knot *(Calidris canutus)*. As shown in *Figure 3*, different sub-populations exist, with some specific migration patterns and some limited or variable exchanges. The area covered, and of concern, is really huge.

This leads to the idea that, in the case of epidemiological surveys, the precise identification of the host species and population, from which a virus strain has been isolated, where and when, are as important as the sub-typing of the virus strain itself. As bird taxonomy is still moving, any change should also be considered for its possible epidemiological consequences.

It could even be of importance to know the age of the birds collected or sampled, as all age classes will not necessarily follow the same migration patterns, cross the same areas or even be present in the same regions. Our temperate Western European migratory breeding birds, for instance, are never present as nestlings or fledglings in African wintering wetlands. However, nestlings or fledglings could show a particular sensitivity

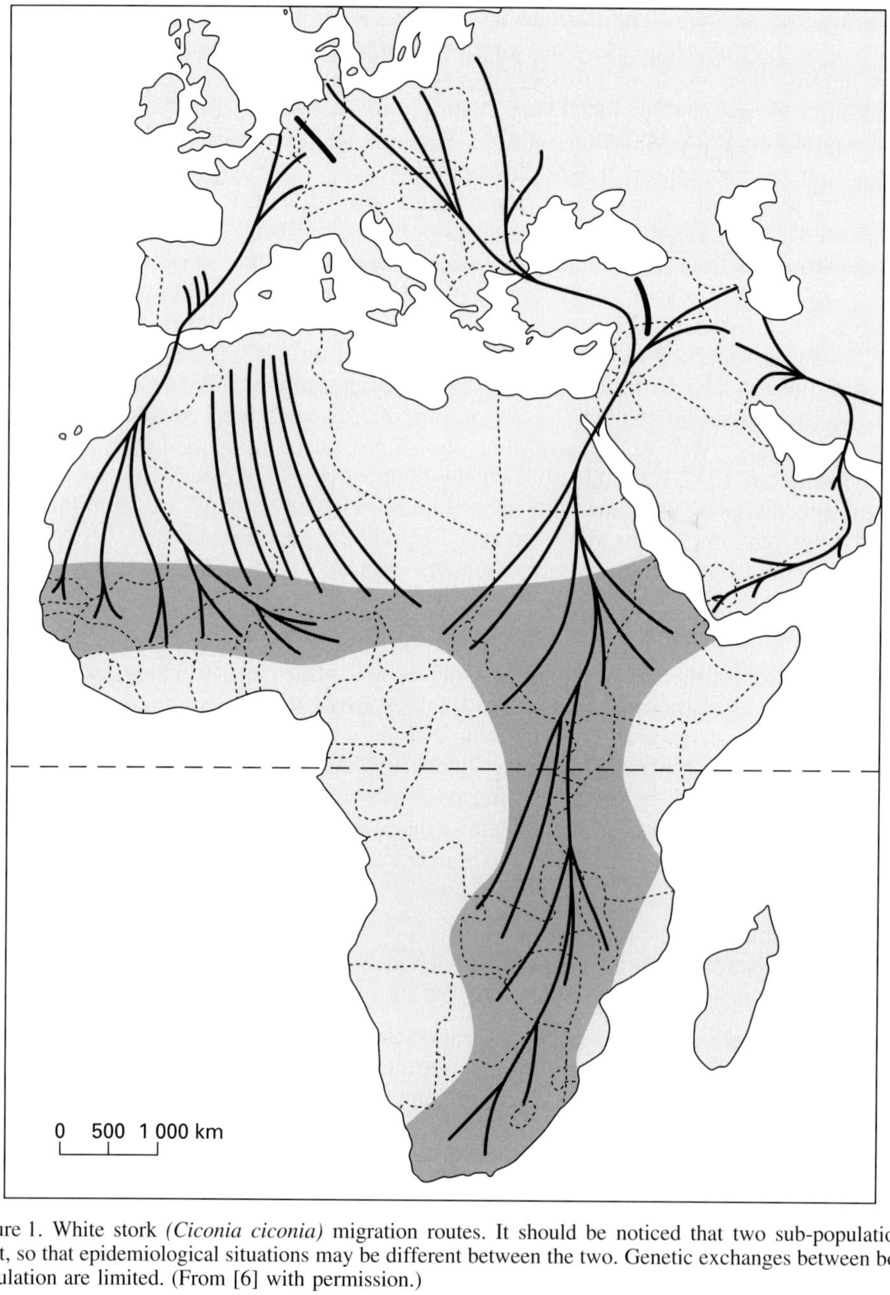

Figure 1. White stork *(Ciconia ciconia)* migration routes. It should be noticed that two sub-populations exist, so that epidemiological situations may be different between the two. Genetic exchanges between both population are limited. (From [6] with permission.)

to the virus, because of specific immunity capabilities, and thus be especially important as a cohort for epidemiological studies. Sanitary consequences may be dissimilar. They certainly depend on the virus but they are also linked to the actual host population, and

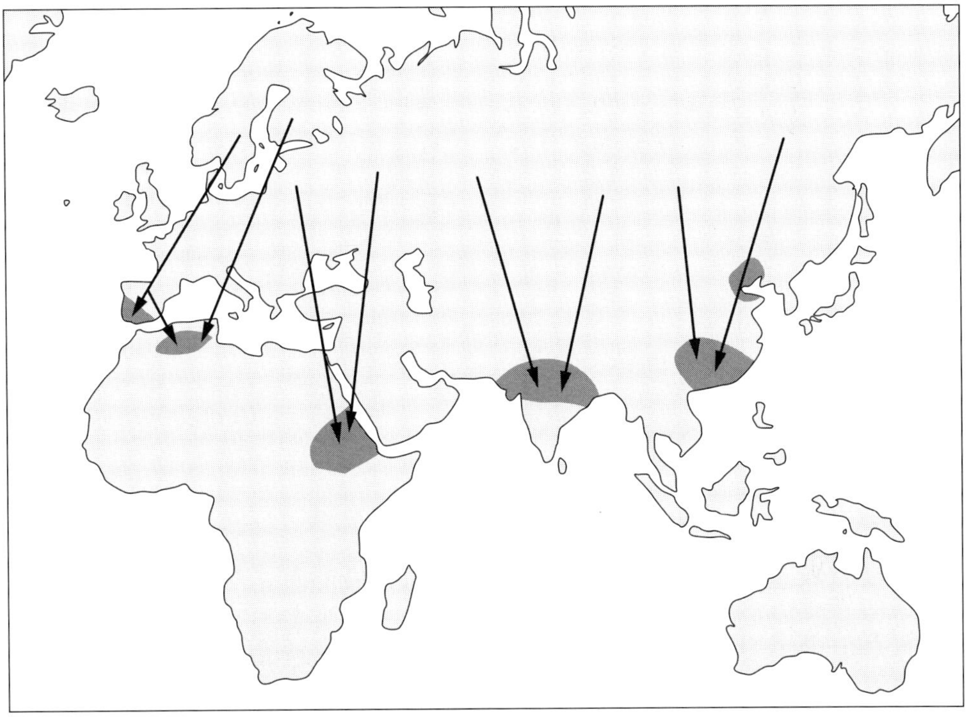

Figure 2. Common crane *(Grus grus)* migration routes. Whereas the birds are dispersed over a huge area in the summer time, they spend the wintertime in discrete, more concentrated, sub-populations. Very young birds are only present in the North. (From [6] with permission.)

the same degree of precision should be expected in molecular virology as in ornithology. Virologists, epidemiologists and ornithologists have to work together.

It must also be recalled that as many as 3.75 billion birds, all species together, aquatic and terrestrial, are supposed to cross the Mediterranean sea every fall, from Europe, on their way to Africa, from North to South. How many viruses are travelling with them? The spring return is less numerous as many individuals, especially yearlings, will not survive the winter. The two movements are not completely symmetrical, as some species will use a circle road, or follow different patterns on their way back. Similar patterns can be found in America and in Asia.

Physiological, behavioural and sanitary consequences of migration

Some global information on the importance of wild and feral birds in human and animal epidemiology can be found in [9] and [10]. Here, we will, of course, speak mostly of influenza and aquatic birds.

As mentioned above, explaining migrations is not easy. As some viruses, like influenza, seem to be well-adapted to birds, even to migrating birds, one question is to look for the possible adaptation of these viruses to migration. It is known that birds enter some physiological changes before the long journey. Not all species or families will

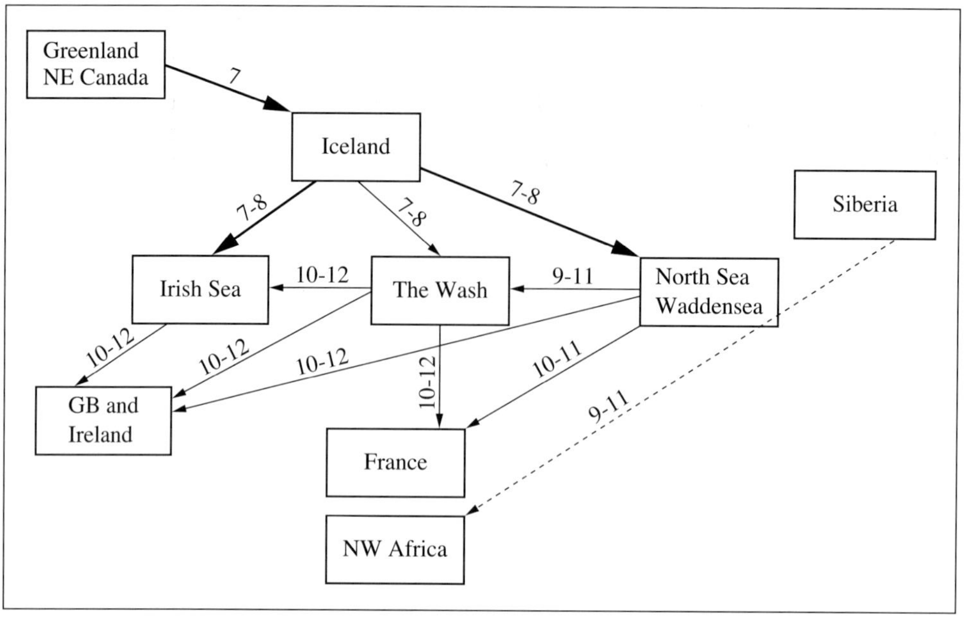

Figure 3. Schematic representation of the knot migration routes of the knot *Calidris canutus* over the Western Palearctic. The time schedule (number for months) and the quantification (thickness of arrows) of all movements would be important to be determined for all species. (From [6] with permission.)

undergo the same preparation, but usually this includes gain of weight, as fat builds up and flight muscles are reinforced, whereas some organs like the digestive tract may undergo some reduction of volume and function, so that only useful weight is kept. Birds will also loose water and glycogen, as water and energy will originate from lipid metabolism.

As in the case of ducks (Anatidae) the virus is carried within intestinal cells, it could be interesting to know how it faces all these modifications. Some species of ducks *(Anatidae)* will fly South quite straight and quite rapidly, and may be only partly concerned by these modifications. However, it is also known that ducks will spread many influenza viruses at the end of the summer, just before beginning their fall migration, when all the ducklings of the year are present, in their largest numbers and highest density. Viruses may then be carried by water and may survive for a while in cold fresh water [1]. The fact that most young birds get infected just before their first South or South/West migration could be seen as an adaptation of the virus to survive from one generation to the next and from one location to the other. Each individual duck may be a short time carrier, but populations as a whole may be seen as a reservoir for influenza viruses.

One other question would be to know if migrations, either fall, spring, or both, may have an immunological impact on some bird species, linked to these physiological changes, and could explain some specific timing of virus dissemination or transmission. A garganey teal *(Anas querquedula)* may loose 50% of its weight between Europe and Mali, in Western Africa, and song birds will loose 1% of their body weight for every hour of (night) flight. Metabolism could be quite disturbed by such modifications.

Following the localisation of the virus within the bird, it may have developed specific strategies to survive migrations or to take advantage of behavioural modifications.

Physiological changes are, effectively, also linked to behavioural changes. Some migratory species will travel in very large groups, gathering for variable periods of time. Others will gather only on their breeding grounds, in huge rookeries, travelling alone most of their lives. Some are highly social all year long. In terms of epidemiological consequences, these situations represent different risk factors for virus transmission. If the birds meet every year at the same season, this is when the virus transmission seems to have the highest probability of occurrence. What happens with influenza and ducks at the end of the summer seems to fit well with virus dispersion and survival, knowing also that the virus may survive for some time in the water, where many birds will meet during the early migration period.

Discussion

Meteorological broadcasts are useful to foresee not only weather conditions, but also the localisation of migrating birds according to the season or the weather, as well as some of their flight habits [11]. This is why some of the first water birds influenza virus monitoring surveys in France were performed in the Baie de Somme during the winter. This location, not too far from the Institut Pasteur laboratories in Paris, is well known for the high numbers of waders and ducks wintering there. If the winter gets very cold, they will fly south again, but if it remains mild, they can spend most of it there. The knowledge of where aquatic birds will stop, given the weather conditions, is important when trying to monitor virus movements, as well as for disease prevention.

This may have some implications when thinking of controlling the transmission of viruses from waterfowl to domestic stock or human beings. It is well known that domestic ducks may induce their wild relatives to stop next to them. Decoys of wildfowl hunters play just the same role. This may have some consequences in term of virus transmissibility. This is why bird farms that are located along the traditional flyways may be a cause for concern. In any given region, the locations of the main wetlands should be taken into account when choosing a site for an open air duck yard.

One specific situation that could be tested is the importance of urban lakes and ponds, with ornamental swans and ducks or any aquatic birds, as they can act as live decoys for their passing wild relatives. They may be seen as sentinel birds to monitor virus circulation.

Another situation that could be investigated is the importance of captive bred mallards used for hunting purposes. In some regions they may represent a high number of all mallards and their sanitary status is not always known.

Lands where ducks, both domestic and wild, domestic pigs and human beings can live close together or mix freely, like in some regions of China, are thought to present a classical risk situation. This is certainly true. At the same time, it could be important to know if some relatively new factors, or factors of increasing importance, such as ornithological collections, ornamental aquatic birds close to or within cities, wildfowl breeding and trading for hunting purposes, and wildlife rescue centres could also constitute locations to monitor.

Migration is not a new phenomenon, neither are its sanitary consequences. As these are well-known, they should be taken care of. We also have to remember that birds are at the origin of Hamilton's and Zuk's hypothesis linking bright colours and ornamental long feathers to the presence of high levels of antibodies against micro-parasites [12]. Birds offer a good support for the theoretical approach of host/parasite relationships as an evolutionary process. The idea that viruses like influenza are well-adapted to birds (higher internal temperature than mammals, transmission process, physiological and behavioural adaptations), when they so often mean diseases in mammals, man included, could lead to the proposition that some viruses are so well-adapted to birds that they could be seen as "Biboviruses" for "bird-borne viruses". The influenza virus, the Newcastle disease virus *(Rubulavirus)*, or even arboviruses like the West Nile virus could be considered as belonging to this category.

Note: English and scientific names of birds mentionned in the text are as in: Commission internationale des noms français des oiseaux. *Noms Français des Oiseaux du Monde*. Sainte-Foy (Québec, Canada): Éditions MultiMondes; Bayonne (France): Editions Chabaud, 1993, 452 p. This book includes a list of English, French and scientific names of all birds of the world.

References

1. Webster RG. Influenza: an Emerging Disease. *Emerg Infect Dis* 1998; 4 (3): www.cdc.gov/
2. Lesaffre G. *Le manuel d'ornithologie*. Lausanne et Paris: Delachaux et Niestlé, 2000, 271 p.
3. Dorst J. *Les oiseaux ne sont pas tombés du ciel*. Paris: Jean-Pierre de Monza, 1995, 375 p.
4. Stallknecht DE, Shane SM. Host range of avian influenza virus in free-living birds. *Vet Res Com* 1988; 12: 125-41.
5. Webster RG, Kawaoka Y. Influenza, an emerging and re-emerging disease. *Semin Virol* 1994; 5: 103-11.
6. Berthold P. *Bird migration. A general survey*. Oxford: Oxford University Press, 1993: 63, 64, 69.
7. Bell CP. Process in the evolution of bird migration and pattern in avian ecogeography. *J Avian Biol* 2000; 31: 258-65.
8. Fouque C, Barthe C, Dej F, Tesson JL. Dénombrement hivernaux d'anatidés et de foulques macroules en France: synthèse de l'hiver 1997-1998. *Bull Mens Off Natl Chasse* 1999; 249: 4-11.
9. Guiguen C, Camin AM. Le rôle des oiseaux en pathologie humaine. In: Clergeau P, ed. *Oiseaux à risque en ville et en campagne*. Paris: INRA Editions, 1997: 233-61.
10. Moutou F. Place des oiseaux sauvages en épidémiologie animale. In: Clergeau P, ed. *Oiseaux à risque en ville et en campagne*. Paris: INRA Editions, 1997: 263-78.
11. Elkins N. *Les oiseaux et la météo*. Lausanne et Paris: Delachaux et Niestlé, 1996, 220 p.
12. Zuk M. Parasites and bright birds: new data and new prediction. In: Loye JE, Zuk M, eds. *Bird-parasite interactions*. Oxford: Oxford University Press, 1991: 317-27.

Emergence and Control of Zoonotic Ortho- and Paramyxovirus Diseases
B. Dodet, M. Vicari, eds.

Ecology of avian influenza in domestic birds

Dennis J. Alexander
Central Veterinary Laboratory Agency, Weybridge, Addlestone, Surrey, United Kingdom

A disease known as "fowl plague" that caused up to 100% mortality in domestic fowl was first distinguished from bacterial diseases in 1878. Since 1981 this disease has been termed highly pathogenic avian influenza (HPAI). It was not until 1955 that the virus responsible for HPAI and a few other viruses isolated from birds that caused much milder disease were shown to be influenza A (AI) viruses [1]. Only type A influenza viruses are known to cause natural infections of birds, but all 15 (H1-H15) haemagglutinin and all 9 (N1-N9) neuraminidase influenza A subtypes recognised currently have been found in avian species and in the majority of possible combinations.

In the surveys of wild birds listed by Stallknecht and Shane [2], a total of 21,318 samples from all species resulted in the isolation of 2,317 (10.9%) viruses. Of these samples 14,303 were from birds of the order *Anseriformes* and yielded 2,173 (15.2%) isolates. The next highest isolation rates were 2.9% and 2.2% from the *Passeriformes* and *Charadriiformes* respectively and the overall isolation rate from all birds other than ducks and geese was 2.1%. Each year waterfowl congregate in huge flocks before migratory flights are undertaken. Data from the 3-year study by Hinshaw *et al.* [3] on ducks congregating on lakes in Alberta, Canada, prior to their southern migration showed that AI virus isolation rates from juvenile ducks may exceed 60%. This reservoir of AI viruses is extremely important in the ecology of AI in domestic birds.

Phylogenetic studies [*e.g.* 4-6] of AI viruses show that lineages and clades of isolates are more related to geographical and temporal parameters than the host from which they were isolated and that there is no distinction between wild and domestic bird isolates.

Disease in domestic poultry

AI viruses can be divided into two groups on their ability to cause disease in poultry. The very virulent viruses that cause HPAI are restricted to subtypes H5 and H7, although not all viruses of these subtypes cause HPAI. There have been 18 reported primary isolates of such viruses from domestic poultry since 1959 *(Table I)*. All other

Table I. Reported HPAI isolates from poultry* since 1959.

1. A/chicken/Scotland/59 (H5N1)
2. A/turkey/England/63 (H7N3)
3. A/turkey/Ontario/7732/66 (H5N9)
4. A/chicken/Victoria/76 (H7N7)
5. A/chicken/Germany/79 (H7N7)
6. A/turkey/England/199/79 (H7N7)
7. A/chicken/Pennsylvania/1370/83 (H5N2)
8. A/turkey/Ireland/1378/83 (H5N8)
9. A/chicken/Victoria/85 (H7N7)
10. A/turkey/England/50-92/91 (H5N1)
11. A/chicken/Victoria/1/92 (H7N3)
12. A/chicken/Queensland/667-6/94 (H7N3)
13. A/chicken/Mexico/8623-607/94 (H5N2)
14. A/chicken/Pakistan/447/94 (H7N3)
15. A/chicken/NSW/97 (H7N4)
16. A/chicken/Hong Kong/97 (H5N1)
17. A/chicken/Italy/330/97 (H5N2)
18. A/turkey/Italy/99 (H7N1)

* Where outbreaks were widespread and affecting more than one species, the isolate from the first outbreak identified is listed.

viruses cause a much milder disease consisting primarily of respiratory disease and depression with egg production problems in laying birds; in this review, infections with these viruses will be termed low pathogenicity avian influenza (LPAI). Concurrent infections with other organisms or environmental conditions may cause exacerbation of LPAI leading to much more serious disease. For example in outbreaks of LPAI in Italy in 1999, high mortality was often recorded in young turkeys, reaching 97% in one flock [7].

Current theories suggest that AI subtype H5 and H7 viruses of high virulence emerge from viruses of low virulence by mutation [8, 9]. This is supported by phylogenetic studies of H7 subtype viruses, which indicate that HPAI viruses do not constitute a separate phylogenetic lineage or lineages, but appear to arise from non-pathogenic strains [4, 5] and the *in vitro* selection of mutants virulent for chickens from an avirulent H7 virus [10]. It appears that such mutations occur only after the viruses have moved from their natural host to poultry.

Infections of domestic poultry

Introduction to poultry

Primary introduction of AI viruses to poultry depends chiefly on contact with free-living birds, especially migratory waterfowl, so that outbreaks occur more frequently when farming practices increase the direct or indirect contact [*e.g. via* infective faeces] with free-living birds. AI infections of domestic poultry are more likely to occur in geographical areas on migratory routes than in those that are not. This is certainly true for infections in turkeys, which occur particularly in areas on migratory waterfowl flyways, *e.g.* Norfolk in England, and more frequently at some stages of the migratory route than others, *e.g.* Minnesota, USA, compared to other states on the Mississippi flyway

[11]. In addition, there is a marked similarity between the subtypes prevalent in the local waterfowl population and those infecting turkeys [12, 13].

The higher incidence of influenza virus infections in domestic ducks than in turkeys, and in turkeys than in chickens is compatible with introductions being made by wild birds. Domestic ducks, particularly fattening birds, are usually raised in fields or on ponds and are open to contact with wild birds. In some countries, turkeys are raised on open range, as practised in Minnesota, USA, during May to November. Lang [14] concluded that the major reason for the decline in AI infections in turkeys in Canada was the move to keeping the birds in doors all year. Pomeroy [15] contrasted the incidence of AI infections in chickens and turkeys kept in confinement to that in turkeys reared on open range. Chickens are reared mostly in substantial houses that resist wild bird invasion and this may account for the relatively low incidence of AI in chickens.

Secondary spread

The principal method of spread of AI viruses is by mechanical transfer of infective faeces, in which virus may be present at concentrations as high as 10^7 infectious particles/gram and may survive for longer than 44 days [16]. Birds or other animals that are not themselves susceptible to infection may become contaminated and spread the virus. Shared water or food may also become contaminated. However, for domestic poultry the main agent of secondary spread is man. In several specific accounts strong evidence implicated the movements of caretakers, farm owners and staff, trucks and drivers moving birds or delivering food, and artificial inseminators in the spread of the virus both on to and through a farm. Following studies during the devastating epizootic in chickens in Pennsylvania in 1983-1984, King [17] listed 6 types of fomite that may be moved from farm to farm and 11 types of personnel that may be in contact with two farms or more; Utterback [16] produced even longer lists.

Avian influenza in commercial ducks

The influenza status of commercial ducks in most countries is poorly understood or has not been investigated. When surveillance of commercial ducks has been undertaken, AI virus has been readily isolated and many subtype combinations have been detected, especially from birds reared on open fields. For example, Alexander [18] reported the isolation of 32 viruses from 60 pools of cloacal swabs taken from ducks at slaughter. Studies in Hong Kong in the late 1970s and early 1980s isolating virus from carcases at duck dressing plants or on duck farms indicated about 6% of the ducks were infected with AI viruses of various subtypes [19]. In 1997, H5 viruses were isolated from 2.5% of ducks sampled in Hong Kong [20] in contrast to an H5 virus isolation rate from ducks of 0.25% five years earlier. In 1997, H9 viruses were also isolated from 0.9% of ducks compared to 0.19% five years earlier.

Avian influenza in turkeys

Since 1963, when the first reported influenza isolation was made from turkeys, most of the major turkey-producing countries have had disease problems associated with AI infections. In the USA, since 1964, influenza outbreaks in turkeys have been reported from 19 different states spread across the country. In the majority of these states outbreaks have been infrequent, but in California and Minnesota, where turkey farms are heavily concentrated and situated on migratory waterfowl flyways, AI virus infections have been seen more consistently. In Minnesota, AI outbreaks in turkeys have occurred every year since 1966, occasionally reaching particularly severe proportions [11, 21]. In 1995, two separate, major, outbreaks caused by LPAI viruses occurred in turkeys in the USA [21]. A virus of H7N3 subtype affected turkeys in Utah and was associated with about 40% mortality in 0- to 4-week-old birds. In most cases mortality was associated with dual infections with *Escherichia coli* or *Pasteurella multocida*. The other outbreak, caused by an H9N2 virus, occurred in Minnesota; 178 turkey farms were infected resulting in the worst economic loss to AI infections (approximately $6,000,000) recorded in one year in Minnesota [21].

A different pattern has been seen in countries like Great Britain where influenza outbreaks in turkeys have been restricted to one or two isolated incidents in the years recorded, except in 1979 when 16 farms were affected [18]. Of the 22 separate introductions recorded in turkeys in Great Britain between 1963 and 1993, 17 were on farms in the county of Norfolk, an important "stop-over" area for migratory waterfowl.

In 1999, LPAI virus of H7N1 subtype caused 199 outbreaks in Northern Italy, 170 were in turkey flocks with mortality rates in birds up to 40 days old of 40-97% [7]. HPAI emerged in the same region in December 1999 and of the 413 outbreaks confirmed, the last in April 2000, 177 were in meat turkeys and 5 in breeder turkeys.

Despite the frequency of isolations of LPAI viruses from turkeys, HPAI has been reported rarely. Excluding spread to turkeys during epizootics that affected mainly chickens, of the 18 reported isolations of HPAI since 1959 only 6 were primarily from turkeys *(Table I)*. In contrast to the high incidence of LPAI infections in turkeys in North America, only one HPAI outbreak has been reported, in 1966 in Ontario, Canada.

Avian influenza in chickens

In the second half of the 20th century reports of AI infections of chickens were relatively rare compared to infections of domestic turkeys or ducks, even though there are much higher populations of chickens throughout the world. For example in the USA, despite frequent AI epizootics in turkeys in some states, between 1964 and 1982 only three outbreaks in chickens were recorded [11]. Despite the low incidence of AI infections, 12 of the 18 primary HPAI outbreaks since 1959 were in chickens. Significant spread in chickens occurred in Pennsylvania and neighbouring states in the USA during 1983-1984 [22], Mexico [23, 24] and Pakistan [25] in 1994/95 and Italy in 1999/2000 with huge losses of birds.

In Pennsylvania, outbreaks of LPAI due to H5N2 subtype virus began in April 1983 and spread throughout the state before HPAI virus emerged in October 1983 [22]. By the last outbreak, in July 1984, over 17,000,00 birds had died or been slaughtered.

In Mexico, a similar pattern of events was seen. H5N2 LPAI virus was isolated from outbreaks of respiratory disease in May 1994 and during 1994 spread through 11 states

[24]. HPAI virus was first isolated in January 1995 and resulted in a complicated situation in which both HPAI and LPAI viruses circulated.

This was repeated in NE Italy in 1999/2000. Between March and December 1999 LPAI outbreaks due to H7N1 virus were recorded (27 in chickens). HPAI emerged by virus mutation in December 1999 and 413 HPAI outbreaks were recorded up to April 2000, 189 in chickens [7]. The losses in poultry exceeded 13,000,000 birds.

The accumulating evidence that HPAI viruses arise from LPAI H5 or H7 viruses infecting chickens and turkeys suggests that only when viruses of these subtypes spread from free-living birds is there a potential that they may become virulent. If mutation to virulence is a random event, the longer the presence and greater the spread in poultry, as occurred in Pennsylvania, Mexico and Italy, the more likely it is that HPAI virus will emerge. However, when and if this will occur remain unpredictable. Presumably in outbreaks of HPAI such as that in England in 1991 [26], which affected only a single house of turkeys, the mutation happened very quickly after introduction. Most countries have control measures for HPAI but not LPAI; so where HPAI outbreaks have occurred with limited spread, as in Italy in 1997-1998 [27, 28] and the 5 outbreaks in Australia [29], this has been aided by the application of strict control measures without the complication of the presence of LPAI.

Outbreaks of H5N1 HPAI occurred on three farms in Hong Kong during March-May 1997 with mortality rates of 70-100% [30] and subsequent spread to live bird markets. As a result of the spread of this virus to humans [30], the entire chicken population of Hong Kong of over 1,000,000 birds was slaughtered.

One feature in the USA has been the maintenance of H5 viruses in live bird markets since 1983. In 1986, a survey showed that 38 of 70 live bird markets in New York and New Jersey had birds which were positive for H5N2 virus [31]. The number of live bird markets has grown over the intervening years and remains a source of H5 viruses [32].

Avian influenza in ratites

The first AI viruses isolated from ratites were of H7N1 subtype, but of low pathogenicity in chickens, obtained as a result of an epizootic in ostriches in South Africa in 1991 with high mortality in young birds [33]. In 1994, AI viruses of H5N9 were isolated from ostriches in South Africa, and from emus and casowaries in The Netherlands [34]. H5N2 subtype viruses were isolated from ostriches in Zimbabwe in 1995 and 1996 and also in ostriches imported into The Netherlands and Denmark in 1996. In Denmark, the isolations were associated with 146/506 deaths within 23 days of importation; however, the virus was LPAI in chickens [35]. H9N2 virus was isolated from ostriches in South Africa in 1995. In the USA, LPAI viruses of the following subtypes were isolated from rheas and emus [36]: H3N2 in 1992, H4N2, H5N2 and H7N1 in 1993, H4N6, H5N9 and H10N4 in 1994, H7N3 in 1995 and H7N3 and H10N7 in 1996. The HPAI epizootic in Italy in 2000 included spread to ostrich flocks [37].

Avian influenza in other domestic poultry

Other birds reared commercially represent a very small proportion of domestic poultry in most countries. Some such birds (*e.g.* pheasants and geese) are reared under semi-wild conditions. Isolations of AI viruses have been reported from muscovy ducks *(Cairinia moschata)*, mallard ducks *(Anas platyrhyncos)*, pheasants *(Phasianus* spp.), Japanese quail *(Coturnix coturnix japonica)*, chukars *(Alectoris chukar)*, guinea fowl *(Numida meleagris)*, and various types of geese. In the 1997/98 H5N2 outbreaks in Italy guinea fowl were infected and in the 1999/2000 H7N1 outbreaks guinea fowl, quail and pheasants were infected [28, 37].

H9 subtype infections

In the 1990s, infections of poultry, mainly chickens, with H9 AI viruses reached almost panzootic proportions. Outbreaks, due to H9N2 AI, occurred in domestic ducks, chickens and turkeys in Germany during 1995-97 and in 1998 [38, 39]; in chickens in Italy in 1994 and 1996 [27], pheasants in Ireland in 1997 [40], ostriches in South Africa in 1995 [6], turkeys in the USA in 1995 and 1996 [21] and in chickens in Korea in 1996 [41]. Outbreaks due to H9N3 subtype virus were reported in China in 1994 [42]. More recently, H9N2 infections have been reported in the Middle East and caused widespread outbreaks in commercial chickens in Iran and Pakistan [25]. Infections of chickens with H9N2 viruses in Korea and China also occurred in this period. Phylogenetic analysis of isolates [6] suggests reports of H9 AI viruses from different parts of the world represent both spread among poultry and separate introductions from feral birds.

Infections of other domestic birds

Avian influenza in caged "pet" birds

Captive caged birds may be important in the ecology of AI because they are often feral birds trapped and exported from the country of origin, usually from tropical and subtropical Asian countries to Western destinations, or Japan, and from the Southern to the Northern hemisphere. AI viruses isolated from imported caged birds have been reported from countries such as Great Britain, USA, Austria and Japan [43]. The isolates have been mainly of H4 or H3 subtypes usually with N6 or N8 subtypes, although N1-N3 have also been reported [36, 43, 44]. Panigrahy and Senne [36] noted that the majority of AI viruses from caged birds came from passerine species.

AI isolations from caged birds are notable for the changes from H4 to H3 as the prevalent subtype and the periods, often lasting several years, when no isolations have been made. Alexander [44] suggested that these may reflect epizootics in feral birds in the countries of origin, but stressed that there was little evidence confirming this.

Avion influenza in falcons

Hunting with falcons is practised in a number of countries around the world. The birds have close contact with humans and are highly domesticated and yet the nature of the purpose for which they are kept means they also have contact with feral birds. There have been two recent reports of AI infections of falcons. Manvell *et al.* [45] isolated an HPAI virus of H7N3 subtype from a peregrine falcon *(Falco peregrinus)* dying in the United Arab Emirates. The virus showed close homology with the H7N3 viruses responsible for the outbreaks in Pakistan four years earlier [5]. During the HPAI outbreaks in Italy in 2000, an H7N1 virus was isolated from a saker falcon *(Falco cherrug)* that died three days after normal hunting activity [46].

Conclusion

The principal reservoir for AI viruses that infect domestic birds is wild birds. Nowhere is AI considered to be enzootic in domestic poultry or other birds. However, the situation in Mexico, where extensive vaccination against H5 subtype AI has been practised since 1995, remains unclear. Also, the perpetuation of AI viruses in live bird markets in the USA represents a potential source for other domestic birds. Apart from these, even where outbreaks occur regularly, *e.g.* Minnesota, USA, the considerable variation in virus subtype, the differences in the number of outbreaks seen each year, and the seasonal relationship of outbreaks all suggest that the AI epizootics are brought about as a result of new primary introductions. This knowledge should allow the development of farming practices that will minimise the risk of primary introduction of AI virus. However, in many countries practices likely to encourage wild birds to poultry farms, such as surface storage of drinking water, rearing mixed species on the same farm, failure to bird-proof food stores and even the construction of artificial ponds to attract waterfowl are common place.

Once AI virus is introduced into commercial poultry modern management systems that are now practised world wide and involve multiple visits of a variety of personnel to poultry farms mean that AI virus can be spread *via* contaminating infective faeces extremely quickly and efficiently. This was demonstrated particularly by the HPAI outbreaks in Mexico, Pakistan and Italy and the LPAI H9N2 outbreaks throughout Asia.

Failure to control AI in poultry and other domestic birds rapidly represents not just disease problems and economic loss in commercial poultry, but, in view of the reports of direct spread from birds to humans, may have much more serious consequences.

References

1. Schafer W. Vergleichende sero-immunologischs Untersuchungen uber die viren der influenza und klassichen Geflugelpest. *Zeits Naturforsch* 1955; 10b: 81-91.
2. Stallknecht DE, Shane SM. Host range of avian influenza virus in free-living birds. *Vet Res Commun* 1988; 12: 125-41.
3. Hinshaw VS, Webster RG, Turner B. The perpetuation of orthomyxoviruses and paramyxoviruses in Canadian waterfowl. *Can J Microbiol* 1980; 26: 622-9.

4. Rohm C, Suss J, Volker P, Webster RG. Different hemagglutinin cleavage site variants of H7N7 in an influenza outbreak in chickens in Leipzig, Germany. *Virology* 1996; 218: 253-7.
5. Banks J, Speidel EC, McCauley JW, Alexander DJ. Phylogenetic analysis of H7 haemagglutinin subtype influenza A viruses. *Arch Virol* 2000; 145: 1-12.
6. Banks J, Speidel EC, Harris PA, Alexander DJ. Phylogenetic analysis of influenza A viruses of H9 haemagglutinin subtype. *Avian Pathol* 2000; 29: 353-60.
7. Capua I, Mutinelli F, Marangon S, Alexander DJ. H7N1 avian influenza in Italy (1999-2000) in intensively reared chickens and turkeys. *Avian Pathol* 2000; 29: 537-43.
8. Garcia M, Crawford JM, Latimer JW, Rivera-Cruz E, Perdue ML. Heterogeneity in the haemagglutinin gene and emergence of the highly pathogenic phenotype among recent H5N2 avian influenza viruses from Mexico. *J Gen Virol* 1996; 77: 1493-1504.
9. Perdue M, Crawford J, Garcia M, Latimer J, Swayne D. Occurrence and possible mechanisms of cleavage site insertions in the avian influenza hemagglutinin gene. *Proc 4th Intl Symp Avian Influenza, Athens, Georgia 1997.* US Anim Hlth Assoc 1998: 182-93.
10. Li S, Orlich MA, Rott R. Generation of seal influenza virus variants pathogenic for chickens, because of hemagglutinin cleavage site changes. *J Virol* 1990; 64: 3297-303.
11. Pomeroy BS. Avian influenza in the United States (1964-1980). *Proc 1st Intl Symp Avian Influenza,* 1981. Carter Comp Corp Richmond USA 1982: 13-7.
12. Halvorson DA, Karunakaran D, Senne D, Kelleher C, Bailey C, Abraham A, Hinshaw V, Newman J. Epizootiology of avian influenza – simultaneous monitoring of sentinel ducks and turkeys in Minnesota. *Avian Dis* 1983; 27: 77-85.
13. Halvorson DA, Kelleher CJ, Pomeroy BS, Sivanandan V, Abraham AS, Newman JA, Karunakaran D, Poss PE, Senne DA, Pearson JE. Surveillance procedures for avian influenza. *Proc 2nd Intl Symp Avian Influenza,* 1986. Univ Wisconsin, Madison 1987: 155-63.
14. Lang G. A review of influenza in Canadian domestic and wild birds. *Proc 1st Intl Symp Avian Influenza, 1981.* Carter Comp Corp, Richmond, USA 1982: 21-7.
15. Pomeroy BS. Avian influenza in turkeys in the USA. *Proc 2nd Intl Symp Avian Influenza, 1986.* Univ Wisconsin, Madison 1987: 14-21.
16. Utterback W. Update on avian influenza through February 21, 1984 in Pennsylvania and Virginia. *Proc 33rd West Poult Dis Conf* 1984: 4-7.
17. King LJ. How APHIS'war room' mobilized to fight AI. *Broil Ind* 1984; 47: 44-51.
18. Alexander DJ. Current situation of avian influenza in poultry in Great Britain. *Proc 1st Intl Symp Avian Influenza, 1981.* Carter Comp Corp, Richmond 1982: 35-45.
19. Shortridge KF. Avian influenza A viruses of Southern China and Hong Kong: ecological aspects and implications for man. *Bull WHO* 1982: 60: 129-35.
20. Shortridge KF. Poultry and the influenza H5N1 outbreak in Hong Kong, 1997: Abridged chronology and virus isolation. *Vaccine* 1999; 17: S26-S29.
21. Halvorson DA, Frame DD, Friendshuh AJ, Shaw DP. Outbreaks of low pathogenicity avian influenza in USA. *Proc 4th Intl Symp Avian Influenza.* Athens, Georgia 1997. US Anim Hlth Assoc 1998: 36-46.
22. Eckroade RJ, Silverman LA, Acland HM. Avian influenza in Pennsylvania. *Proc 33rd West Poult Dis Conf* 1984: 1-2.
23. Campos-Lopez H, Rivera-Cruz E, Irastorza-Enrich M. Situacion y perspectivas del programa de erradicacon de la influenza aviar en Mexico. *Proc 45th West Poult Dis Conf,* May 1996, Cancun, Mexico, 13-16.
24. Villarreal CL, Flores AO. 1997. The Mexican avian influenza H5N2 outbreak. *Proc 4th Intl Symp Avian Influenza.* Athens Georgia 1997. US Anim Hlth Assoc 1998; 18-22.
25. Naeem K. The avian influenza H7N3 outbreak in South Central Asia. *Proc 4th Intl Symp Avian Influenza.* Athens Georgia 1997. US Anim Hlth Assoc 1998: 31-35.
26. Alexander DJ, Lister SA, Johnston MJ, Randall CJ, Thomas PJ. An outbreak of highly pathogenic avian influenza in turkeys in Great Britain in 1991. *Vet Rec* 1993; 132: 535-6.
27. Fioretti A, Menna LF, Calabria M. The epidemiological situation of avian influenza in Italy during 1996-1997. *Proc Joint 4th Ann Meet Natl Newcastle Disease and Avian Influenza Labs Countries EU, Brussels, 1997.* 1998: 17-22.
28. Capua I, Marangon S, Selli L, Alexander DJ, Swayne DE, Dalla Pozza M, Parenti E, Cancellotti FM. Outbreaks of highly pathogenic avian influenza (H5N2) in Italy during October (1997) to January (1998). *Avian Pathol* 1999; 28: 455-60.
29. Westbury HA. History of high pathogenic avian influenza in Australia and the H7N3 outbreak (1995). *Proc 4th Intl Symp Avian Influenza, Athens, Georgia 1997.* US Anim Hlth Assoc 1998: 23-30.

30. Claas CJ, Osterhaus ADM, Beek R, De Jong J, Rimmelzwaan GF, Senne DA, Krauss S, Shortridge KF, Webster RG. Human influenza A H5N1 virus related to a highly pathogenic avian influenza virus. *Lancet* 1998; 351: 472-7.
31. Garnett WH. Status of avian influenza in poultry: 1981-1986. *Proc 2nd Intl Symp Avian Influenza, 1986*. Univ Wisconsin, Madison 1987: 61-66.
32. Trock SC. Epidemiology of influenza in live bird markets and ratite farms. *Proc 4th Intl Symp Avian Influenza, Athens, Georgia 1997.* US Anim Hlth Assoc 1998: 76-8.
33. Allwright DM, Burger WP, Geyer A, Terblanche AW, 1993. Isolation of an influenza A virus from ostriches (Struthio camelus). *Avian Pathol* 1993; 22: 59-65.
34. Koch G. Report of disease incidence of avian influenza in The Netherlands in 1994. *Proc Joint 2nd Ann Meets Natll Newcastle Disease & Avian Influenza Labs Count EU, Brussels, 1994.* 1995: 11-2.
35. Jorgensen PH, Nielsen OL, Hansen HC, Manvell RJ, Banks J, Alexander DJ. Isolation of influenza A virus, subtype H5N2, and avian type 1 paramyxovirus from a flock of ostriches in Europe. *Avian Pathol* 1998; 27: 15-20.
36. Panigrahy B, Senne DA. Subtypes of avian influenza virus isolated from exotic birds and ratites in the United States, 1992-1996. *Proc 4th Intl Symp Avian Influenza, Athens, Georgia 1997.* US Anim Hlth Assoc 1998: 70-5.
37. Capua I, Moreno-Martin A, Mutinelli F, Cordioli P Alexander DJ. The 1999-2000 avian influenza (H7N1) epidemic in Northern Italy. *Proc ESVV Congr Vet Virol in the New Millennium, Brescia, Italy* 2000: 301-2.
38. Werner O. Avian influenza – Situation in Germany 1995-1997. *Proc Joint 4th Ann Meets Natl Newcastle Disease & Avian Influenza Labs Count EU Brussels, 1997.* 1998: 9-10.
39. Werner O. Avian influenza – situation in Germany 1997/98. *Proc Joint 5th Ann Meets Natl Newcastle Disease & Avian Influenza Labs Count EU Vienna, 1998.* 1999: 10-1.
40. Campbell G. Report of the Irish national reference laboratory for 1996 and 1997. *Proc Joint 4th Ann Meets Natl Newcastle Disease & Avian Influenza Labs Count EU, Brussels, 1997.* 1998: 13.
41. Mo IP, Song CS, Kim KS, Rhee JC. An occurrence of non-highly pathogenic avian influenza in Korea. *Proc 4th Intl Symp Avian Influenza, Athens, Georgia. 1997.* US Anim Hlth Assoc, 1998: 379-83.
42. Yingjie S, Avian influenza in China. *Proc 4th Intl Symp Avian Influenza, Athens, Georgia 1997.* US Anim Hlth Assoc, 1998: 47-9.
43. Alexander DJ. Isolation of influenza A viruses from exotic birds in Great Britain. *Proc 1st Intl Symp Avian Influenza, 1981.* Carter Comp Corp, Richmond, USA, 1982: 79-92.
44. Alexander DJ. Influenza A isolations from exotic cage birds. *Vet Rec* 1988; 123: 442.
45. Manvell RJ, McKinney P, Werney U, Frost K. Isolation of a highly pathogenic influenza A virus of subtype H7N3 from a peregrine falcon *(Falco peregrinus). Avian Pathol* 30: in press.
46. Magnino S, Fabbi M, Moreno A, Sala G, Lavazza A, Ghelfi E, Gandolfi L, Pirovona G, Gasperi E. Avian influenza virus (H7 serotype) in a saker falcon in Italy. *Vet Rec* 2000: 740.

Emergence and Control of Zoonotic Ortho- and Paramyxovirus Diseases
B. Dodet, M. Vicari, eds.

Evolution and pathobiology of avian influenza virus virulence in domestic birds

David E. Swayne, David L. Suarez
Southeast Poultry Research Laboratory, Agricultural Research Service, United States Department of Agriculture, Athens, Georgia, USA

Summary – Avian influenza (AI) viruses have infected a variety of domestic and wild birds. Most AI viruses have produced subclinical infections or, less frequently, mild disease characterized by respiratory or urogenital problems. Rarely, some H5 and H7 subtypes of AI virus have produced severe, systemic disease with mortality rates approaching 100%. Pathogenicity studies in chickens and *in vitro* tests have been used to assess the virulence potential of individual AI viruses for regulatory purposes. Viruses causing low mortality rates have been categorized as mildly pathogenic (MP) or of low pathogenicity while those producing high mortality rates as highly pathogenic (HP). Those AI viruses that do not produce disease or death are sometimes termed "not pathogenic". Since 1959, 18 outbreaks of HPAI have occurred: 17 in domestic poultry and 1 in wild birds. The virus strain and host species both impact the virulence of AI.

In 3 of the 18 outbreaks of HPAI (North-East United States in 1983-84, Mexico in 1994-95 and Italy in 1999-2000), documentation demonstrated widespread circulation of MP H5 or H7 AI viruses in domestic poultry before the appearance of HPAI viruses in the field. The HPAI viruses emerged 6-12 months after the MPAI viruses and caused major economic losses to the commercial poultry industries and increased consumer costs. Replication of the MPAI virus in large numbers of AI naive domestic poultry resulted in host adaptation and efficient transmission. Subsequent RNA mutations in the hemagglutinin resulted in an abrupt change in virulence from MP to HP. The virulence change did not result from reassortment of gene segments.

Several model systems have been developed to predict emergence of HPAI viruses from MPAI viruses of the H5 and H7 subtypes. Our laboratory has developed a 14-day-chicken-embryo-adult-laying-hen modeling system. Nineteen MP H5 and ten H7 AI viruses isolates obtained from poultry and ratites were tested in the model system. Eight H5 and one H7 AI virus isolates changed from producing a few deaths (MP) to killing 75% of chickens (HP) in an intravenous pathogenicity test. Lesions in the chickens that died were consistent with naturally occurring HPAI viruses and the viruses caused cytopathic effect in tissue culture without exogenous trypsin. Some of these viruses had changes in the proteolytic cleavage site of the hemagglutinin such as substitution or insertion of additional basic amino acids and/or loss of a glycosylation site. Such changes were similar to those reported in field AI viruses.

Using the Hong Kong H5N1 HPAI virus of 1997, host impact on virulence has been assessed in experimental models. The Hong Kong AI virus was highly pathogenic for seven species in the order *Galliformes*, and a single species in each of the orders *Passeriformes* and *Psittaciformes*. Although, the Hong Kong AI virus infected birds in the orders *Anseriformes* and *Rheiformes*, the virus was mildly pathogenic or not pathogenic for the birds. The virus did not infect birds of the order *Columbiformes*. Other highly pathogenic AI viruses have shown varying abilities to infect and cause disease and death in diverse bird species.

Avian influenza (AI) viruses are type A orthomyxoviruses that have infected a variety of domestic and wild birds [1]. Most AI viruses have produced subclinical infections, usually in wild birds of the orders *Anseriformes* or *Charadriiformes*. Less frequently, AI viruses have produced mild disease, typically in domestic poultry, characterized by respiratory or urogenital problems. Rarely, some AI viruses of the H5 and H7 subtypes have produced severe, multi-systemic disease with mortality rates approaching 100%. For national and international regulations, virulence potential of the AI viruses are assessed by pathogenicity studies conducted in chickens and *in vitro* tests. Viruses producing less than 75% mortality are categorized as mildly pathogenic (MP) or of low pathogenicity while those producing mortality rates greater than or equal to 75% are highly pathogenic (HP) [2]. Those AI viruses that do not produce disease or death are sometimes called "not pathogenic" or "non-pathogenic". Presence of multiple basic amino acids at the hemagglutinin proteolytic cleavage site of H5 and H7 AI viruses or the ability to plaque in tissue culture without exogenous trypsin are criteria for high pathogenicity and would result in eradication efforts.

Historical background of avian influenza virus virulence

HPAI was first recognized as a distinct disease in Italy by Perroncito in 1878 and was called fowl plague [3]. Fowl plague was a severe, rapidly spreading disease that produced high mortality in chickens. In 1901, the etiology was determined by Centanni and Savonuzzi to be a filterable agent or a virus. This highly virulent disease spread throughout Europe in the late 1800s and early 1900s *via* poultry exhibitions and shows, where it was endemic in domestic poultry until the 1930s. However, fowl plague virus (FPV) was not taxonomically classified until 1955 when Schafer determined that FPV was a type A influenza virus related to other influenza viruses that commonly infected humans, pigs and horses [4]. Up until the late 1950s and early 1960s, fowl plague was considered a unique disease of high virulence for poultry. Today, these original FPV are serologically categorized as the H7 subtype of the hemagglutinin surface glycoprotein, but since 1959, highly virulent avian influenza viruses of the H5 subtype have been identified and have produced clinical disease indistinguishable from fowl plague [1]. In 1981, at the First International Symposium on Avian Influenza, Beltsville, Maryland, USA, the term "fowl plague" was abandoned for the more accurate term "highly pathogenic avian influenza" [5].

Beginning in the mid 1900s, hints were unearthed of less virulent forms of influenza infections in birds [6]. These less virulent influenza viruses included the Dinter agent from chickens (A/chicken/Germany/49), the influenza virus from Manitoba ducklings (A/duck/Canada/52) and influenza viruses from ducks in England and Czechoslovakia from 1956. In the 1960s, various different hemagglutinin subtypes of influenza viruses were isolated from turkeys with mild respiratory and reproductive diseases (*i.e.* non-fowl plague syndromes). Interestingly, a MPAI virus serologically identical to FPV, *i.e.* H7, was isolated from turkeys in Oregon in 1971 [7]. In 1972, wild waterfowl of the order *Anseriformes* (ducks and geese) were demonstrated to be a principal reservoir and the natural host for MPAI viruses [8]. These findings suggested that AI viral infections have been more widespread than fowl plague, were usually non-pathogenic or mildly pathogenic for birds, and infected a variety of poultry and non-poultry species.

Influenza viruses isolated from birds are diverse, representing hemagglutinin serotypes 1-15, but only a small number of the H5 and H7 subtypes are HPAI viruses [1].

Highly pathogenic avian influenza or fowl plague

HPAI has been reported in North and South America, Africa, Asia, Europe and Australia [1]. Since 1959, 18 outbreaks of HPAI have been reported in the English literature; 17 in domestic poultry and 1 in wild birds *(Table I)*. The virus strain and host species both impact the virulence of AI. HPAI is an epizootic and not endemic disease of various domestic poultry species. The most frequently affected species, in decreasing order, are chickens, turkeys, guinea fowl and quail. Ducks have been infected with HPAI viruses, but such infections have been subclinical or produced only mild disease.

With 15 outbreaks, HPAI appeared suddenly as a severe multi-systemic disease with high mortality rates *(Table I)*. In three of the 18 outbreaks of HPAI (United States in 1983-84, Mexico in 1994-95 and Italy in 1999-2000), MP H5 or H7 AI viruses circulated widely in domestic poultry for 6-12 months before HPAI viruses appeared. Replication of the MPAI viruses in large numbers of AI-susceptible domestic poultry resulted in host adaptation and efficient transmission. Subsequent RNA mutations in the hemagglutinin resulted in an abrupt change in virulence from MP to HP and not from reassortment of gene segments. The reservoir for HPAI viruses are not wild birds as with MPAI virus [9]. The HPAI viruses appear to arise from MPAI viruses that circulate in large populations of AI-susceptible poultry.

Table I. HPAI outbreaks since 1955.

1959-Scotland, H5N1	1991-England, H5N1
1961-S. Africa, H5N3	1992-Australia, H7N3
1963-England, H7N3	1994-Australia, H7N3
1966-Canada, H5N9	*1994-95-Mexico, H5N2
1975-Australia, H7N7	1995-Pakistan, H7N3
1979-England, H7N7	1997-Australia, H7N4
*1983-84-U.S., H5N2	1997-Italy, H5N2
1983-Ireland, H5N8	1997-Hong Kong, H5N1
1985-Australia, H7N7	*1999-2000-Italy, H7N1

* Change from MP to HPAI in the field.

Emergence of highly pathogenic avian influenza viruses in the field

Cleavability of the hemagglutinin (HA) protein has been identified as the major determinant of virulence in HPAI viruses [10]. In addition, a proper constellation of all eight gene segments is essential for full expression of virulence potential. Mildly pathogenic H5 AI viruses have a consensus sequence at hemagglutinin proteolytic cleavage site (PCS) of ...Pro-Gln-Basic-Glu-Thr-Basic/Gly... which requires a trypsin-like enzyme to cleave the HA0 to HA1 and HA2 to produce infectious viral particles. This restricts replication to a few cell types and tissues, usually epithelial cells in the respiratory and gastrointestinal tracts, and occasionally the kidney and pancreas. By contrast, HP H5 AI viruses have an altered hemagglutinin PCS with additional basic amino acids, as either substitutions or insertions, and/or loss of glycosylation sites [11]. This allows cleavage and virus replication by ubiquitous proteases present in many cell and tissue types throughout the body. The majority of HPAI viruses isolated in the past 40 years have insertions of one-four basic amino acids in the hemagglutinin proteolytic cleavage site *(Figure 1)* [12].

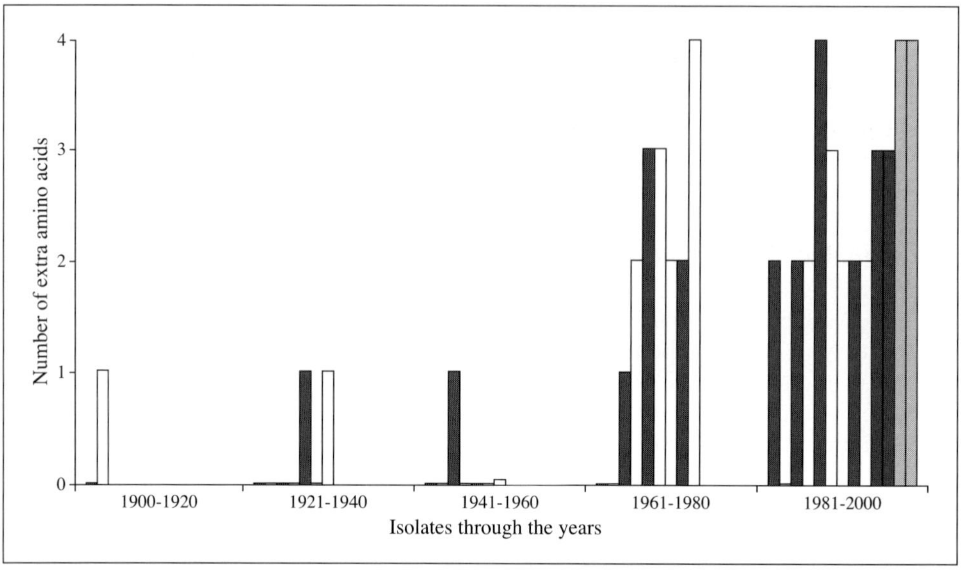

Figure 1. Proteolytic cleavage site insertions in HPAI viruses from outbreaks [12].

Evolution of virulence from MP to HPAI viruses has been seen through changes in hemagglutinin sequence data, *in vitro* characteristics and pathobiology in field outbreaks. The 1994-95 Mexican HP H5 AI outbreak is a good case study. Mildly pathogenic AI appeared as an undiagnosed respiratory disease in the fall of 1993 in broilers of central Mexico [12]. When virus isolation and identification were made in May 1994, most of broiler production areas were affected. The AI viruses isolated from May to December 1994 plaqued inefficiently in chicken embryo fibroblast cultures without exogenous trypsin, and had a hemagglutinin PCS and produced clinical disease typical of an MPAI virus *(Table II)*. This included respiratory disease and mortality between 12-18%. Experimentally, the AI viruses produced interstitial pneumonia, nephrosis and nephritis, and lymphocyte deletion in multiple lymphoid organs. In other studies, MPAI viruses have caused some diarrhea, mild drops in egg production, production of soft shelled eggs, rhinitis, sinusitis, blepharitis, air sacculitis, involution of ovaries with hemorrhagic follicles and “egg yolk peritonitis”. Occasionally, swollen kidneys and visceral urate deposition have been reported.

In late November in Puebla, Mexico, chickens on three layer farms were experiencing less severe respiratory disease, but the appearance of new clinical features including depression, precipitous drops in egg production and some neurological signs were reported. This AI virus had an insertion of two basic amino acids and one substitution of a basic amino acid in the hemagglutinin PCS, and had high plaquing efficiency in cell culture without exogenous trypsin similar to previous HPAI viruses *(Table II)*.

Table II. Pathogenicity characteristics of Mexican avian influenza viruses.

Virus	PE (%)	HA Sequence
Hidalgo 5/94	1-10	Pro-Gln-Arg-Glu-ThrArg/Gly
Mexico 5/94	1-10	Pro-Gln-Arg-Glu-ThrArg/Gly
Jalisco 12/94	< 1	Pro-Gln-Arg-Glu-ThrArg/Gly
Puebla 11/94	100	Pro-Gln-Arg-Lys-Arg-Lys-ThrArg/Gly
Queretaro 19/95	100	Pro-Gln-Arg-Lys-Arg-Lys-ThrArg/Gly
Queretaro 20/95	100	Pro-Gln-Arg-Lys-Arg-Lys-Arg-Lys-ThrArg/Gly

However, in experimental studies, initial pathogenicity tests did not have high mortality rates, typical of HPAI viruses, but passage in chickens resulted in the emergence of derivatives that caused high mortality and caused severe necrosis in heart muscle and pancreatic acinar epithelium. In January 1995, an influenza virus was identified in Queretaro, Mexico in broiler breeders which caused complete cessation of egg production and other clinical signs of HPAI *(Table II)*. These signs included high mortality, depression, edematous and necrotic combs and wattles, edema of the head and legs, subcutaneous hemorrhages of feet, pulmonary edema, congestion, hemorrhage of lungs and hemorrhages in multiple visceral organs. This virus had a cleavage site identical to the Puebla virus and experimentally was highly lethal for chickens. Another AI virus from Queretaro in June had an insertion of four basic amino acids and a single basic amino acid substitution *(Table II)*. This virus was biologically identical to the January 1995 Queretaro 19/95 HPAI virus.

Predicting potential for the emergence of highly pathogenic avian influenza viruses

Several model systems have been developed to predict emergence of HPAI viruses from MPAI viruses of the H5 and H7 subtypes [13]. Our laboratory has developed a 14-day-chicken-embryo-adult-laying-hen modeling system. Nineteen H5, ten H7, an H10 and an H4 MPAI virus isolates obtained from poultry and ratites were tested in the model system *(Table III)*. Eight H5 and one H7 AI virus isolates changed from producing low mortality rates (MP) to killing 75% of chickens (HP) in an intravenous

Table III. Acquisition of high pathogenicity by AIVs after passage in 14-day-old embryos and adult hens.

YES	NO	
H5	H5	H7
A/ck/PA/83 (H5N2)	A/ck/TX/82 (H5N2)	A/sb/IL/92 (H7N1)
A/ck/VA/83 (H5N2)	A/ck/FL/89 (H5N2)	A/rhea/NC/93 (H7N1)
A/ck/VA/84 (H5N2)	A/ck/NY/93 (H5N2)	A/sb/CA/94 (H7N1)
A/ck/NJ/86 (H5N2)	A/ck/HID/94 (H5N2)	A/ck/Italy/99 (H7N1)
A/ck/FL/86 (H5N2)	A/ck/MEX/94 (H5N2)	A/ck/NY/95 (H7N2)
A/emu/TX/93 (H5N2)	A/ck/JAL/94 (H5N2)	A/ck/PA/97 (H7N2)
A/ck/PA/93 (H5N2)	A/ck/CHIS/97 (H5N2)	A/quail/PA/98 (H7N2)
A/ck/FL/93 (H5N2)	A/ph/NJ/98 (H5N2)	A/ck/NY/00 (H7N2)
H7	A/env/NY/98 (H5N2)	A/ty/OR/71 (H7N3)
A/PR/CA/94 (H7N1)	A/av/NY/00 (H5N2)	Other
	A/rhea/NC/94 (H5N9)	A/ck/AL/75 (H4N8)
		A/ty/VA/91 (H10N7)

chicken pathogenicity test. Lesions in the chickens that died were consistent with naturally occurring HPAI viruses and the viruses caused cytopathic effect in tissue culture without exogenous trypsin. The original H5 MPAI isolates had two, three or four basic amino acids at the hemagglutinin PCS, but only H5 MPAI viruses with the latter two PCS resulted in emergence of HPAI viruses *(Table IV)*. Seven of the H5 HPAI viruses emerged after loss of a glycosylation site at amino acid position 11 and one HPAI virus emerged after insertion of two basic amino acids at the PCS *(Table IV)*. Such hemagglutinin PCS changes were similar to those reported in field AI viruses. Based on phylogenetic analysis of the hemagglutinin gene sequence, the derivatives that gave rise to HPAI viruses clustered into two sublineages: 1) 1983-89 H5 MPAI virus lineage containing the USA 1983 HPAI virus from the Pennsylvania outbreak, and 2) 1993 H5 MPAI viruses *(Figure 2)*. The former lineage has not been seen since 1989, but the latter continues to be perpetuated in the live-bird-markets of the Northeastern USA and poses a risk for emergence of HPAI viruses.

Table IV. Emergence of H5 HP from MPAI viruses in an experimental model.

Hemagglutinin proteolyic cleavage site	# Tested	Highly pathogenic
Pro – Gln – Basic – Glu – Thr – Basic/Gly	9	0
Pro – Gln – Basic – Basic – Thr – Basic/Gly	4	3
Pro – Gln – Basic – Basic – Basic – Basic/Gly	6	5

The H7 MPAI that gave rise to an HPAI virus did not require passage in the experimental model *(Table V)*. At the reference laboratory, the original isolated was MP, but the same vial of virus in our laboratory pathogenicity tests was highly lethal. This may have resulted from the isolate being a mixture of H7 MP and HPAI virus strains. We have been unsuccessful in obtaining a H7 HPAI virus from other H7 MPAI isolates.

Table V. Emergence of H7 HP from MPAI viruses in an experimental model.

Hemagglutinin proteolyic cleavage site	# Tested	Highly pathogenic
Pro – Basic – Pro – Basic/Gly	3	0
Pro – Basic – Gly – Basic/Gly	4	0
Pro – Basic – Thr – Basic/Gly	4	0
Pro – Basic – Basic – Basic – Basic/Gly	1	1

The experimental model was successful in producing HP from MPAI viruses in some lineages of H5 AI viruses. These derivatives had changes in the hemagglutinin PCS consistent with field H5 HPAI viruses, caused cytopathic effect in tissue culture without exogenous trypsin, were highly lethal in chickens, and produced gross and histologic lesions identical to HPAI field outbreaks. However, attempts to reproduce emergence of HP from MPAI viruses from lineages of MPAI viruses that gave rise to field outbreaks in Mexico and Italy were not successful. This indicates that the emergence of HP derivatives in the 14-day-chicken-embryo-adult-laying-hen model system is variable depending on the individual H5 and H7 AI virus isolates. The model may be a

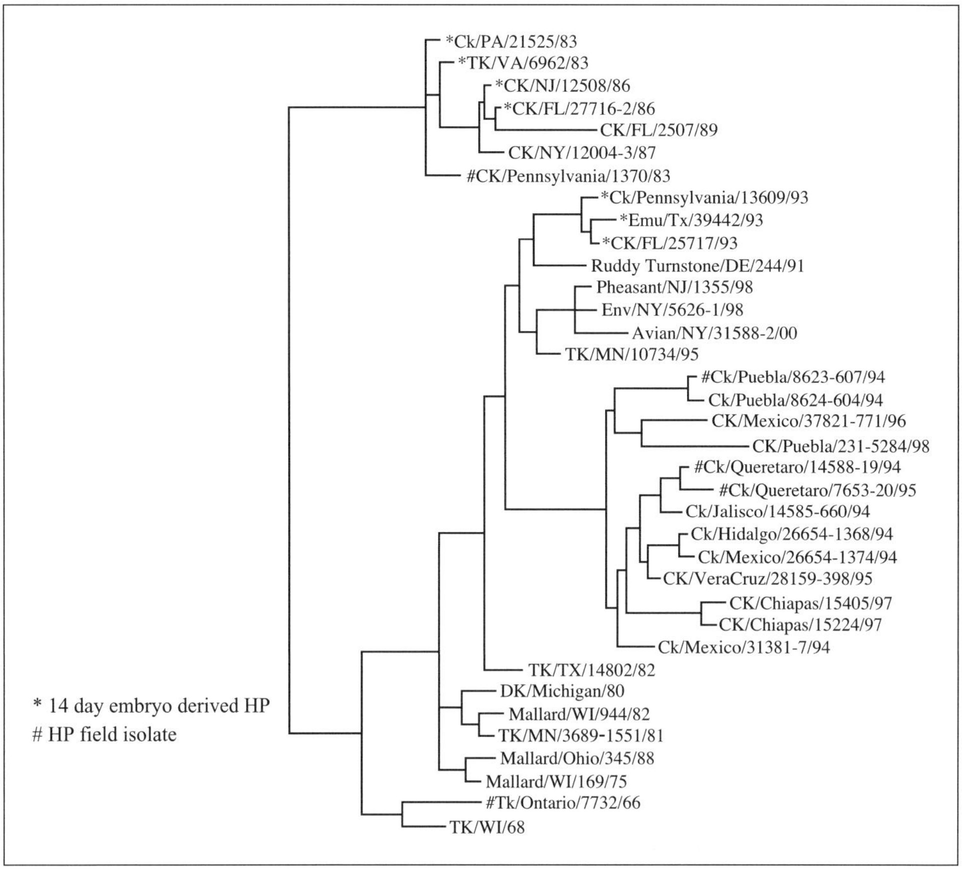

Figure 2. H5 HA1 nucleotide phylogenetic tree.

tool for predicting emergence of HPAI viruses in the field. However, lack of HP emergence in the current model system may not be totally predictive of the field situation where passage of MP H5 and H7 AI viruses in millions of susceptible chickens may result in the emergence of HPAI viruses, as occurred in central Mexico in 1994-95 and Italy in 1999-2000. For H5 MPAI viruses, the best predictor is the presence of three or more basic amino acids at the hemagglutinin PCS. Additional research is needed to refine the model such that better prediction of emergence of HP viruses can result. Additional sequence work is needed on other genes, especially the polymerase genes to determine their impact on emergence of HPAI viruses.

Impact of host species on virulence

Using the Hong Kong H5N1 HPAI virus of 1997, host impact on virulence has been assessed in experimental models. The Hong Kong AI virus was highly pathogenic for seven species in the order *Galliformes* [14], and a single species in each of the orders *Passeriformes* and *Psittaciformes* as measured by 75% or greater mortality rates. Although the Hong Kong AI virus infected birds in the orders *Anseriformes* and *Rheiformes*, the virus was mildly pathogenic or not pathogenic for the birds. The virus did not infect birds of the order *Columbiformes*. Other highly pathogenic AI viruses have shown varying abilities to infect and cause disease and death in diverse bird species.

References

1. Swayne DE, Suarez DL. Highly pathogenic avian influenza. *Rev Sci Tech Off Int Epiz* 2000; 19: 463-82.
2. Pearson JE. Report of the Committee on Transmissible Diseases of Poultry and Other Avian Species. Avian influenza in ratites. In: *Proc 98th Ann Meet US Animal Health Assoc*. Richmond, Virginia: US Animal Health Association, 1994: 519-21.
3. Stubbs E. Fowl pest. In: Biester HE, Schwarte LH, eds. *Diseases of poultry*. Iowa: Iowa State University Press, 1948: 603-14.
4. Schafer W. Vergleichende sero-immunologische untersuchungen uber die viren der influenza unf klassichen geflugelpest. *Z Naturforsch* 1955; 10B: 81-91.
5. Bankowski RA. Introduction and objectives of the symposium. In: Bankowski RA, ed. *Proc 1st Intl Symp Avian Influenza*. Richmond, Virginia: US Animal Health Association, 1981: vii.
6. Easterday BC, Tumova B. Avian influenza. In: Hofstad MS, Calnek BW, Helmbolt CF, Reid WM, Yoder HW, eds. *Diseases of poultry*. 7 ed. Ames, Iowa: Iowa State University Press, 1978: 549-73.
7. Beard CW, Easterday BC. A-Turkey-Oregon-71, an avirulent influenza isolate with the hemagglutinin of fowl plague virus. *Avian Dis* 1973; 17: 173-81.
8. Slemons RD, Johnson DC, Osborn JS, Hayes F. Type-A influenza viruses isolated from wild free-flying ducks in California. *Avian Dis* 1974; 18: 119-24.
9. Rohm CT, Horimoto T, Kawaoka Y, Suss J, Webster RG. Do hemagglutinin genes of highly pathogenic avian influenza viruses constitute unique phylogenetic lineages? *Virology* 1995; 209: 664-70.
10. Bosch FX, Orlich M, Klenk HD, Rott R. The structure of the hemagglutinin, a determinant for the pathogenicity of influenza viruses. *Virology* 1979: 95: 197-207.
11. Perdue ML, Suarez DL, Swayne DE. Avian influenza in the 1990s. *Avian Poult Biol Rev* 2000; 11: 1-20.
12. Perdue ML. How can a virus suddenly become very pathogenic? *World Poultry Special Issue* 2000; 2000 (November): 9-10.
13. Swayne DE, Beck JR, Garcia M, Perdue ML, Brugh M. Pathogenicity shifts in experimental avian influenza virus infections in chickens. In: Swayne DE, Slemons RD, eds. *Proc 4th Intl Symp Avian Influenza*. Richmond, Virginia: US Animal Health Association 1998: 171-81.
14. Perkins LEL, Swayne DE. Pathobiology of A/chicken/Hong Kong/220/97 (H5 NI) avian influenza virus in seven gallinaceous species. *Vet Pathol* 2001; 38: 149-64.

Emergence and Control of Zoonotic Ortho- and Paramyxovirus Diseases
B. Dodet, M. Vicari, eds.

The epidemiology and evolution of influenza viruses in pigs

Ian H. Brown
Virology Department, Veterinary Laboratories Agency-Weybridge, Addlestone, United Kingdom

Abstract – Swine influenza (SI) was first observed at the time of the pandemic in humans in 1918 and since that time subtypes H1N1 and H3N2 have been widely reported in pigs, frequently associated with respiratory disease. These include classical swine H1N1, avian-like H1N1 and human- and avian-like H3N2 viruses. Swine husbandry practises influence directly the evolution of SI viruses through reduced immune pressure and constant availability of susceptible hosts. The classical H1N1 viruses have remained largely conserved both genetically and antigenically. Influenza A viruses of H3N2 subtype related closely to early human strains circulate widely in pigs, particularly in Europe and Asia where they continue to persist long after their disappearance from the human population. These viruses have evolved more slowly than their human counterparts and now form distinct lineages related to geographical location. The pig has been the leading contender for the role of intermediate host for reassortment of influenza A viruses since they are the only mammalian species which are susceptible to, and allow productive replication of avian and human influenza viruses due to the presence of receptors for both virus types (α2,3 and α2,6 respectively) and this can result in modification of the receptor binding specificities of avian influenza viruses from α2,3 to α2,6 linkage thereby providing a potential link from birds to humans. Adaptation of a "newly" transmitted influenza virus to pigs can take many years unless it is able to reassort with an endemic strain which provides the "genetic backbone" of the new virus. Several independent introductions of avian viruses to pigs have occurred, primarily involving H1N1, which has led to the establishment of stable lineages, but more recently with H4N6 virus in North America and H9N2 viruses in Asia. The prevailing human viruses primarily of H3N2 subtype continue to transmit frequently to pigs and may be able to establish stable lineages without genetic reassortment in contrast to human H1N1 viruses. Reassortant viruses of H3N2 and H1N2 subtype derived from mixed lineages and usually containing genes encoding surface glycoproteins from human viruses, have been reported widely in pigs. Numerous transmissions of virus from pigs to humans have occurred but without apparent secondary spread. Pigs may be important in the generation of "new" strains, some of which may have the potential to transmit to other species including humans.

Reservoirs of influenza A viruses

Influenza A viruses infect a large variety of animal species [1, 2] including humans, pigs, horses, sea mammals and birds. Given the worldwide interaction between humans, pigs, birds and other mammalian species, there is a high potential for cross-species transmission of influenza viruses in nature. Phylogenetic studies of influenza A viruses have revealed species-specific lineages of viral genes and have demonstrated that the prevalence of interspecies transmission depends on the animal species [2]. Aquatic birds are known to be the source of all influenza viruses for other species. Pigs are an important host in influenza virus ecology since they are susceptible to infection with both avian and human influenza A viruses, often being involved in interspecies transmission, facilitated by regular close contact with humans or birds. Following the transmission to, and independent spread of avian or human influenza A viruses in pigs, these viruses are generally referred to as "avian-like" swine or "human-like" swine, reflecting their previous host. Following genetic reassortment with other influenza A viruses, some of the genes of these viruses may be maintained in the resulting progeny viruses. Therefore, the evolution of influenza genes in species-specific gene lineages is an invaluable characteristic in studying influenza virus epidemiology.

Early history of swine influenza

Swine influenza (SI) was first observed in 1918 in the United States, Hungary and China [3, 4]. It coincided with an influenza pandemic in humans, which was the most severe of modern times, accounting for at least 20 million deaths worldwide. Those who first noticed the disease in pigs, recognised similarities between the porcine and human disease and suggested they had a common aetiology. Later retrospective serological investigations confirmed that the disease in humans and pigs had been caused by closely related influenza A viruses in both cases. The causative agent was an H1N1 influenza A virus which had possibly derived from a common ancestor [5, 6]. Genetic sequencing studies of the haemagglutinin (HA) and neuraminidase (NA) genes of the human virus revealed that the virus most probably spread from humans to pigs [6, 7], which is supported by observations from veterinarians who did not describe the disease in pigs until just after its appearance in humans. Although the disease in pigs was described during the following years, it was not until 1930 that the virus was isolated and identified [8].

Outbreak course and persistence in pigs

Swine husbandry practises influence directly the evolution of influenza viruses in pigs leading generally to reduced genetic drift, particularly in the genes encoding HA and NA, compared to those of similar viruses in the human population. SI generally appears with the introduction of new pigs into a herd, thereby being related to the movement of animals from infected to susceptible herds. Once a herd is infected, the virus is likely to persist through the production of young susceptible pigs and the introduction of new stock. Complete depopulation is the only effective measure for eliminating the disease. Once a herd becomes infected with SI, it is likely to be maintained with annual episodes of acute disease. There may be differences in the epizootiology of SI between the United States and Europe. In Europe many herds may harbour virus without showing clinical signs [9].

The disease often appears simultaneously on several farms within an area. Such multicentric outbreaks are not necessarily the result of recent movement of infected animals, but due to the widespread distribution of the virus among herds in an area. The primary route of virus transmission is through pig to pig contact *via* the nasopharyngeal route, the virus being shed in nasal secretions and disseminated through droplets or aerosols. Close contact between pigs (often enhanced through husbandry practises), stressful situations, meteorological and environmental factors are conducive to the spread of influenza viruses.

Outbreaks of disease occur throughout the year but usually peak in the colder months [10]. Infection with swine influenza H1N1 virus is frequently subclinical, and typical signs are seen often in only 25 to 30 per cent of a herd. Blaskovic *et al.* [11] showed that swine influenza H1N1 virus was excreted from one infected pig for over four months, although 7 to 10 days is typical. Continuous circulation of influenza viruses within a herd without the apparent need for an intermediate host has been shown by the isolation of virus from a herd the year round [12]. Furthermore, swine influenza H1N1 virus has been recovered from pigs with no signs of disease [13].

The interepizootic survival and the potential existence of reservoirs for the virus have been studied extensively. There are no clear data to support or reject the existence of a long-term true carrier state of influenza viruses in pigs, but the widespread occurrence of the virus in pigs themselves and the methods of swine husbandry make it likely that the virus is maintained by continual passage to young susceptible pigs.

Epidemiology

Influenza A viruses of subtypes H1N1 and H3N2 have been reported widely in pigs, associated frequently with clinical disease. These include classical swine H1N1, "avian-like" H1N1 and "human"- and "avian-like" H3N2 viruses. These viruses have remained largely endemic in pig populations worldwide and have been responsible for one of the most prevalent respiratory diseases in pigs. Although usually regarded as an endemic disease, epidemics may result when influenza infection occurs in an immunologically naive population (which can be linked to significant antigenic drift) or through exacerbation by a variety of factors such as poor husbandry, secondary bacterial or viral infections and cold weather. Serosurveillance results in Great Britain indicated that more than half of adult pigs in the national population had been infected with one or more influenza A viruses during their lifetime, including 14 per cent of pigs which had been infected with influenza viruses of both human and swine origin [14].

Classical H1N1

Following the reported occurrence of influenza in pigs at the time of the 1918 pandemic, SI was for a long time apparently confined to the United States, where, after its first appearance, annual outbreaks occurred during the winter months. These and viruses closely related are termed classical viruses. Elsewhere SI was observed much later with the situation being frequently complicated by the association of other agents with respiratory disease. However, classical swine influenza viruses, or their antibodies, have been reported from many parts of the world including North and South America, Asia, and Africa [reviewed 15]. In Europe, the first isolations of influenza virus from pigs probably related to recent transmissions of virus from humans. After these episodes the virus apparently disappeared and there was no evidence of infection in Europe for nearly twenty years, until 1976 when classical swine influenza virus was isolated from disease outbreaks in Northern Italy. The viruses isolated were closely related to classical swine influenza virus from the United States [16], and it is probable that the virus was introduced *via* imported pigs from the United States. The infection was limited to Northern Italy until 1979, when the virus spread to Northern Europe. The disease spread rapidly to the rest of Europe including Sweden and the United Kingdom. This virus became endemic in pigs throughout Europe with a seroprevalence of 20 to 25 per cent [14] but following the emergence of "avian-like" H1N1 virus its has apparently disappeared.

Easterday [10] considered that the natural history of SI has remained largely stable for a period of at least sixty years, the virus being maintained relatively unchanged both antigenically and genetically through this period of time. Serological studies of pigs in the United States have shown that classical swine H1N1 influenza virus was prevalent throughout the pig population, with approximately 25 per cent of fattening pigs having evidence of infection [13] whilst amongst the longer lived breeding population this figure rises to 45%. In Asia, classical H1N1 viruses are apparently the predominant influenza virus infecting pigs [17].

"Human-like" viruses

Infections of pigs with the prevailing human subtypes also occur under natural conditions. Shope [18] presented serological evidence that human to pig transmission could occur, but it was not until the isolation of Hong Kong H3N2 virus from pigs in Taiwan in 1970 [19] that investigations began to examine the potential transmission of human strains to pigs. Although no disease was reported among infected pigs, in the next several years H3N2 viruses were isolated regularly from pigs and/or antibody was in swine populations throughout the world [reviewed 15]. H3N2 influenza A viruses related to a human strain from 1973, continued to circulate in European pig populations long after their disappearance from the human population. Since 1984, outbreaks of clinical influenza in pigs due to an H3N2 influenza A virus, related antigenically to human strains from the early to mid 1970's, have been observed throughout Europe with infections frequently characterised by high seroprevalence. Until 1998 H3N2 virus was rarely detected in pigs in the United States [20] but subsequently the emergence of an H3N2 virus derived following genetic reassortment (*see* "Genetic reassortment in the pig", *p. 49*) resulted in rapid spread, and the virus was often associated with outbreaks of clinical disease [21, 22].

Human H1N1 viruses can also infect pigs, but although pig to pig transmission has been demonstrated under experimental conditions, most strains are not readily transmitted among pigs in the field [13]. Serological surveillance studies worldwide suggest that the prevailing human H1N1 strains are readily transmitted to pigs [14] and have resulted occasionally in the isolation of virus [23] but are not apparently maintained in pigs independently of the human population.

"Avian-like" viruses

In Eurasia, there have been several introductions of avian H1N1 viruses to pigs that have led to the establishment of stable lineages. These viruses have spread widely in pigs in this region and are often associated with disease epizootics. Since 1979 these viruses have become the dominant strain in European pigs and are antigenically and genetically distinguishable from classical swine H1N1 influenza viruses, but related closely to H1N1 viruses isolated from ducks [24]. All of the gene segments of the prototype viruses were of avian origin indicating that transmission of a whole avian virus into pigs had occurred, and as a result have been implicated as the possible precursors of the next human pandemic virus [25]. These "avian-like" viruses appear to have a selective advantage over classical swine H1N1 viruses which are related antigenically, since in Europe they have replaced classical swine influenza virus [9, 26]. Within two years of the introduction of "avian-like" viruses into pigs in Great Britain, classical swine H1N1 apparently disappeared as a clinical entity. More recently an independent introduction of H1N1 virus from birds to pigs has occurred in Southern China and these viruses have been detected in pigs in South-East Asia since 1993 [17] where they are currently cocirculating with classical H1N1 viruses. Phylogenetic analysis of the genes of these viruses has revealed that they form an Asian sublineage of the Eurasian avian lineage. In addition, some of the H3N2 viruses isolated from pigs in Asia since the 1970's have been entirely "avian-like" and have been introduced apparently from ducks, although their association with epizootics of respiratory disease in pigs is unproven.

H1N2 viruses

Influenza A H1N2 viruses, derived from classical swine H1N1, and "human-like" swine H3N2 viruses have been isolated in Japan and France. In Japan, these viruses appear to have spread widely within pigs and are associated frequently with respiratory disease [27]. Subsequently an H1N2 influenza virus (*see* "Genetic reassortment", *p. 49*) related antigenically to human and "human-like" swine viruses has emerged and become endemic in pigs in Great Britain [28] often in association with respiratory disease. These viruses have subsequently spread to pigs in the rest of Europe.

Avian influenza viruses newly detected in pigs

Recently, H9N2 viruses have apparently been introduced into pigs in South-East Asia, possibly from poultry [29]. Influenza viruses of H9N2 subtype have become increasingly widespread in bird populations presumably facilitating transmission through frequent contact. In 1999, an avian H4N6 virus was isolated from pigs in Canada with respiratory symptoms. There was local spread on the farm which was located next to an area of open water where waterfowl congregate. The genotype of the virus was entirely avian, indicating in-toto transmission from a bird [30]. The potential of H9N2 or H4N6 avian viruses novel to pigs, to spread and persist within pigs remains unknown, substantiating the need for good surveillance of swine populations worldwide.

The pig as an intermediate host for influenza A viruses?

Given the worldwide interaction between humans, pigs, birds and other mammalian species there is a high potential for cross-species transmission of influenza viruses in nature. Pigs are an important host in influenza virus ecology since they are susceptible to infection with both avian and human influenza A viruses, often being involved in interspecies transmission, facilitated by regular close contact with humans or birds. Pigs serve as major reservoirs of H1N1 and H3N2 influenza viruses and the maintenance of these viruses in pigs and the frequent introduction of viruses from other species may be important in the generation of "new" strains of influenza, some of which may have the potential to transmit to other species including humans.

The pig has been the leading contender for the role of intermediate host for influenza A viruses. Pigs are the only mammalian species which are domesticated, reared in abundance and are susceptible to, and allow productive replication of avian influenza viruses. This susceptibility is due to the presence of both α2,3- and α2,6-galactose sialic acid linkages in cells lining the pig trachea which can result in modification of the receptor binding specificities of avian influenza viruses from α2,3 to α2,6 linkage [31], which is the native linkage in humans, thereby providing a potential link from birds to humans.

It has been shown that humans occasionally contract influenza viruses from pigs. The internal protein genes of human influenza viruses share a common ancestor with the genes of some swine influenza viruses. A number of authors have proposed the nucleoprotein (NP) gene as a determinant of host range which can restrict or attenuate virus replication thereby controlling the successful transmission of virus to a "new" host. These observations support the potential role of the pig as a mixing vessel of influenza viruses from avian and human sources. The pig appears to have a broader host range in the compatibility of the NP gene in reassortant viruses [32] than both humans and birds. Studies by Kida *et al.* [33], investigating experimentally the growth potential of a wide diversity of avian influenza viruses in pigs, indicate that these viruses (including representatives of subtypes H1 to H13), with or without HA types known to infect humans, can be transmitted to pigs. Therefore the possibility for the introduction of avian influenza virus genes to humans *via* pigs could occur. Furthermore, these studies showed that avian viruses which do not replicate in pigs can contribute genes in the generation of reassortants when coinfecting pigs with a swine influenza virus. Constant cocirculation of viruses of different genotype and phenotype results in continual genetic exchange amongst these viruses which may give rise to a novel virus with the potential to spread to other species.

Pigs in the "influenza epicentre"

The majority of pandemic strains have apparently originated in China raising the possibility that this region is an influenza epicentre. In China, influenza viruses of all subtypes are prevalent in ducks and in water frequented by ducks. This region accounts for over sixty per cent of the world pig population and agricultural practices provide that there is close contact between wild aquatic birds, domestic ducks, pigs and humans, thereby presenting the opportunity for interspecies transmission and genetic exchange among influenza viruses, with the pig acting as an intermediary between domestic ducks and humans. However, the interface between pigs and other species particularly humans is also significant in many other parts of the world (*see* "Pig to human transmission").

Genetic reassortment in the pig

Eurasia

Evidence for the pig as a mixing vessel of influenza viruses of non swine origin has been demonstrated in Europe by Castrucci *et al.* [34], who detected reassortment of human and avian viruses in Italian pigs. Phylogenetic analyses of human H3N2 viruses circulating in Italian pigs revealed that genetic reassortment had been occurring between avian and "human-like" viruses since 1983. The unique co-circulation of influenza A viruses within European swine may lead to pigs serving as a mixing vessel for reassortment between influenza viruses from mammalian and avian hosts with unknown implications for both humans and pigs. It would appear that human H1 viruses are able to perpetuate in pigs following genetic reassortment. Furthermore, these viruses may be maintained in pigs long after one or both of the progenitor viruses have disappeared from their natural hosts. Reassortant viruses of H1N2 subtype derived from human and avian viruses [35] or H1N7 subtype derived from human and equine viruses [36] have been isolated from pigs in Great Britain. The H1N2 viruses derived from a multiple reassortant event, spreading widely within pigs in Great Britain and subsequently to other parts of Europe. Viruses of H1N2 subtype have also been derived from genetic reassortment of strains endemic in pigs, and have been established in pigs in Japan since 1978 [37]. Similar viruses were detected in France but apparently failed to become established.

North America

Since 1998 H3N2 viruses isolated from pigs in the USA have contained combinations of human, swine and avian genes. Furthermore, the HA gene of these viruses was derived from a human virus circulating in the human population in 1995 [21]. These newly emerged triple reassortant H3N2 viruses appear to be established in pigs in North America and are able to reassort with classical H1N1 viruses producing another unique genotype of H1N2 virus [38].

Transmission between pigs and other species

Pigs serve as major reservoirs of H1N1 and H3N2 influenza viruses and are often involved in interspecies transmission of influenza viruses. The maintenance of these viruses in pigs and the frequent introduction of new viruses from other species could be important in the generation of pandemic strains of human influenza.

Transmission between pigs and humans

Transmission of influenza A viruses from pigs to humans occurs on a regular basis, however subsequent transmission of these viruses within the human population is very rare. Serological studies of people having occupational contact with pigs support frequent transmissions, through the detection of antibodies, to swine influenza viruses. Pigs were implicated as the source of infection when an H1N1 virus was isolated from a soldier who had died of influenza at Fort Dix, New Jersey, USA. The virus was identical to viruses isolated from pigs in the USA. Furthermore, five other servicemen were shown to be infected by virus isolation, and serological evidence suggested that some 500 personnel at Fort Dix were, or had been, infected with the same virus. Subsequently there have been several reports of classical swine H1N1 influenza virus being isolated from humans with respiratory illness, occasionally with fatal consequences. All cases examined followed contact with sick pigs. Perhaps of greater significance for humans is a report of two distinct cases of infection of children in the Netherlands during 1993 with H3N2 viruses whose genes encoding internal proteins were of avian origin [39]. Genetically and antigenically related viruses had been detected in European pigs [24] raising the possibility of potential transmission of avian influenza virus genes to humans following genetic reassortment in pigs. These concerns were substantiated further by the results of serological studies in Italy which indicated that these "swine" H3N2 viruses had apparently been transmitted to young, immunologically naive persons [26].

The prevailing strains in the human population transmit to pigs frequently but it would appear that only H3N2 viruses can establish stable lineages without genetic reassortment. Human H3N2 viruses are endemic in most pig populations worldwide, where they persist many years after their antigenic counterparts have disappeared from humans and therefore present a reservoir of virus which may in the future infect a susceptible human population. However, there is no apparent evidence of pigs being infected with this subtype prior to the pandemic in humans in 1968.

Transmission between pigs and birds

The probable introduction of classical swine H1N1 influenza viruses to turkeys from infected pigs has been reported from North America and in some cases influenza-like illness in pigs has been followed immediately by disease signs in turkeys. Serological studies have revealed antibodies to classical swine H1 influenza virus in both turkeys and pigs. Genetic analyses of H1N1 viruses from turkeys in the United States has revealed a high degree of genetic exchange and reassortment of influenza A viruses from turkeys and pigs, in the former species. Hinshaw *et al.* [40] report the isolation of swine H1N1 virus from turkeys and the subsequent transmission to a laboratory technician who displayed fever, respiratory illness, virus shedding and seroconversion. These findings raise the possibility that viruses from pigs, humans, turkeys and ducks may serve as a source of virus for the other three. In Europe, avian H1N1 viruses were transmitted to pigs (*see* "Avian-like H1N1 viruses"), established a stable lineage and have subsequently been reintroduced into turkeys from pigs causing economic losses. *See also* "Avian influenza viruses newly detected in pigs", *p. 47.*

Adaptation of "new" influenza viruses to pigs

Following interspecies transmission and/or genetic reassortment an influenza virus may undergo many pig to pig transmissions because of the continual availability of susceptible pigs. The mechanisms whereby an avian virus is able to establish a new lineage in pigs remain unclear; although following the introduction of an avian virus into European pigs in 1979, the virus was relatively unstable for approximately ten years [25], but the mutation rate of this virus did not subsequently increase [41]. Furthermore, adaptation of this virus to pigs, resulted in the virus acquiring altered receptor specificity, preferentially recognising receptors with α2,6 linkage [31], the native linkage in humans (*see* "The pig as an intermediate host for influenza A viruses?"). The avian H4N6 virus detected in pigs in 1999 had some modifications in the receptor binding pocket on the HA gene which may have facilitated binding to receptors with α2,6 linkage [30]. Furthermore, the continual genetic exchange between viruses is likely to result in the emergence of "genetic variants" with a higher fitness and therefore potential selective advantage. It would appear that the adaptive processes can take many years as occurred following transmission of both avian H1N1 and human H3N2 viruses to pigs. Following new introductions of influenza A virus to pigs, close monitoring of the epizootiology of SI in a population is essential to determine the rate of change, which, if elevated, may facilitate further transmissions across the species barrier with potential implications for disease control in a range of other species including humans.

Genetic variation

Phylogenetic analyses of influenza virus genes have revealed that they have evolved broadly in five major host-specific pathways comprising early and late equine viruses, human/classical swine viruses, H13 gull viruses and all other avian viruses. Geographic patterns of evolution occur amongst bird populations forming sublineages relating to North America, Eurasia and Australasia. Following transmission to pigs, influenza virus genes evolve in the pathway of the host of origin but diverge forming a separate sublineage [5]. All of the genes of human and classical swine viruses form a sister group since they share a common ancestor and the comparable rate of change in some genes such as NP is very similar [5]. However, analyses of the genes of avian viruses following their transmission to pigs in Europe revealed the highest evolutionary rates for influenza genes for a period of approximately ten years, and may be due to the virus possessing a mutator mutation in the polymerase complex [25].

Genes that code for the surface proteins HA and NA are subjected to the highest rates of change. The HA gene of both the classical and "avian-like" swine H1N1 viruses is undergoing genetic drift, being more marked in the latter. However, genetic drift in the HA gene of swine H1N1 viruses is confined generally to regions unrelated to antigenic sites, which is in marked contrast to genetic drift in the HA gene of human H1N1 viruses. The limited antigenic variation in the HA gene of swine viruses is probably due to the lack of significant immune selection in pigs because of the continual availability of non-immune pigs. The HA genes of classical swine H1N1 influenza virus isolates in North America have remained conserved both genetically and antigenically over a period of at least 25 years, but viruses distinguishable antigenically, although closely related, have been detected. Following new introductions of influenza A virus to pigs, as occurred in South-East Asia in 1993, close monitoring of the epizootiology of SI in a population is essential to determine the rate of change, which, if elevated, may facilitate further transmissions across the species barrier with potential implications for disease control in a range of other species including humans.

Influenza viruses of H3N2 subtype continue to circulate widely in pigs worldwide. The majority of these virsues are antigenically, closely related, to early human strains such as A/Port Chalmers/1/73. The limited immune selection in pigs facilitates the persistence of these viruses, which may in the future transmit to a susceptible human population. However, some viruses although related closely to the prototype human viruses have antigenic differences in the surface glycoproteins and may cocirculate with the former strains [28]. "Human-like" swine H3N2 viruses appear to be evolving independently in different lineages to those of human and avian strains [42, 43]. The rates of genetic drift in HA and NA genes is equivalent to those of H3N2 viruses in the human population but in contrast to the latter the changes are not generally associated with antigenic sites [44]. However, marked genetic drift resulting in considerable antigenic variation in the HA gene of "human-like" H3N2 viruses in European pigs has led to an apparent increase in epizootics attributable to this virus. In addition, the prevailing epidemic strains in the human population are transmitted frequently to pigs [44] and these viruses are clearly distinguishable antigenically from the early human viruses established in pigs.

References

1. Alexander DJ. Ecological aspects of influenza A viruses in animals and their relationship to human influenza: a review. *JR Soc Med* 1982; 75: 799-811.
2. Webster RG, Bean WJ, Gorman OT, Chambers TM, Kawaoka Y. Evolution and ecology of influenza A viruses. *Microbiol Rev* 1992; 56: 152-79.
3. Chun J. Influenza including its infection among pigs. *Nat Med J China* 1919; 5: 34-44.
4. Koen JS. A practical method for the field diagnosis of swine diseases. *Am J Vet Med* 1919; 14: 468.
5. Gorman OT, Bean WJ, Kawaoka Y, Donatelli I, Guo YJ, Webster RG. Evolution of influenza A virus nucleoprotein genes: implications for the origins of H1N1 human and classical swine viruses. *J Virol* 1991; 65: 3704-14.
6. Reid AH, Fanning TG, Hultin JV, Taubenberger JK. Origin and evolution of the 1918 "Spanish" influenza virus hemagglutinin gene. *Proc Natl Acad Sci USA* 1999; 96: 1651-6.
7. Reid AH, Fanning TG, Janczewski TA, Taubenberger JK. Characterization of the 1918 "Spanish" influenza virus neuraminidase gene. *Proc Natl Acad Sci USA* 2000; 97: 6785-90.
8. Shope RE. Swine influenza. III. Filtration experiments and etiology. *J Exp Med* 1931; 54: 373-85.
9. Bachmann PA. Swine influenza virus. In: Pensaert MB, ed. *Virus infections of porcines*. Amsterdam: Elsevier Science Publishers, 1989: 193-207.
10. Easterday BC. Animals in the influenza world. *Philosophical Transactions of the Royal Society, London* 1980; B288: 433-7.
11. Blaskovic D, Jamrichova D, Rathova V, Kocisckova D, Kaplan MM. Experimental infection of weanling pigs with A/swine/influenza virus. 2. The shedding of virus by infected animals. *Bull WHO* 1970; 42: 767-70.
12. Nakamura RM, Easterday BC, Pawlisch R, Walker GL. Swine influenza: epizootiological and serological studies. *Bull WHO* 1972; 47: 481-7.
13. Hinshaw VS, Bean J Jr, Webster RG, Easterday BC. The prevalence of influenza viruses in swine and the antigenic and genetic relatedness of influenza viruses from man to swine. *Virology* 1978; 84: 51-62.

14. Brown IH, Harris PA, Alexander DJ. Serological studies of influenza viruses in pigs in Great-Britain 1991-2. *Epidemiol Infect* 1995; 114: 511-20.
15. Brown IH. The epidemiology and evolution of influenza viruses in pigs. *Vet Microbiol* 2000; 74: 29-46.
16. Nardelli L, Pascucci S, Gualandi GL, Loda P. Outbreaks of classical swine influenza in Italy in 1976. *Zentralblatt fur Veterinarmedizin* 1978; 25B: 853-7.
17. Guan Y, Shortridge KF, Krauss S, Li PH, Kawaoka Y, Webster RG. Emergence of avian H1N1 influenza viruses in pigs in China. *J Virol* 1996; 70: 8041-6.
18. Shope RE. Serological evidence for the occurrence of infection with human influenza virus in swine. *J Exp Med* 1938; 67: 739-48.
19. Kundin WD. Hong Kong A2 influenza virus infection among swine during a human epidemic in Taiwan. *Nature* 1970; 228: 857.
20. Chambers TM, Hinshaw VS, Kawaoka Y, Easterday BC, Webster RG. Influenza viral infection of swine in the United States 1988-1989. *Arch Virol* 1991; 116: 261-5.
21. Zhou NN, Senne DA, Landgraf JS, Swenson SL, Erickson G, Rossow K, Liu L, Yoon KJ, Krauss S, Webster RG. Genetic reassortment of avian, swine and human influenza A viruses in American pigs. *J Virol* 1999; 73: 8851-6.
22. Karasin AI, Schutten MM, Cooper LA, Smith CB, Subbarao K, Anderson GA, Carman S, Olsen CW. Genetic characterization of H3N2 influenza viruses isolated from pigs in North America, 1977-1999: evidence for wholly human and reassortant virus genotypes. *Virus Res* 2000; 68: 71-85.
23. Katsuda K, Sato S, Shirahata T, Lindstrom S, Nerome R, Ishida M, Nerome K, Goto H. Antigenic and genetic characteristics of H1N1 human influenza virus isolated from pigs in Japan. *J Gen Virol* 1995; 76: 1247-9.
24. Pensaert M, Ottis K, Vandeputte J, Kaplan MM, Bachmann PA. Evidence for the natural transmission of influenza A virus from wild ducks to swine and its potential importance for man. *Bull WHO* 1981; 59: 75-8.
25. Ludwig S, Stitz L, Planz O, Van H, Fitch WM, Scholtissek C. European swine virus as a possible source for the next influenza pandemic? *Virology* 1995; 212: 555-61.
26. Campitelli L, Donatelli I, Foni E, Castrucci MR, Fabiani C, Kawaoka Y, Krauss S, Webster RG. Continued evolution of H1N1 and H3N2 influenza viruses in pigs in Italy. *Virology* 1997; 232: 310-8.
27. Ouchi A, Nerome K, Kanegae Y, Ishida M, Nerome R, Hayashi K, Hashimoto T, Kaji M, Kaji Y, Inaba Y. Large outbreak of swine influenza in southern Japan caused by reassortant (H1N2) influenza viruses: its epizootic background and characterisation of the causative viruses. *J Gen Virol* 1996; 77: 1751-9.
28. Brown IH, Chakraverty P, Harris PA, Alexander DJ. Disease outbreaks in pigs in Great Britain due to an influenza A virus of H1N2 subtype. *Vet Rec* 1995; 136: 328-9.
29. Peiris JSM, Guan Y, Ghose P, Markwell D, Krauss S, Webster RG, Shortridge KF. H3N2, H9N2 and H1N1 subtype influenza viruses co-circulate in pigs in south eastern China. *Proc Options Control Influenza* IV, Hersonissos, Crete, Greece, 23-28 September, 2000, p. 40.
30. Karasin AI, Brown IH, Carmen S, Olsen CW. Isolation and characterization of H4N6 avian influenza viruses from pigs with pneumonia in Canada. *J Virol* 2000; 74: 9322-7.
31. Ito T, Nelson J, Couceiro SS, Kelm S, Baum LG, Krauss S, Castrucci MR, Donatelli I, Kida H, Paulson JC, Webster RG, Kawaoka Y. Molecular basis for the generation in pigs of influenza A viruses with pandemic potential. *J Virol* 1998; 72: 7367-73.
32. Scholtissek C, Burger H, Kistner O, Shortridge KF. The nucleoprotein as a possible major factor in determining host specificity of influenza H3N2 viruses. *Virology* 1985; 147: 287-94.
33. Kida H, Ito T, Yasuda J, Shimizu Y, Itakura C, Shortridge KF, Kawaoka Y, Webster RG. Potential for transmission of avian influenza viruses to pigs. *J Gen Virol* 1994; 75: 2183-8.
34. Castrucci MR, Donatelli I, Sidoli L, Barigazzi G, Kawaoka Y, Webster RG. Genetic reassortment between avian and human influenza A viruses in Italian pigs. *Virol* 1993; 193: 503-6.
35. Brown IH, Harris PA, McCauley JW, Alexander DJ. Multiple genetic reassortment of avian and human influenza A viruses in European pigs, resulting in the emergence of an H1N2 virus of novel genotype. *J Gen Virol* 1998; 79: 2947-55.
36. Brown IH, Alexander DJ, Chakraverty P, Harris PA, Manvell RJ. Isolation of an influenza A virus of unusual subtype (H1N7) from pigs in England, and the subsequent experimental transmission from pig to pig. *Vet Microbiol* 1994; 39: 125-34.
37. Sugimura T, Yonemochi H, Ogawa T, Tanaka Y, Kumagai T. Isolation of a recombinant influenza virus (Hsw1N2) from swine in Japan. *Arch Virol* 1980; 66: 271-4.

38. Karasin AI, Olsen CW, Anderson GA. Genetic characterization of an H1N2 influenza virus isolated from a pig in Indiana. *J Clin Micro Biol* 2000; 38: 2453-6.
39. Claas ECJ, Kawaoka Y, De Jong JC, Masurel N, Webster RG, De Jong JC. Infection of children with avian-human reassortant influenza virus from pigs in Europe. *Virology* 1994; 204: 453-7.
40. Hinshaw VS, Webster RG, Bean WJ, Downie J, Senne DA. Swine influenza like viruses in turkeys: potential source of virus for humans? *Science* 1983; 220: 206-8.
41. Stech J, Xiong X, Scholtissek C, Webster RG. Independence of evolutionary and mutational rates after transmission of avian influenza viruses to swine. *J Virol* 1999; 73: 1878-84.
42. Castrucci MR, Campitelli L, Ruggieri A, Barigazzi G, Sidoli L, Daniels R, Oxford JS, Donatelli I. Antigenic and sequence analysis of H3 influenza virus haemagglutinins from pigs in Italy. *J Gen Virol* 1994; 75: 371-9.
43. DeJong JC, van Nieuwstadt AP, Kimman TG, Loeffen WLA, Bestebroer TM, Bijlsma K, Verweij C, Osterhaus ADME, Claas ECJ. Antigenic drift in swine influenza H3 haemagglutinins with implications for vaccination policy. *Vaccine* 1999; 17: 1321-8.
44. Nerome K, Kanegae Y, Shortridge KF, Sugita S, Ishida M. Genetic analysis of porcine H3N2 viruses originating in southern China. *J Gen Virol* 1995; 76: 613-24.

Emergence and Control of Zoonotic Ortho- and Paramyxovirus Diseases
B. Dodet, M. Vicari, eds.

Equine influenza outbreaks in China, including Hong Kong, 1989-94. A review

Thomas M. Chambers[1], Kennedy F. Shortridge[2], Alexander C.K. Lai[3], David G. Powell[1], Keith L. Watkins[4]

[1] *Gluck Equine Research Center, University of Kentucky, Lexington, KY, USA*
[2] *Department of Microbiology, Queen Mary Hospital, The University of Hong Kong, Hong Kong SAR, China*
[3] *Department of Microbiology and Molecular Genetics, Oklahoma State University, Stillwater, OK, USA*
[4] *The Hong Kong Jockey Club, Veterinary Department, Sha Tin Racecourse, New Territories, Hong Kong SAR, China*

Abstract – Since 1989, the largest outbreaks of equine influenza worldwide have occurred in China. These included outbreaks in 1989-90 whose cause was determined to be a novel equine agent, a genetically avian-like subtype H3N8 influenza virus (equine/Jilin/1/89). Research established that conventional equine influenza vaccines were unlikely to have protected against this virus. Thus arose concern that subsequent outbreaks in this part of the world might represent the establishment and spread of this virus. In 1993 another outbreak of H3N8 influenza did occur in China that, although of the established equine-2 H3N8 virus lineage, was atypical in its severity and range of epizootic spread. Also in 1992 an outbreak occurred in Hong Kong, which was shown to be caused not by the avian-like virus but by an equine-2 influenza virus similar to those circulating in England and Ireland, from whence it was probably introduced in imported horses. This last-named outbreak was among an equine population that received regular, close veterinary scrutiny; thus the origin and course of this outbreak could be documented with unusual clarity. This population was well vaccinated, yet that did not prevent 75% from becoming infected. The investigation produced insights into the effectiveness of the usual standard of equine quarantine protocols in protecting against imported infectious diseases; the time course of an epizootic starting from virus introduction; the routes by which equine influenza viruses could spread within a controlled-environment equine facility; the limitations of conventional diagnostic methodologies and applicability of new ones; the effectiveness of conventional vaccination; the evolution of equine-2 influenza viral hemagglutinin worldwide and also within an outbreak; and not least the economic costs of such an outbreak. These insights have since led to considerably altered protocols for quarantine testing and vaccination in Hong Kong, and their lessons should be applied in other developed countries if similar outbreaks are to be avoided.

Equine influenza worldwide

Equine influenza is not a new disease, though its history prior to the twentieth century is clouded. Descriptions of influenza-like illness in horses can be found in military literature from the Roman Empire. One historical epizootic of equine respiratory disease with the hallmarks of influenza, *i.e.* coughing, nasal discharge, and extremely rapid spread, originated in Toronto at the end of September 1872, and spread across the North American continent to Cuba by November 1872, to California by April 1873, and to British Columbia, Mexico, and Guatemala during the summer of 1873. During the six weeks of its prevalence in New York City, the excess deaths of horses attributed to influenza were estimated to be 1,412, or 3.7% of the entire horse population of the city [1], a mortality rate that may have been higher than the overall rate for the human 1918 pandemic. This epizootic was never reported in Europe, probably because the duration of a sea voyage effectively quarantined any infected horses for several weeks of recovery.

The modern history of equine influenza began in 1955 when the influenza virus was first associated with equine respiratory disease [2], and shortly thereafter the first equine influenza virus isolate, influenza A/equine/Prague/56 (H7N7) was obtained from Czechoslovakia [3]. Subsequent serological studies suggested this virus, now known as the equine-1 subtype, might have circulated in horses in England as early as 1948 [4] or in the USA by the mid-1950's [5]. But, as nucleotide sequencing has established, the Prague/56 strain is, evolutionarily, remarkably primitive. Except for the hemagglutinin (HA) and neuraminidase (NA) genes that undergo antigenic drift, the genes of Prague/56 virus are more similar in sequence to their counterparts in influenza B viruses than are those of any other influenza A virus isolate. Thus, the evolutionary distance from the hypothetical common ancestor of influenza A and B viruses to Prague/56 virus is less than for any other influenza A virus [6]. Whence this virus originated and how long it was maintained in horses are unknown – ca. 1800 has been estimated – but the general susceptibility of horses worldwide to equine-1 influenza in the 1950's and early 1960's suggests its surface antigens were recently acquired.

A second subtype, now called equine-2 (H3N8) influenza virus, was first isolated in the United States in 1963 [7] and spread rapidly around the world. Nucleotide sequencing has revealed a heterogeneous origin for this virus subtype. The genes encoding its HA and NA surface antigens seem to have co-evolved from a hypothetical ancestral equine-2 virus of ca. 1952 [8, 9], but their divergence from common avian ancestral genes was much earlier. The HA and also PB1, PA, and NP genes seem to have diverged from ancestral avian lineages coincidentally at ca. 1870, although any connection with the equine epizootic event of 1872-73 [1] can only be speculative. The PB2, M, and NS genes diverged from avian ancestors more recently; this is estimated at 1952 in the case of the NS [10]. Thus the equine-2 subtype apparently arose from a reassortment event of ca. 1952 in which one of the parents was a contemporary avian influenza virus, whereas the other had previously diverged from avian lineages and, although unrelated to the equine-1 subtype, was possibly already being maintained in horses.

Both subtypes co-circulated in horses from 1963 to approximately 1979, and reassorted with each other sometime during 1964-1973, so that later equine-1 viruses possessed equine-2 genes for all segments except HA, NA, and M [11]. Since 1980 there has not been a confirmed outbreak of wild-type equine-1 influenza [12], although unconfirmed outbreaks were reported from India and Egypt [13, 14]. Equine-2 influenza has circulated widely: most parts of the world have experienced at least one outbreak, and the disease has been enzootic in the USA, Western Europe, and Scandinavia. Equine-1 and equine-2 viruses have not been reported from Australia and New Zealand.

Recent evolution of equine-2 influenza viruses will be discussed elsewhere in these proceedings.

Outbreaks in China

China has been the subject of much recent study by human influenza virologists as a result of 1) the frequent appearance of new antigenic variants in China and East Asia before they become predominant in the Western hemisphere; 2) the observation that the last two major pandemics resulting from antigenic shift both originated in Southern China; 3) the Hong Kong "bird flu" event of 1997 which was considered to be an incipient pandemic; and 4) the "mixing vessel" hypothesis ascribing the advent of pandemic influenza viruses to reassortment between avian and human strains, most likely in the pig. The last, if true, would seem to be most favored or promoted by the agricultural practices of China which favor a close association between humans and animals [15, 16]. For these reasons the region has been recognized for the last 20 years as a hypothetical influenza epicenter for the emergence of pandemic viruses [17].

The equine population of China is mostly in the north and are mostly working animals often receiving relatively little veterinary care or vaccination. Thus in retrospect it should be no surprise that major outbreaks of equine influenza have occurred in China, or that one of these involved a novel avian-derived agent. But importantly there has been no observed reassortment or antigenic shift. Equine influenza is enzootic in the Autonomous Region of Inner Mongolia (Nei Mongol), commonly arising at the end of winter. Equine-1 influenza was reported in 1974 [18] causing 30% morbidity. The outbreaks of 1989-90, 1992 in Hong Kong, and 1993-94 are discussed below.

1989 outbreak of avian-like virus

In March 1989 a novel strain of equine influenza appeared in horses in China, triggering a massive outbreak from March to June involving over 20,000 horses, of which some 400 (2%) perished. This outbreak occurred in the Jilin and Heilongjiang Provinces of North-East China, and apparently did not spread further *(Figure 1)*. Overall morbidity was reported as 81%, and mortality in some herds was as high as 20%. Symptoms were typical of severe equine influenza: fever exceeding 40 °C, coughing, bronchitis, mucoid nasal and sometimes ocular discharge, and pneumonia, with the typical course of disease lasting 5-6 days [19, 20].

A second outbreak of this novel strain occurred in April 1990 in the Heilongjiang province, causing 41% morbidity but no mortality. No subsequent outbreaks have been reported [19, 20]. No humans are known to have contracted disease from these outbreaks.

The agents of these outbreaks were studied by Guo *et al.* [20]. The isolated virus strains included influenza A/equine/Jilin/1/89, A/equine/Heilongjiang/89, and A/equine/Heilongjiang/90. These were H3N8 viruses, but further analysis revealed they were antigenically, by both hemagglutination- and neuraminidase-inhibition tests, more similar to duck H3N8 than to classical equine-2 influenza viruses. Nucleotide sequence

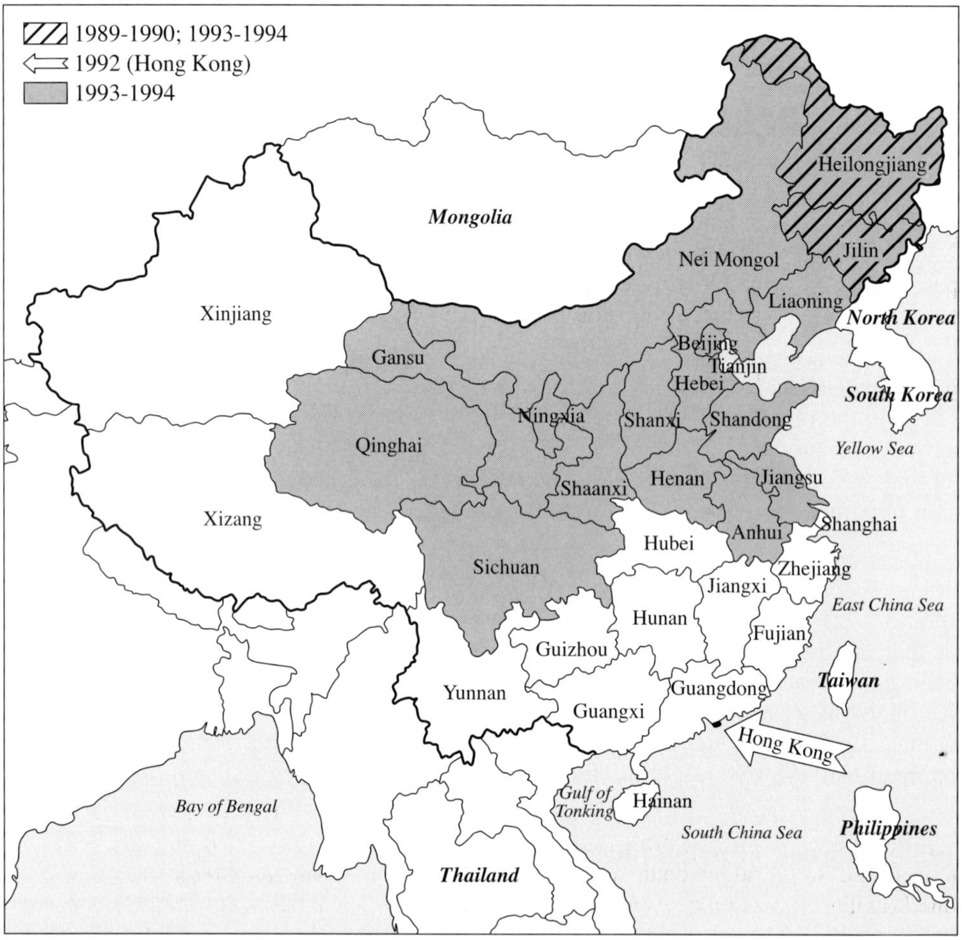

Figure 1. Equine flu outbreaks.

analysis showed that six of the eight gene segments of each virus (PA, HA, NP, NA, M, NS) were more similar to avian (duck) influenza virus genes than to either equine-1 or equine-2 influenza genes, or to the counterpart genes of gull, pig, and human influenza viruses. The Eq/Jilin/89 H3 HA was most similar to the HA of the H3 prototype Duck/Ukraine/3/63 virus. The origin of the remaining two genes, PB1 and PB2, was equivocal as these are highly similar among the influenza A viruses of different hosts. The Jilin and Heilongjiang isolates were nearly identical, indicating that the 1989 and 1990 outbreaks resulted from a single virus introduction.

Despite its apparently recent avian origin, Eq/Jilin/89 virus failed experimentally to replicate in ducks, while in chickens it replicated efficiently only when inoculated intravenously. In contrast, it did replicate efficiently in both mice and ferrets following intranasal inoculation [20]. Thus significant viral adaptation to growth in mammals had already occurred, and indeed five unique amino acid substitutions were identified in the Eq/Jilin/89 NP gene that may possibly be associated with adaptation to horses. The significance of this adaptation may be of relevance to understanding how pandemic influenza viruses arise.

Since no reassortment was involved, the outbreak this most closely parallels is the "bird flu" outbreak of avian H5N1 virus in humans, in Hong Kong in 1997 [21]. The Jilin outbreak posed a risk that the novel virus strain might spread to other parts of the world, or it might reassort with the established (equine-2) influenza virus strain to solidify its adaptation to the equine host, and start a panzootic of equine "bird flu". Unlike the H5N1 virus, however, the new equine virus seems intrinsically no more pathogenic than the existing equine-2 subtype aside from its antigenic difference, as evidenced by the reduced morbidity of its 1990 recurrence. Equine influenza vaccines then commercially available in the USA were weakly cross-reactive but not highly immunogenic, and would not have provided complete protection against the Eq/Jilin/89 virus [22, 23]. Indeed, that generation of vaccines did not completely protect against contemporaneous classical equine-2 strains either as suggested by the 1992 Hong Kong outbreak *(see below)* among others (*e.g.* Binns *et al.* [24]; Chambers *et al.*, [25]).

This Northern Chinese outbreak represents a second, independent introduction of avian-like H3N8 influenza virus into horses. Why H3N8? It remains unclear whether the H3N8 subtype has unique properties facilitating virus growth in horses. Unpublished results from one of us (TMC) suggest that some other avian influenza subtypes are able to replicate in equine tracheal cells.

Horses, however, do not appear to be mixing vessels as pigs are thought to be. While it has been previously suggested that equine-2-like viruses may have been involved in the human pandemic of ca. 1890 [26, 27], no equine influenza outbreak, including the Eq/Jilin/89 outbreak, is known to have caused disease in humans. Also there is no evidence that equines are susceptible to human influenza viruses. A recent study by Suzuki *et al.* [28] demonstrates that differences in the predominating structure of epithelial cell sialyl sugar chain receptors between horses and humans are an effective block against replication of human H3 influenza viruses in horses. Similarly, we have been unable to transmit equine-2 influenza virus to cattle (Lin *et al.*, unpublished data). So, despite their frequent close contact with other influenza-susceptible species, horses appear not to be sources for interspecies transmission of influenza.

1993-94 outbreak

A new outbreak of equine influenza was first detected in Inner Mongolia in May 1993. It is believed to have been derived from an outbreak in Northwest China during the autumn of 1992, then spread eastward through Mongolia, crossing border checkpoints by way of mounted soldiers (Shortridge *et al.*, in preparation). It gradually spread as far Northeast as Heilongjiang, eastward to Hebei Province and Beijing, and Southwest through Gansu and Qinghei Provinces during early 1994. In April 1994 the outbreak spread to horses in Sichuan and Anhui Provinces, where it finally abated soon after *(Figure 1)*. From May 1993 to mid-April 1994 about 2.25 million horses were clinically affected with a mortality of about 1% [29]. Donkeys and mules were also affected, but not humans or other domestic animals. This outbreak did not spread beyond the Yangtze River into Southern China, where equine populations were much lower.

The concern raised by this outbreak was the threat mentioned above, that either the avian-like Eq/Jilin/89 virus was becoming established, or a reassortant of that virus with equine-2 virus was emerging. In fact, antigenic and partial sequence analyses demonstrated that the Eq/Gansu/94 virus isolates were most similar to recent equine-2 viruses in all their gene segments and so were not reassortants [30]. The HA gene was similar to that of other Eurasian strains then in circulation. Horses in Heilongjiang Province had lower convalescent titers to the Eq/Gansu/94 virus than horses elsewhere. This, together with higher than expected titers against Eq/Jilin/89 virus, suggested either that Eq/Jilin/89 virus was still in circulation or that previously infected horses had responded to the 1994 outbreak by producing antibodies against the earlier strain, *i.e.* "original antigenic sin".

Outbreak in Hong Kong, 1992

Although chronologically earlier, the Hong Kong outbreak is discussed last because its circumstances of scale and scrutiny yield a clearer picture of its course from beginning to end than virtually any other outbreak, save for that in South Africa in 1986 [31]. As in 1993-94 the initial fear was that it represented reemergence of the Eq/Jilin/89 virus, but instead a classical equine-2 influenza virus was responsible. The first isolate, Eq/Hong Kong/1/92, was most similar to recent equine-2 strains in all its genes. Its HA gene was almost identical to a contemporaneous strain isolated in England, Eq/Lambourn/22778/92, differing only at a single amino acid (Thr-244) [32]. In addition to the index virus, 15 more isolates were collected during this outbreak. Sequence analysis of the HA genes direct from the initial swab samples indicates there is heterogeneity, either C or T, sometimes both in the same sample, at nucleotide position 805, the second base of codon 244. Thus some "earlier" isolates code for Met-244, as in Eq/Lambourn/92. Some later isolates code for Thr-244 as in the index virus (Lai, unpublished data). Codon 244 is at antigenic site D in the human H3 HA structure, so this appears to signify the start of antigenic drift within a 2-week period including the height of the outbreak.

In Hong Kong all horses are imported (249 during the 1992/93 racing season) and there is no horse breeding in the SAR. In this respect, the Hong Kong horse population is unlike those of the rest of China or, indeed, in most parts of the world. The Hong Kong equine population in November 1992 totaled 1,311 horses and ponies at 10 locations, of which 955 Thoroughbreds were stabled at the Sha Tin Racecourse in the New Territories, the racing facility of the (then) Royal Hong Kong Jockey Club. These racehorses were all on an equine influenza vaccination program: either a primary course administered when arriving unvaccinated from influenza-free countries, Australia and New Zealand; or an annual booster administered as scheduled if their certification showed prior vaccination. All the racehorses were boosted annually in June at the end of the racing season, which ran from September to June. The most updated commercially available vaccine at that time contained the Kentucky/81 and Miami/63 strains of the equine-2 influenza virus. The racehorses were stabled in a modern, controlled high-density complex of either two or three story air-conditioned stables, with separate quarantine blocks nearby. Designated trainers and veterinary surgeons were responsible for these animals, observed them daily, and kept records that have allowed reconstruction of the sequence of events in some detail [33].

Although the first clinical cases were not reported until November 16, the outbreak undoubtedly originated with the October importation of horses from the United Kingdom or Ireland. One such group (6 horses) arrived by air and was quarantined from October 15 to October 29. A second group of 8 imported horses arrived by air and was quarantined in a separate building from October 22 to November 5. All 14 imported horses had been vaccinated at least twice (primary course) and most had been boosted during the previous year. Following quarantine, the imported horses were released into the main stables, although individuals in both groups had significant rises in antibody titers to equine-2 influenza. Of three isolated cases of ill horses in the main stables reported prior to November 16, two were in proximity to the new arrivals. Influenza virus was probably introduced in the first group of imported horses, if not in both groups. On November 16, 17 horses from at least five different stable buildings were reported with fever. At least 10 cases were reported each day from November 18-27, with the peak of 69 cases on November 23, and total cases were 352, or 37% of the Sha Tin population. The only fatality was a horse which raced with no apparent signs of disease, but subsequently developed severe bronchopneumonia and pleuritis and was euthanized. This case caused the Jockey Club to cancel all racing for 32 days, which undoubtedly was beneficial for the recovery of the horses. The Jockey Club would have potentially lost some $1 billion (HK) in betting turnover; consequently Hong Kong would have lost about 10% of its tax revenue during this period, and donations from the Jockey Club to various community and charity projects would also have been adversely affected. Potential losses are recorded since the seven cancelled race meetings were subsequently rescheduled throughout the remainder of the racing season.

The 11-18 day period between introduction of virus into the population and incidence of multiple cases is longer than the 5-10 day period estimated from previous outbreaks [34], and much longer than the usual 1-3 day incubation period [35]. It suggests a prolonged "seeding" of virus through subclinical cases in a population with variable levels of immunity. Retrospectively, about 70% of horses without clinical disease still had serological evidence of infection. Recent vaccination alone did not protect, but the disease incidence in horses imported during 1992 from Australia and New Zealand, where equine influenza is not known to be present and vaccination is not carried out, was significantly greater than that in horses imported during 1992 from North America or Europe where the disease is enzootic and vaccination is common (52% *vs* 20%, $p < 0.001$). In older horses imported prior to 1992 there was little difference [33].

Powell *et al.* [33] noted several environmental factors that could have contributed to the seeding and eventual explosion of this outbreak. These include the density of about 40 horses per acre in stable buildings served by air conditioning that would have facilitated dissemination of virus aerosols, close contact between groups of horses in the confined exercise area, and daily contact with both sick and healthy horses by grooms, trainers, farriers, and veterinary surgeons which could have facilitated virus transmission through fomites.

Laboratory confirmation of the presumptive diagnosis was delayed because initially herpesvirus was suspected due to almost annual minor outbreaks of this disease, while the influenza virus grew poorly in embryonated hens' eggs. Nasopharyngeal swab samples were taken from 65 horses, but no swab was positive on first egg passage. Each of the first 16 isolates required from 2 to 5 "blind" passages before virus was detected, leading to doubt and delay. We retrospectively reanalyzed this sample set using the Directigen Flu-A test (Becton Dickinson Corporation) as a rapid diagnostic test, and found that it detected equine influenza virus in the original swab samples with high sensitivity and predictive value [36]. Thus the diagnosis could have been confirmed almost immediately had the appropriate test been available.

The failure of existing quarantine procedures to prevent this outbreak, coupled with this demonstration of a reliable and much faster detection method for equines influenza, prompted the Royal Hong Kong Jockey Club to change its horse importation requirements to what are now some of the most strict anywhere. These requirements, for permanently importing horses from all countries, now call for pre-export isolation (minimum 21 days), and post-arrival quarantine (minimum 14 days) at a new facility with dedicated quarantine staff located 1 km from the resident population of horses. Directigen testing is performed at the beginning and end of both periods (waived pre-export for equine influenza free countries) and anytime for horses with signs of respiratory disease. A primary course of equine influenza vaccination is given upon arrival, irrespective of previous vaccination history, followed by biannual boosters using a vaccine containing updated virus strains [33]. Australia, a country never apparently exposed to equine influenza, adopted similar regulations for the importation of horses for the equestrian competitions of the 2000 Olympics.

Conclusion

The study of equine influenza in China provides an alternative perspective on the ecology of influenza in lower animals. It reminds that outbreaks can spread explosively and over long distances and periods of time within populations much less dense overall than those of humans, but lacking good immunity. Many thousands of horses are flown around the world every year for competition and production. Hong Kong alone imported 382 horses and exported 167 horses between July 1999 and June 2000. Air transport is an excellent way for these viruses to spread, and the updated Hong Kong importation rules for equines are an example of what would be needed to effectively reduce the chance of their international transmission – an issue that few countries have seriously engaged. It is relevant to note that the incidence of international horseracing has "exploded" in the last 10 years and all the signs are that this trend will continue. In addition racehorses now take in several international racing events on one travel circuit, *e.g.*, the Breeders Cup USA, the Japan Cup, and the Hong Kong International Races or the Singapore Cup, the Dubai World Cup, the Audemars Piguet Cup, Queen Elizabeth II Cup, Hong Kong and the Singapore Airlines International Cup with horses from 11 or more countries involved. Some countries, notably the Hong Kong SAR China, have endeavored to facilitate these international events by modifying horse import protocols to permit continued training of these elite equine athletes competing at the very top level. To do this, pre-export isolation/quarantine periods for most countries, including equine influenza endemic countries, have been waived. Although clinical monitoring, testing and post arrival isolation/quarantine are maintained, a calculated sacrifice to prevention of international equine influenza transmission has been made.

Horses are the third mammalian species, behind humans and pigs, that serve as common hosts for influenza A viruses. Because of the general similarity of equine and human influenza A viruses and disease, equine influenza virologists can take advantage of advances in the human field – such as in diagnostic technologies, as described – or sometimes equine practice can serve as a testing ground for new advances, such as in vaccine technologies. The Eq/Jilin/89 outbreak is a reminder that, like humans and pigs, horses can be recipients for interspecies transmission of influenza A viruses. But so far this appears to be a one-way street. Whether horses can also be sources for interspecies transmission of influenza viruses, and thus potentially be reservoirs for virus genomes not found in other mammals (such as H7N7), remains uncertain. The scale of virological surveillance for outbreaks of novel equine influenza virus strains is still too small to be expected to provide advance warning.

Acknowledgements

The authors wish to thank the Hong Kong Jockey Club, the University of Kentucky Equine Research Foundation, The University of Hong Kong, and the late Mr. Paul Mellon for financial support for the Hong Kong studies, and Ms. Diane Furry for assistance in preparing the presentation and manuscript.

References

1. Judson A. Report on the origin and progress of the epizootic among horses in 1872, with a table of mortality in New York. *Veterinarian* 1874; 47: 492-521.
2. Heller L, Espmark A, Viriden P. Immunological relationship between the infectious cough in horses and human influenza A. *Arch Gesamte Virusforschung* 1957; 7: 120-4.
3. Sovinova O, Tumova B, Pouska F, Nemec J. Isolation of a virus causing respiratory diseases in horses. *Acta Virol* 1958; 1: 52-61.
4. Beveridge W, Mahaffey L, Rose M. Influenza in horses. *Vet Rec* 1965; 77: 57-9.
5. Doll E. Influenza of horses. *Am Rev Respir Dis* 1961; 83: 48-50.
6. Webster R, Bean W, Gorman O, Chambers T, Kawaoka Y. Ecology and evolution of influenza A viruses. *Microbiol Rev* 1992; 56: 152-79.
7. Waddell G, Teigland M, Sigel M. A new influenza virus associated with equine respiratory disease. *J Am Vet Med Assoc* 1963; 143: 587-90.
8. Bean W, Schell M, Katz J, Kawaoka Y, Naeve C, Gorman O, Webster R. Evolution of the H3 influenza virus hemagglutinin from human and nonhuman hosts. *J Virol* 1992; 66: 1129-38.
9. Saito T, Kawaoka Y, Webster R. Phylogenetic analysis of the N8 neuraminidase gene of influenza A viruses. *Virology* 1993; 193: 868-76.
10. Kawaoka Y, Gorman O, Ito T, Wells K, Donis R, Castrucci M, Donatelli I, Webster R. Influence of host species on the evolution of the nonstructural (NS) gene of influenza A viruses. *Vir Res* 1998; 55: 143-56.
11. Ito T, Kawaoka Y, Ohira M, Takakuwa H, Yasuda J, Kida H, Otsuki K. Replacement of internal protein genes, with the exception of the matrix, in equine 1 viruses by equine 2 influenza genes during evolution in nature. *J Vet Med Sci* 1999; 61: 987-9.
12. Webster R. Are equine 1 influenza viruses still present in horses? *Equine Vet J* 1993; 25: 537-8.
13. Ismail T, Sami A, Youssef H, Zaid A. An outbreak of equine influenza type 1 in Egypt in 1989. *Vet Med J Giza* 1990; 38: 195-206.
14. Singh G. Characterization of A/eq-1 virus isolated during the equine influenza epidemic in India. *Acta Virol* 1994; 38: 25-6.
15. Shortridge K. Pandemic influenza: a zoonosis? *Semin Resp Infect* 1992; 7: 11-25.

16. Shortridge K, Gao P, Guan Y, Ito T, Kawaoka Y, Markwell D, Takada A, Webster R. Interspecies transmission of influenza viruses: H5N1 virus and a Hong Hong SAR perspective. *Vet Microbiol* 2000; 74: 141-7.
17. Shortridge K, Stuart-Harris C. An influenza epicentre? *Lancet ii* 1982: 812-3.
18. Deng G, Zhang L, Li S, Shu J, Ren G. Epidemiological surveys of equine influenza epidemic in Inner Mongolia and Beijing. *Chinese J Epidemiol* 1980; 1: 19-22.
19. Guo Y, Guo Z, Pan X, Guo C, Wang M, Liu X, Dong C, Li S, Zhang S, Wang P, Ji W, Chen Q. Etiologic and seroepidemiologic surveys of an equine influenza outbreak in northeast China. *Chinese J Exp Clin Virol* 1990; 3: 318-22.
20. Guo Y, Wang M, Kawaoka Y, Gorman O, Ito T, Saito T, Webster R. Characterization of a new avian-like influenza A virus from horses in China. *Virology* 1992; 188: 245-55.
21. Claas EC, Osterhaus AD, Van Beck R, de Jong JC, Rimmelzwaan GF, Senne DA, Krauss S, Shortridge KF, Webster RG. Human influenza A H5N1 virus related to a highly pathogenic avian influenza virus. *Lancet* 1998; 351: 472-7.
22. Chambers T. Cross-reactivity of existing equine influenza vaccines with a new strain of equine influenza virus from China. *Vet Rec* 1992; 131: 388-91.
23. Webster R, Thomas T. Efficacy of equine influenza vaccines for protection against A/Equine/Jilin/89 (H3N8) – a new equine influenza virus. *Vaccine* 1993; 11: 987-93.
24. Binns M, Daly J, Chirnside E, Mumford J, Wood J, Richards C, Daniels R. Genetic and antigenic analysis of an equine influenza H3 isolate from the 1989 epidemic. *Arch Virol* 1993; 130: 33-43.
25. Chambers T, Lai A, Franklin K, Powell D. Recent evolution of the hemagglutinin of equine-2 influenza virus in the USA. In: Nakajima H, Plowright W, eds. *Equine infectious diseases VII*. Newmarket: R&W Publications Ltd., 1994: 175-80.
26. Kilbourne E. Recombination of influenza A viruses of human and animal origin. *Science* 1968; 160: 74-6.
27. Laver W, Webster R. Studies on the origin of pandemic influenza. 3. Evidence implicating duck and equine influenza viruses as possible progenitors of the Hong Kong strain of human influenza. *Virology* 1973; 51: 383-91.
28. Suzuki Y, Ito T, Suzuki T, Holland R, Chambers T, Kiso M, Ishida H, Kawaoka Y. Sialic acid species as a determinant of the host range of influenza A viruses. *J Virol* 2000; 74: 11825-31.
29. Shortridge K, Chan W, Guan Y. Epidemiology of the equine influenza outbreak in China, 1993-94. *Vet Rec* 1995; 136: 160-1.
30. Guo Y, Wang M, Zheng G, Li W, Kawaoka Y, Webster R. Seroepidemiological and molecular evidence for the presence of two H3N8 equine influenza viruses in China in 1993-94. *J Gen Virol* 1995; 76: 2009-14.
31. Kawaoka Y, Webster R. Origin of the hemagglutinin on A/equine/Johannesburg/86 (H3N8): the first known equine influenza outbreak in South Africa. *Arch Virol* 1989; 106: 159-64.
32. Lai A, Lin Y, Powell D, Shortridge K, Webster R, Daly J, Chambers T. Genetic and antigenic analysis of the influenza virus responsible for the 1992 Hong Kong equine influenza epizootic. *Virology* 1994; 204: 673-9.
33. Powell D, Watkins K, Li P, Shortridge K. Outbreak of equine influenza among horses in Hong Kong during 1992. *Vet Rec* 1995; 136: 531-6.
34. Bryans J, Doll E, Wilson J, Zent W. Epizootiologic features of disease caused by *myxovirus influenzae* A equine. *Am J Vet Res* 1967; 28: 9-17.
35. Gerber H. Clinical features, sequelae, and epidemiology of equine influenza. In: Bryans JT, Gerber H, eds. *Equine infectious diseases II*. Basel: Karger, 1970: 63-80.
36. Chambers T, Shortridge K, Li P, Powell D, Watkins K. Rapid diagnosis of equine influenza by the Directigen FLU-A enzyme immunoassay. *Vet Rec* 1994; 135: 275-9.

Emergence and Control of Zoonotic Ortho- and Paramyxovirus Diseases
B. Dodet, M. Vicari, eds.

Risk factors for recent influenza virus disease outbreaks in animals

Thierry Chillaud
Office International des Epizooties (OIE), Paris, France

Abstract – Although the various animal diseases grouped together under the heading "influenza" are all caused by influenza viruses, the relevant governmental authorities do not grant them all the same level of priority. This is because their potential economic impact varies considerably depending on the species affected.

When an epizootic of avian influenza occurs, an entire sector of the agricultural economy of the affected country is threatened. Recent epizootics have not, however, resulted from international trade in live domestic birds or their products. Wild birds are accused of being the source of the virus but, to date, there has been little research to evaluate the risk of virus transmission from wild birds present in a given region. Once the disease has become established in a territory there are very many possible routes of transmission, leading countries to considerably restrict their imports of poultry products from infected countries. The question of the definition of avian influenza arises as, in several recent epizootics, outbreaks clearly resulted from a deficiency in controlling the circulation of viral strains of low pathogenicity in large-scale commercial poultry units. The application of vaccination also poses a problem in the absence of international recommendations on its use and on the sanitary precautions to be taken by importing countries.

Equine influenza circulates in various regions of the world and, in practice, those countries that are infected have learned to live with the disease, leaving it up to the national equestrian authorities to encourage the regular vaccination of competition horses, which, due to their movements, are the most likely to come into contact with and spread the influenza virus. This helps to avoid epizootics, which would otherwise lead to the cancellation of equestrian events and training activities. However, vaccination can only be effective if field strains of the virus are continuously monitored and vaccines adapted accordingly. Some of countries currently enjoying equine influenza-free status previously experienced epizootics due to the application of inappropriate import quarantine measures. The recommendations of the Office International des Epizooties on this subject are contained in the *International Animal Health Code*.

Swine influenza is present in many countries with commercial swine production. Its persistence or control is highly dependent on husbandry practices, and the responsibility for control operations is usually left to the discretion of individual producers. Veterinary administrations do not conduct official monitoring of disease as they do not consider it serious enough to justify the setting-up of a full-scale reporting system, despite its potential public health implications.

Animal influenza particularly attracted the attention of the international community when cases of human influenza in Hong Kong at the end of 1997 were found to be directly related to contamination by poultry. The event was, however, confined to Hong

Kong and was short-lived. Generally speaking, the diseases grouped under the heading of animal influenza have been known for a long time, and although they are all caused by influenza viruses, they are not given equal importance by governmental authorities, and notably the national veterinary authorities, as demonstrated by the fact that highly pathogenic avian influenza (fowl plague) is included in List A of the Office International des Epizooties (OIE), whereas equine influenza is in List B, and swine influenza is in neither of these lists. This is due to the very different impact that these diseases can have on a country's agricultural economy, and the animal health status of importing countries in respect to each of these diseases.

Highly pathogenic avian influenza

Avian influenza (referred to as highly pathogenic avian influenza at the OIE) is a disease of paramount importance for all countries with a highly developed poultry production sector. This explains why it is included among the diseases on OIE List A (those considered to be the most highly contagious). The definition of the disease is given in the *Manual of Standards for Diagnostic Tests and Vaccines* [1]. When an epizootic occurs, an entire sector of the agricultural economy of the infected country is threatened by the resulting direct (morbidity, mortality, production losses) and indirect losses (trade restrictions imposed by importing countries on poultry products from the infected country).

Yet, such epizootics are rare. *Table I* gives a list of all the reports submitted to the OIE since 1990 relating to highly pathogenic avian influenza in poultry and avian influenza of low pathogenicity in ratites. This table should not be considered as a complete list of all avian influenza episodes observed worldwide during the past decade, since only outbreaks of highly pathogenic avian influenza have to be reported to the OIE. Consequently, episodes of avian influenza that laboratory tests have shown not to be highly pathogenic are not brought to the attention of the OIE, except when they cause deaths in ratites (Netherlands, South Africa) or when they have been preceded by an epizootic of avian influenza, as was the case in Mexico in 1994-1995 [2] and Italy in 1999-2000 [3].

The economic losses resulting from an outbreak of avian influenza of low pathogenicity are far from negligible. For example, they were estimated to amount to 3.5 million dollars for the episode that occurred in Pennsylvania in 1997-1998, taking into account both losses in flocks before and after depopulation of infected farms and the loss of revenue following the application of this measure [4]. Losses stemming from an epizootic of highly pathogenic avian influenza are even greater, and may even become catastrophic if it occurs in a developing country, since there might be a delay in diagnosing the disease and the necessary funds might not be available to compensate owners whose flocks have had to be slaughtered to stop the virus from spreading [5].

It should be noted that international trade in birds and their products is never cited as the source of the disease. Whenever a hypothesis regarding the source is proposed, it is of infection from wild birds, and principally aquatic birds. While this has not been definitively proved, there is often strong circumstantial evidence, as in the outbreak that occurred in December 1994 near Lowood, in the State of Queensland, Australia

Table I. Outbreaks of highly pathogenic avian influenza in poultry or of avian influenza in ratites reported to the OIE since 1990.

Country	Date	Location	Species	No. of outbreaks	No. of birds destroyed	Subtype	Origin
United Kingdom	12/91-01/92	Norfolk	Turkeys	1	624	H5N1	Unknown
Australia	07/92	Victoria	Broilers; breeding poultry; ducks	1	22,808 birds; 36,536 day-old chicks; 434,000 hatching eggs	H7N3	Unspecified
Netherlands	04/94	Northern Brabant	Ratites	1	...	H5N9	Unknown
South Africa	05/94	Cape province	Ostriches	1	0		Unspecified
Australia	12/94	Queensland	Layers and pullets; geese	1	20,457	H7N3	Watercourse used by wild water fowl
Mexico	06/94-06/95	Puebla; Querétaro	Poultry	2	4,320,000	H5N2	Unspecified
Pakistan	1995	Rawalpindi; Islamabad	...	80	...	H7N2	Unspecified
Hong Kong	04-06/97	–	Poultry	3	1,600,000	H5N1	Unspecified
Australia	11-12/97	New South Wales	Layers; chicks; emus	1	310,000 birds + hatching eggs	H7N4	Watercourse used by wild water fowl
Italy	11/97-01/98	Venezia; Friuli-Venezia Julia	Backyard poultry	8	5,406	H5N2	Probably wild birds
Italy	03/99-04/00	26 provinces	Turkeys; layers...	399	...	H7N1	Unspecified

[6]. Surveillance of viral activity in wild birds is particularly difficult as they do not present clinical signs, and random surveys are out of the question as they would be too expensive and complicated. This situation has led researchers to develop quantitative risk evaluation techniques to try to identify which wild birds are the most likely reservoir of the virus [7].

Once avian influenza has become established in a given area, there are many possible secondary routes of viral transmission, generally involving the mechanical movement of infective faeces. A list of these can be drawn up based on the control measures implemented in Italy [8]:
- movement of birds from infected premises;
- poultry markets;
- dead birds;

– hatching eggs;
– humans (poultry production personnel, veterinarians);
– vehicles;
– litter.

To this list can also be added less important factors of spread, namely water and foodstuff, wind (transmission between neighbouring farms) and insects.

This multiplicity of spreading routes leads most importing countries to prohibit the importation of poultry and poultry products from infected countries. When trade relations are nevertheless maintained, as is the case within the European Union, an infected exporting country is required to implement drastic controls. Details are given in Council Directive 92/40/EEC of 19 May 1992, introducing Community measures for the control of avian influenza (Official Journal of the European Communities (OJEC) No. L167 of 22 June 1992).

The epizootics that occurred in Mexico and Italy resulted from inadequate control of the circulation of low pathogenicity viral strains. This led the European Union's Standing Veterinary Committee to consider a new definition of avian influenza and to propose that one of the following three strategies be adopted [9]:

1) retain the definition in force within the European Union with a recommendation that Member States impose restrictions to limit the spread of low pathogenic avian influenza viruses;

2) define avian influenza as an infection of poultry with any virus of H5 or H7 subtype;

3) define avian influenza as any infection with a virus of H5 or H7 subtype, but modify the control measures imposed for different categories of virus and/or different types of host.

To date, the definition of highly pathogenic avian influenza within the European Union has not been amended. Nevertheless, in view of the fact that during the epidemiological investigations conducted in Italy the presence of low pathogenic viruses was detected in a region with a high density of poultry production (province of Verona), the European Commission authorised the use of vaccination in 42 municipalities of that province to supplement control measures and movement restrictions (see Commission Decision 2000/721/EC of 7 November 2000 on introducing vaccination to supplement the measures to control avian influenza in Italy and on specific movement control measures – OJEC No. L 291 of 18 November 2000, modified by Decision 2000/785/EC of 6 December 2000 – OJEC No. L311 of 12 December 2000).

To avoid the disease spreading to other countries, this authorisation was accompanied by the following control measures:
– No live birds and hatching eggs coming from and/or originating from the vaccination area in the region of Veneto in the province of Verona shall be dispatched from Italy.
– Live birds and hatching eggs coming from and/or originating from the territory of Italy outside the vaccination area can only be dispatched from Italy if no contacts or other epidemiological links in relation to avian influenza can be established to a holding or a hatchery situated in the vaccination area.

– Fresh poultry meat originating from the vaccination area or produced in slaughterhouses in the vaccination area cannot be dispatched from Italy.

– Table eggs produced in the vaccination area cannot be exported; those produced in the remainder of Veneto must be packed in disposable packaging material or packaging material that can be effectively washed and disinfected.

– All means of transport used for poultry, hatching eggs, table eggs and poultry foodstuff in the vaccination area must be cleaned and disinfected immediately before and after use.

The chapter on avian influenza in the OIE *International Animal Health Code* simply refers to the recommendations of the chapter on Newcastle disease for the animal health precautions to be taken in international trade in live birds and avian products. However, the chapter on Newcastle disease currently in force is out of date and is now being revised. As soon as the revised chapter has been adopted by the OIE (it is due to be presented for adoption for the first time in May 2001), there will be an urgent need to start revising the chapter on highly pathogenic avian influenza, taking into account the latest results of scientific and epidemiological researches on the disease.

Equine influenza

Equine influenza is found in most regions of the world, and while epizootics may occur, it is more frequent in enzootic form, as shown in *Table II*, which includes the only two epizootics reported to the OIE since 1990.

Table II. Equine influenza epizootics reported to the OIE since 1990.

Country	Date	Location	No. of outbreaks	No. of dead horses	Serotype	Origin
Colombia	06-07/91	8 departments	1,935	41	A-equi 2 (Miami)	Indigenous
Hong Kong	10/92	Shatin race course	1	7	A-equi 2	Horses imported from two European countries
Jordan	05-06/94	4 districts to the South of Amman	7	0	?	Annual gathering for the racing season

Of approximately 120 countries or territories that submitted information to the OIE on equine influenza in 1999, only 27 mentioned that the disease had been present, and, among these, few indicated the number of outbreaks. This would seem to imply that the official Veterinary Services do not conduct effective surveillance of the disease (it is a notifiable disease in only 37 of the 120 countries or territories). The only conclusions that can be drawn from the available data are that Oceania is free of the disease, and that this is probably the case for the countries of the Caribbean (the most recent episode was in Trinidad and Tobago in 1994 [10], at a period when the country was not a member of the OIE) and the majority of African countries.

International movements of horses, especially competition horses, only serve to increase the risk of spread of the influenza virus, which is already highly contagious. Paradoxically, incidents attributable to such movements are rare: examples are the episode that occurred in Hong Kong in 1992 [11], and the epizootic that occurred in South Africa in 1986 following the importation of horses from the United States of America [12]. In each of these cases, transmission of the disease from the imported horses to other horses was made possible by inappropriate animal health importation procedures. The 1986 episode in South Africa is particularly demonstrative. At that time, vaccination was not required prior to importation. Some of the horses imported from the United States of America in December 1986 presented signs of a respiratory disease, yet no suspicion was raised. During the same period, horses from other sources were admitted into the quarantine station, while others were released from quarantine and dispatched to different parts of the country. The disease then broke out in horses due to participation in a national equestrian event. Half of the horses were affected, and a number of competitors decided to withdraw their animals in the hope that they would escape the infection, which only served to exacerbate the spread of the disease. Furthermore, one of the trainers visited a sick horse in the quarantine station without taking the necessary precautions, and then returned to the horses in his care, resulting in the appearance of other cases of the disease.

In both South Africa and Hong Kong, these events led to a major revision of quarantine procedures: for example, in South Africa, the following measures were introduced: compulsory vaccination 30 to 60 days before dispatch to South Africa, post-arrival quarantine on an all-in all-out basis, restrictions on entry to the quarantine station, wearing of protective clothing and disinfection of equipment.

The conditions recommended by the *International Animal Health Code* for the importation of horses from an infected country to an equine influenza-free country are drastic. They include the following measures:

– isolation for four weeks prior to shipment;

– no new animal has been introduced into the isolation facilities during this period;

– no animal in the isolation facilities showed clinical signs of equine influenza during the isolation period;

– animals have been vaccinated against both subtypes of equine influenza virus, and have received a booster dose of vaccine no less than two weeks and no more than eight weeks prior to shipment.

In September 2000, the Olympic Games were held in Australia, an equine influenza-free country not vaccinating its equine population against the disease and anxious to protect its status due to the economic losses that would result from any incursion of the disease [13]. For the equestrian competitions held during this international event, Australia applied the general importation measures provided for in its sanitary regulations for the temporary importation of horses (which are slightly less stringent than those recommended by the OIE), namely:

– pre-export quarantine for 14 days;

– a further 14-day quarantine period on an all-in all-out basis on arrival in Australia, during which the animals are subjected to a twice daily clinical examination including temperature measurement;

– wearing of protective clothing by the personnel, and specific equipment at the quarantine station, to reduce the risk of spreading the virus by fomites;

– thereafter, the horses are to be kept under surveillance (in practice they remained on the site of the Olympic Games) until their re-exportation.

For the movement of competition horses between infected countries, the OIE, in association with the International Equestrian Federation, has developed a specific model passport (Appendix 4.1.5. of the *International Animal Health Code*), which has a special section to record vaccinations against equine influenza. It is generally left up to the national equestrian authorities to encourage regular vaccination of competition horses. In Europe, the prevalence of the disease has shown a marked decline over the past ten years or more, thanks to the vaccination of these animals at high risk. However, vaccination can only remain effective if field strains of the influenza virus are continuously monitored by the OIE World Reference Laboratories, of which there are currently three:
– Institute for Medical Microbiology, Infectious and Epidemic Diseases, Veterinary Faculty, Ludwig-Maximilians-University, Munich (Germany);
– Animal Health Trust, Lanwades Park, Kentford, Newmarket, Suffolk (United Kingdom);
– Maxwell H. Gluck Equine Research Center, Department of Veterinary Science, University of Kentucky, Lexington, Kentucky (United States of America).

Monitoring allows any new variants to be detected, meaning that vaccine producers can be advised in good time of the changes to be made to their products. The latest conclusions and recommendations on this subject issued by the WHO/OIE Expert Surveillance Panel on Equine Influenza Vaccine Strain Selection were published in the July-August 1998 issue of the OIE *Bulletin*, following a meeting of the Panel held in Dubai (United Arab Emirates) the previous month. An updated version of these conclusions and recommendations is due to be published in the near future.

Swine influenza

Swine influenza exists in many countries with large-scale commercial pig production. The influenza virus is usually transmitted by direct contact between infected pigs and susceptible animals, though fomites may play a role, as may the wind over short distances.

The responsibility for controlling the disease is left up to pig producers, and the official veterinary authorities do not normally conduct any surveillance in this matter. Swine influenza is considered to be a production disease, with only limited consequences which do not justify the implementation of a heavy administrative system of reporting and intervention. This is also the reason why it appears in neither List A or List B of the OIE.

Good animal health management of the various categories of animals (gilts, sows) and stocking procedures in production units is essential in order to reduce the losses due to swine influenza. Consideration also needs to be given to the risks of virus circulation relating to gathering points, through which pigs of widely differing influenza status transit. Some producers in Europe and North America see vaccination as a solution. While this option has the effect of reducing losses, the only way to stop the virus circulating is to apply purely sanitary measures (depopulation of units, changing the flow of fattening pigs, etc.), but their effective implementation is often confronted by insurmountable problems caused by the size of the farm and lack of space.

Conclusion

This study of animal influenza from an international point of view highlights several key issues for which no straightforward solution currently exists. The term "highly pathogenic avian influenza" poses a problem of definition, the consequences of applying vaccination have yet to be clearly defined, and concerted recommendations on international trade in live poultry, poultry meat and eggs, aimed at avoiding the spread of the disease from one country to another, have yet to be developed. Effective control of equine influenza presupposes continuous monitoring of field virus strains circulating in equids in infected countries. Monitoring of this kind can only be achieved through close working relationships between veterinary administrations, equestrian authorities, national and international reference laboratories, and vaccine producers, which in many countries is still far from being the case. Lastly, it might be opportune to establish truly national surveillance systems for swine influenza, due to potential public health implications of influenza viruses circulating in pigs.

References

1. OIE. *Manual of Standards for Diagnostic Tests and Vaccines*, 4th Edition. OIE, 2000.
2. Highly pathogenic avian influenza in Mexico. *Foreign Animal Disease Report* 1995; 22-4: 7-9.
3. OIE. *World Animal Health in 1999*. OIE, 2000.
4. Davison S, Galligan D, Eckert TE, Ziegler AF, Eckroade RJ. Economic analysis of an outbreak of avian influenza, 1997-1998. *J Am Veter Med Assoc* 1999; 214 (8): 1164-7.
5. Ziggers D. Avian influenza in Iran: unpredictable outbreak with serious losses. *World Poultry* 1999; 15 (4): 49-50.
6. OIE. *Disease Information* 1994; 7 (50): 209-10.
7. McClintock CH, More S, Baldock CH. The development of a qualitative risk assessment model to estimate the probability of disease risk (avian influenza) to the commercial poultry flocks from the activities of wild birds. *Proc OIE/FAVA Epidemiology Programme: special session on emerging diseases*, Cairns, Australia, 28 August 1997, 1998: 13-24.
8. Cahen P. L'Italie lutte contre un influenzavirus depuis mars dernier. *Semaine Vétérinaire* 2000; n° 961, IV.
9. The definition of avian influenza – The use of vaccination against avian influenza. Scientific Committee on Animal Health and Animal Welfare, adopted 27 June 2000 (Sanco/B3/AH/R17/2000). European Commission, Scientific Committee on Animal Health and Animal Welfare, 2000: 37.
10. Harper WR. Update on the equine influenza outbreak in Trinidad. *Caraphin News* 1994; 10: 6.
11. OIE. *Bulletin* 1193; 105 (2): 116-7.
12. Guthrie AJ, Stevens KB, Bosman PP. The circumstances surrounding the outbreak and spread of equine influenza in South Africa. *Revue scientifique et technique de l'OIE* 1999; 18 (1): 179-85.
13. Clement RF, Doyle KA, Murray JG. The significance of a major outbreak of quarantinable disease to the Australian horse industries. *Austr Vet J* 1990; 67: 77-8.

Emergence and Control of Zoonotic Ortho- and Paramyxovirus Diseases
B. Dodet, M. Vicari, eds.

Growth restriction in mammalian cells of influenza A virus possessing the nucleoprotein of A/gull/Maryland/77 (H13N6)

Masato Hatta[1], Peter Halfmann[1], Yoshihiro Kawaoka[1, 2]
[1] *Department of Pathobiological Sciences, School of Veterinary Medicine, University of Wisconsin-Madison, Madison, USA*
[2] *Institute of Medical Science, University of Tokyo, Japan*

Abstract – Influenza A viruses are classified into subtypes based on the antigenicity of their hemagglutinin (HA; H1-H15) and neuraminidase (NA; N1-N9). Of all subtypes, H13 viruses have a unique host range; they have only been isolated from shorebirds, gulls, and whales. Furthermore, H13 viruses do not replicate in the intestinal tracts of ducks, unlike the majority of avian influenza viruses. The M and NP genes have been implicated in the host range restriction of avian influenza A viruses. As an initial step towards understanding the genetic basis for host range restriction of H13 viruses, we generated reassortant viruses between A/gull/Maryland/77 (H13N6; Gull/MD) virus, which replicates poorly in Madin-Darby canine kidney (MDCK) cells and A/WSN/33 (H1N1; WSN), which replicates efficiently in these cells. Using reverse genetics, we generated reassortants possessing the NP or M, or both genes from Gull/MD and the remainder from WSN. The reassortant virus possessing Gull/MD M and other genes from WSN virus replicated similarly to WSN virus, while that with the Gull/MD NP gene replicated appreciably less efficiently. These results suggest that either the NP gene of Gull/MD virus plays a role in host range restriction of Gull/MD virus or is incompatible with the viral proteins of WSN.

Influenza A viruses have been isolated from a variety of animals. They have two surface glycoproteins, hemagglutinin (HA) and neuraminidase (NA), and based on their antigenicity, influenza A viruses are classified into 15 HA and 9 NA subtypes. While only H1, H2, and H3 viruses have been established in humans, all 15 HA subtypes have been isolated from waterfowl, implicating them as the source of viruses in other animals. However, H13 viruses, which have been isolated only from shorebirds, gulls, and whales, have a unique host range [1-3]; they have not been isolated from ducks and do not replicate in the intestinal tract of ducks, unlike the majority of avian influenza viruses of other HA subtypes [1, 4]. The genetic factors associated with this host range restriction, however, remain unknown.

The M and NP genes encode M1 and M2, and NP protein, respectively. Previous studies suggested that these genes may determine the host range of influenza viruses

[5-8]. Phylogenetic studies also indicate that the NP and M genes of H13 viruses form unique lineages distinct from those of other avian viruses, suggesting that H13 NP and M proteins may have adapted in gulls extensively [9, 10].

As an initial step towards understanding the molecular basis for the host range restriction of H13 viruses, we focused on the M and NP genes of A/gull/Maryland/77 (H13N6; Gull/MD) virus and generated reassortant viruses possessing the NP or M or both genes of Gull/MD and the rest from A/WSN/33 (H1N1; WSN) using reverse genetics, and examined their growth properties in Madin-Darby canine kidney (MDCK) cells.

Materials and methods

Cells

293T human embryonic kidney cells and MDCK cells were maintained in DMEM supplemented with 10% FCS and in MEM containing 5% newborn calf serum, respectively. The 293T cell line is a derivative of the 293 line, into which the gene for the simian virus 40 T antigen was inserted [11]. All cells were maintained at 37 °C in 5% CO_2.

Construction of plasmids

The NP and M genes of A/gull/Maryland/77 (H13N6; Gull/MD) virus were synthesized by reverse transcription of viral RNA with an oligonucleotide (Uni 12) complementary to the conserved 3' end of the viral RNA, as described by Katz *et al.* [12]. The cDNA was amplified by PCR with gene-specific oligonucleotide primers containing *BsmBI* sites, and the products were cloned into the pT7Blueblunt vector (Novagen, Madison, WI). After digestion with *BsmBI*, the fragment was cloned into the *BsmBI* sites of a plasmid vector, which contains the human RNA polymerase I promoter and the mouse RNA polymerase I terminator, separated by *BsmBI* sites [13]. The plasmids for expression of vRNA are referred to as "PolI" constructs in this report. All constructs were sequenced in order to ascertain the absence of unwanted mutation.

Plasmid-driven reverse genetics

Transfectant viruses were generated as reported earlier [13]. Briefly, 12 plasmids (eight PolI constructs for eight RNA segments and four protein-expression constructs for polymerase proteins and NP) were mixed with transfection reagent (Trans IT LT-1 [Panvera, Madison, WI]), incubated at room temperature for 10 min, and added to 1×10^6 293T cells cultured in Opti-MEM (GIBCO/BRL) containing 0.3% BSA and 0.01% FCS. Forty-eight hours later, viruses in the supernatant were inoculated onto MDCK cells for the production of stock virus. The NP and M genes of transfectant viruses were sequenced to confirm that they originated from Gull/MD and to ensure that no unwanted mutations were present. In all experiments, the transfectant viruses contained only the NP and/or M gene from Gull/MD and the remaining genes from WSN virus.

Replicative properties of transfectant viruses

MDCK cells were infected with WSN or mutant viruses, overlaid with MEM medium containing 0.5 μg of trypsin per mL, and incubated at 37 °C. At given time intervals, supernatants were assayed for infectious virus by plaque assays in MDCK cells.

Results

Generation of reassortant viruses containing the genes derived from Gull/MD and WSN viruses

To establish an *in vitro* system to study host range restriction of influenza A viruses, we tested the replicative ability of influenza A viruses in MDCK cells. Among the viruses tested, Gull/MD virus consistently showed poor growth in these cells, while WSN virus replicated efficiently. To understand the growth restriction of this virus in MDCK cells, we attempted to generate reassortant viruses between Gull/MD and WSN by plasmid-driven reverse genetics [13]. To this end, we transfected 293T cells with four plasmids for expression of PB2, PB1, PA, and NP and eight plasmids that directed the production of viral RNA segments encoding WSN viral genes, except the NP and/or M gene, which were derived from Gull/MD virus. The transfectant viruses present in the supernatant were amplified in MDCK cells and used as stock viruses. The viruses possessing Gull/MD NP, Gull/MD M, or Gull/MD NP and M genes were designated WSN/GullNP, WSN/GullM, and WSN/GullNP-M, respectively. The titers of the stock viruses (10^7 pfu/ml, WSN/GullNP and WSN/GullM; 10^5 pfu/ml, WSN/GullNP-M) were approximately 1-3 logs lower than that of WSN virus (10^8 pfu/ml).

Growth properties of mutant viruses

We next compared the growth properties of the mutant viruses and WSN virus in MDCK cells. Cells were infected at an MOI of 0.001 and yield of virus in the culture supernatant was determined at different times post-infection at 37 °C. As shown in *Figure 1*, WSN/GullNP and WSN/GullNP-M viruses replicated slower than WSN and WSN/GullM viruses. Similarly, although WSN/GullM virus grew to $10^{7.5}$ PFU/ml, a titre comparable to WSN virus (10^8 pfu/ml), WSN/GullNP and WSN/GullNP-M viruses grew only to 10^6 PFU/ml. By contrast, the plaque sizes of WSN/GullNP and WSN/GullNP-M viruses were similar to that of WSN virus; however, that of WSN/GullM was slightly smaller than that of WSN virus.

Discussion

Because appropriate selection mechanisms are lacking, it has been difficult to address the contribution of genes encoding internal proteins to influenza viral properties. In this

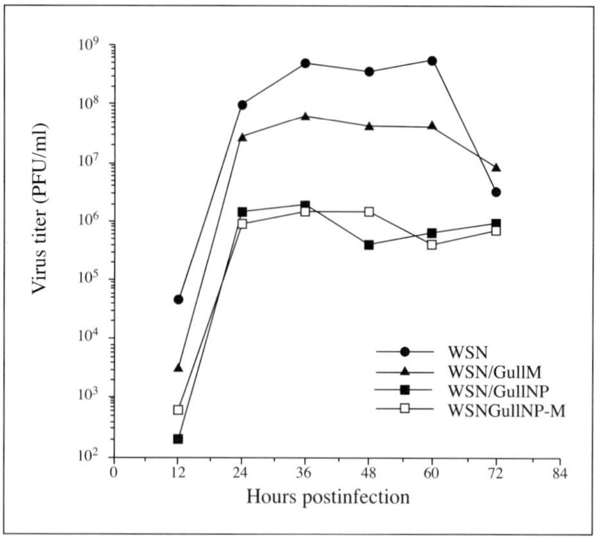

Figure 1. Growth curves of reassortant and wild-type WSN viruses. MDCK cells were infected with virus at an MOI of 0.001. At the indicated time points following infection, the virus titre in the supernatant was determined.

study, we exploited the plasmid-based reverse genetics we recently established to generate reassortant viruses possessing the NP, and/or M genes from Gull/MD virus and the rest from WSN virus.

Our results indicate that the growth of viruses possessing the Gull/MD NP gene is restricted in MDCK cells. Although previous studies implicated the NP gene as a determinant of host range of influenza A viruses, direct evidence to support this was lacking. With plasmid-based reverse genetics, here we unequivocally demonstrated the negative effect of NP on the growth of influenza A virus. Our finding suggests that either the NP of Gull/MD virus plays a role in host range restriction of this virus, or is incompatible with the WSN viral proteins.

Previous studies showed that WSN M1 protein is a determinant for the rapid-growth phenotype and the large plaque size of WSN virus [14, 15]. In this study, the M gene of Gull/MD virus, which grows slower than WSN virus, did not appreciably affect viral growth, although the plaque size of the reassortant virus possessing Gull/MD M gene was smaller than that of WSN virus. There are 6 amino acid differences in the M1 proteins of Gull/MD and WSN virus. The region containing these amino acids may affect the plaque size of the virus. Further analyses of these genes may identify the molecular mechanism of growth-restriction of influenza A virus.

Acknowledgements

We thank Krisna Wells, Martha McGregor, and Nichole Poznik for their excellent technical assistance. Automated sequencing was performed at the University of Wisconsin-Madison, Biotechnology Center. This work was supported by grants from the National Institutes of Health, NIAID.

References

1. Hinshaw VS, Air GM, Gibbs AJ, Graves L, Prescott B, Karunakaran D. Antigenic and genetic characterization of a novel hemagglutinin subtype of influenza A viruses from gulls. *J Virol* 1982; 42: 865-72.
2. Hinshaw VS, Bean WJ, Geraci J, Fiorelli P, Early G, Webster RG. Characterization of two influenza A viruses from a pilot whale. *J Virol* 1986; 58: 655-6.
3. Kawaoka Y, Chambers TM, Sladen WL, Webster RG. Is the gene pool of influenza viruses in shorebirds and gulls different from that in wild ducks? *Virology* 1988; 163: 247-50.
4. Hinshaw VS, Wood JM, Webster RG, Deibel R, Turner B. Circulation of influenza viruses and paramyxoviruses in waterfowl originating from two different areas of North America. *Bull WHO* 1985; 63: 711-9.
5. Murphy BR, Buckler-White AJ, London WT, Snyder MH. Characterization of the M protein and nucleoprotein genes of an avian influenza A virus which are involved in host range restriction in monkeys. *Vaccine* 1989; 7: 557-61.
6. Scholtissek C, Burger H, Kistner O, Shortridge KF. The nucleoprotein as a possible major factor in determining host specificity of influenza H3N2 viruses. *Virology* 1985; 147: 287-94.
7. Snyder MH, Buckler-White AJ, London WT, Tierney EL, Murphy BR. The avian influenza virus nucleoprotein gene and a specific constellation of avian and human virus polymerase genes each specify attenuation of avian-human influenza A/Pintail/79 reassortant viruses for monkeys. *J Virol* 1987; 61: 2857-63.
8. Tian SF, Buckler-White AJ, London WT, Reck LJ, Chanock RM, Murphy BR. Nucleoprotein and membrane protein genes are associated with restriction of replication of influenza A/Mallard/NY/78 virus and its reassortants in squirrel monkey respiratory tract. *J Virol* 1985; 53: 771-5.
9. Ito T, Gorman OT, Kawaoka Y, Bean WJ, Webster RG. Evolutionary analysis of the influenza A virus M gene with comparison of the M1 and M2 proteins. *J Virol* 1991; 65: 5491-8.
10. Gorman OT, Bean WJ, Kawaoka Y, Webster RG. Evolution of the nucleoprotein gene of influenza A virus. *J Virol* 1990; 64: 1487-97.
11. DuBridge RB, Tang P, Hsia HC, Leong PM, Miller JH, Calos MP. Analysis of mutation in human cells by using an Epstein-Barr virus shuttle system. *Mol Cell Biol* 1987; 7: 379-87.
12. Katz JM, Wang M, Webster RG. Direct sequencing of the HA gene of influenza (H3N2) virus in original clinical samples reveals sequence identity with mammalian cell-grown virus. *J Virol* 1990; 64: 1808-11.
13. Neumann G, Watanabe T, Ito H, Watanabe S, Goto H, Gao P, Hughes M, Perez DR, Donis R, Hoffmann E, Hobom G, Kawaoka Y. Generation of influenza A viruses entirely from cloned cDNAs. *Proc Natl Acad Sci USA* 1999; 96: 9345-50.
14. Yasuda J, Toyoda T, Nakayama M, Ishihama A. Regulatory effects of matrix protein variations on influenza virus growth. *Arch Virol* 1993; 133: 283-94.
15. Yasuda J, Bucher DJ, Ishihama A. Growth control of influenza A virus by M1 protein: analysis of transfectant viruses carrying the chimeric M gene. *J Virol* 1994; 68: 8141-6.

Emergence and Control of Zoonotic Ortho- and Paramyxovirus Diseases
B. Dodet, M. Vicari, eds.

Internal genes as determinants of interspecies transmission and host specificity of influenza A viruses

Nadia Naffakh, Pascale Massin, Sylvie van der Werf
Unit of Molecular Genetics of Respiratory Viruses, URA CNRS 1966, Institut Pasteur, Paris, France

Abstract – Experiments on human/avian reassortant viruses have lead to the idea that specific constellations of gene segments encoding the internal proteins could be determining their ability to replicate efficiently in mammalian cells and/or in the respiratory epithelium of primates. This notion was strengthened by the fact that the six internal genes of avian H5N1 and H9N2 viruses that were responsible for outbreaks of respiratory disease in humans in Hong Kong in 1997 and 1999, respectively, were found to be very similar. Residue 627 of PB2 has been shown to be a major determinant for host-specificity. However, the multiple genetic features of internal genes that contribute to host-specificity of influenza A viruses and to their potential for interspecies transmission, and the molecular mechanisms involved, remain to be understood.

Influenza A viruses have been isolated from a wide range of animal species. Aquatic birds, in which all 15 hemagglutinin (HA) subtypes have been found, are believed to be the reservoir of influenza A viruses from which new virus subtypes can episodically be transmitted to a new host and in particular to humans, either directly or indirectly *(Figure 1)* [1]. Generally, avian influenza viruses (AIVs) replicate poorly in humans [2] and in other primates [3]. In contrast, reassortants that derive their gene segments from both human and avian viruses are known to be potentially threatening for humans, such as the viruses responsible for the influenza pandemics in 1957 and 1968 [4]. Several observations suggest that avian and human viruses may have reassorted in pigs and that the resulting reassortants may have been transmitted from pigs to humans [5]. Segments of avian origin not only encoded novel neuraminidase (NA) and/or HA molecules, to which the human population had no immunity, but also an internal protein, the RNA polymerase PB1 [6]. Direct transmission of AIVs to humans can also occur occasionally, as shown by serological data [7] or by the isolation of an H7N7 influenza virus from a patient with severe conjunctivitis [8]. More strikingly, in 1997, a highly pathogenic H5N1 virus that circulated in chickens in Hong Kong was responsible for respiratory disease in at least 18 persons and caused six deaths [9-11]. Each case appeared to result from an independent transmission of the virus from poultry to humans. There was no convincing evidence for human-to-human transmission and since the

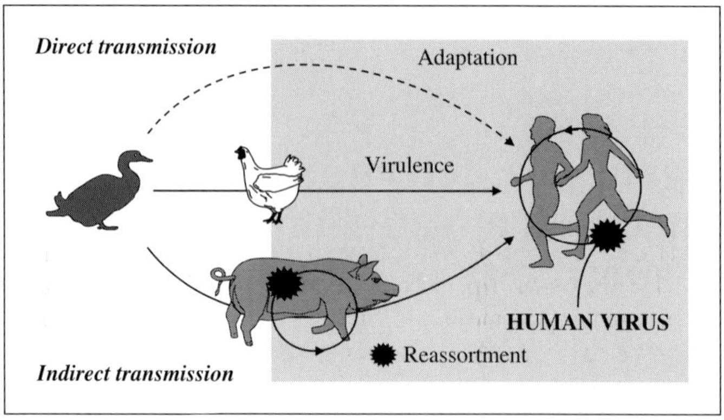

Figure 1. Models for the interspecies transmission and adaptation of influenza viruses. Interspecies transmission of influenza viruses from the wild bird reservoir to humans may occur directly or indirectly. It has been suggested that pigs [5] but also possibly poultry [12] may serve as intermediate hosts in the process of acquisition by avian influenza viruses of the ability to transmit efficiently to humans. Establishment of new influenza viruses in the human population requires full adaptation and the potential for human to human transmission. This may be acquired either progressively upon successive inter-human transmissions, or more readily by reassortment of viruses of avian origin with human influenza viruses circulating in the human or pig population. Along the pathway to adaptation to humans, increased virulence does not seem to be a prerequisite and is likely to involve determinants distinct from those related to species specificity.

mass culling of poultry in Hong Kong, no new human cases of H5N1 virus infection have been recorded. The H5N1 viruses isolated from humans were antigenically and genetically similar to H5N1 viruses circulating at the time in poultry markets in Hong Kong. Zhou *et al.* [12] compared the mean numbers of nucleotide or amino acid changes in genes and encoded proteins of the H5N1 viruses isolated from poultry, of non H5 avian influenza viruses, and of H5N2 influenza viruses that were transmitted from wild aquatic birds to the chicken population of Mexico in 1994 and became highly pathogenic. Surprisingly, in H5N1 viruses isolated from poultry in Hong Kong, the rate of evolution of the HA was an order of magnitude less than that found in H5N2 viruses from chickens in Mexico, and similar to that found in influenza viruses from aquatic birds. In contrast, the rates of coding changes in the NA, PB1, PB2, PA and NP genes in H5 viruses from Hong Kong and Mexico were higher than those found in influenza viruses from aquatic birds [12]. These findings suggested that the Hong Kong H5N1 isolates could be reassortants of which the HA gene was well adapted to domestic poultry, while the rest of the genome came from a different source, and raised the possibility that chickens may be a possible intermediate host in zoonotic transmission. This hypothesis was further confirmed by the phylogenetic analysis of the internal genes of H5N1 viruses and of viruses of different serotypes isolated from various bird species during the Hong Kong outbreak, which indicated that the human and poultry H5N1 influenza viruses in Hong Kong were reassortants that could have obtained internal gene segments from a quail H9N2 virus (A/Qa/HK/G1/97) [13] and the NA gene segment from an H6N1 virus isolated from teal (A/teal/Hong Kong/W312/97) [14]. Viruses of the H9N2 subtype, with internal genes that were shown to be very similar with those of the H5N1 viruses, were responsible for two cases of human infection in Hong Kong in 1999, suggesting that some determinants of their common ability to replicate in humans were contained within their internal genes [15]. Taken together, these observations strongly suggest that the internal genes contain some determinants of interspecies transmission and host specificity of influenza A viruses. Still, the specific genes and molecular mechanisms involved are not well known.

Functions of internal proteins of influenza A viruses

Among internal proteins, the nucleoprotein (NP) and the three subunits of the polymerase complex (PB1, PB2 and PA) have been shown to make up the minimal set of proteins required for the transcription and replication of the viral genome [16]. The molecular assembly of the polymerase complex relies on PB1-PB2 and PB1-PA interactions, whereas no direct PB2-PA interaction has been evidenced [17-20]. Biochemical and genetic data have established that the PB1 subunit displays RNA-dependent RNA polymerase activity [21, 22] and that the PB2 subunit is involved in the cap-snatching mechanism by which viral mRNA synthesis is initiated [21, 23-25], while the only biochemical activity found to be associated with PA is the induction of proteolysis [26]. Beyond its structural role, the NP seems to be involved in the switch from transcription to replication [27], possibly through interactions with the PB1 and PB2 proteins [28]. The RNA segment 7 of influenza A viruses encodes two proteins: the matrix protein M1 which is the most abundant polypeptide in the virion and is thought to be involved in contacts with the RNPs, the membrane, and the cytoplasmic tails of the glycoproteins during virus assembly [29, 30]; and the M2 protein which is a minor component of the virion and has ion channel activity that permits virus uncoating [31]. The RNA segment 8 of influenza A viruses also encodes two proteins, *i.e.* NS1 and NS2. The NS1 protein is abundant in influenza virus infected cells but has not been detected in the virions, hence the designation NS for *non structural*. It has multiple functions including inhibition of the nuclear export of cellular mRNAs [32] and the translational regulation of viral mRNAs [33, 34]. However, recent reports suggest that the major function of NS1 is to counteract or prevent the cellular anti-viral response [35, 36]. The NS2 protein was shown to mediate the nuclear export of virion RNAs by acting as an adaptor between viral ribonucleoprotein complexes and the nuclear export machinery of the cell [37]. Whenever evolutionary rates have been determined for internal protein genes [6, 38-40], they were much lower than those of the surface glycoproteins. However, for each of the internal genes as well as for the HA and NA, human and avian influenza A viruses are associated with distinct evolutionary lineages [1]. Alignment of all available sequences for each of the internal proteins reveals that, at specific positions, some amino acids appear to be characteristic of the human or avian origin of the sequences *(Table I)*, and thus could be involved in the determination of host range.

Host range restriction of avian-human influenza A reassortant viruses

In several experiments involving different virus strains, avian-human influenza A reassortant viruses possessing the HA and NA genes of their human influenza parent and the six internal genes of their avian influenza parent appeared as restricted in replication in squirrel monkeys as was their avian influenza parent [41-45]. These observations clearly indicated that restriction of the replication of the avian viruses was a function of one or more of their internal genes. In order to determine which of the internal genes were responsible for host-restriction, single gene reassortant viruses bearing one avian

Table I. Amino acids characteristic of the human or avian origin of influenza A virus internal proteins.

PB2 AA	**9**	**81**	**199**	**475**	**567**	**588**	**613**	**627**	**674**	**702**
Human	N	M	S	M	N	I	T	K	T	R
HK*	D	T	S/A	L	E	A	V	E/K	A	K
Avian**	D	T	A	L	D/V	A	V	E	A/S	K

PB1 AA	**54**	**473**	**576**	**645**	**741**
Human anterior to 1957	R	L	I	I/M	T
Human posterior to 1957	K	V	L	V	A/S
HK*	R	V	L	V	A
Avian**	K	V	L	V	A

PA AA	**57**	**65**	**100**	**312**	**337**	**382**	**400**	**409**	**552**
Human	Q	L	A	R	S	D	L	N	S
HK*	R	S	V	K	A	E	L	N/S	T
Avian**	R	S	V	K	A/T	E	PQTS	S	T

NP AA	**16**	**31**	**61**	**136**	**283**	**313**
Human	D	K	L	M	P	Y
HK*	G	R	I	M	L	F
Avian**	G	R	I/M	L/I	L	F

NS1 AA	**22**	**81**	**114**	**171**	**216**	**228**
Human	V	M	P	I/N	T	R
HK*	F	I	S	E/D	P	E
Avian**	L/F/V	I/V	G/S	D/T	P	E/G

NS2 AA	**70**
Human	G
HK*	S
Avian**	S

M1 AA	**115**	**121**	**137**	**218**
Human	I	A	A	A > T
HK*	V	T	T	T
Avian**	V	T	T	T

M2 AA	**16**	**28**	**55**	**78**
Human	G > E	V	F	K
HK*	G	V	F	Q
Avian**	E	I	L > F	Q

If only one residue is indicated, the amino acid at the corresponding position is found in more than 90% of the available sequences. If it is followed by > X, the amino acid at this position is found in more than 80% of the available sequences.
* HK: human H5N1 strains isolated in Hong Kong in 1997.
** Avian sequences do not include those from strains isolated from poultry in Hong Kong in 1997 which were found to be very close to the A/Hong Kong/156/97 sequences [64, 13] and could therefore be considered as possible intermediates between pure avian and pure human type.

internal gene and all the remaining genes from a human virus were generated by co-infection of cultured cells, and their ability to replicate *in vitro* and/or *in vivo* was evaluated. Reassortant viruses containing the NP gene from the avian A/Mallard/NY/6750/78 virus and the remaining genes from the human A/Udorn/307/72 virus appeared as restricted in growth in the respiratory tract of squirrel monkeys as was the avian-human reassortant containing each of the six avian influenza internal genes [41]. Similar results were reported by Snyder *et al.* for A/Pintail/Alberta/119/79 × A/Washington/897/80 reassortant viruses [44]. These experiments indicated that the NP gene was the major determinant of the attenuation of avian-human A/Mallard/78 or A/Pintail/79 reassortant viruses in monkeys. They were in agreement with the observation by Scholtissek *et al.* that mutants of the avian A/FPV/Rostock/34 virus with temperature sensitive lesions in the NP could not be rescued by human H3N2 isolates, which suggested that the NP could be a major factor in determining host-specificity of the H3N2 strains [46]. Using A/Mallard/NY/6759/78 × A/Los Angeles/2/87 reassortant viruses, Clements *et al.* confirmed that the NP gene contributed to the attenuation in monkeys, but found that this was not the case in adult human volunteers [45]. These discordant observations indicated that studies of single gene reassortants conducted with monkeys would not necessarily allow the determinants of the attenuation of influenza A viruses for humans to be identified.

The avian M gene appeared to play a major role in the attenuation of the A/Mallard/78 virus and its reassortants in squirrel monkeys in the study of Tian *et al.* [41], but little or no role for the A/Mallard/78 virus or the A/Pintail/79 viruses and their reassortants in the studies of Clements *et al.* [45] and Snyder *et al.* [44], respectively. However in humans, the A/Mallard/78 × A/Los Angeles/87 single gene M reassortant replicated significantly less efficiently than the wild-type human influenza virus parent, suggesting that the M gene contributed to the attenuation phenotype of the avian influenza virus parent [45]. Noticeably, the M single gene reassortant virus formed small plaques in primary chicken kidney (PCK) cells. This *in vitro* phenotype, which was exhibited neither by either parental virus, nor by the other reassortant viruses, indicated that this specific combination of avian and human genes could be responsible for a new phenotype. Thus, it was not possible to determine whether the avian M gene itself or a specific constellation of avian and human influenza A virus genes specified the restriction of virus replication in humans.

Similarly, an unusual *in vitro* host range phenotype was observed by Clements *et al.* for a single gene reassortant that derived its PB2 gene from the avian A/Mallard/NY/6759/78 virus and the remaining genes from the A/Los Angeles/2/87 virus [45]. This reassortant showed efficient replication in PCK cells and restricted replication in mammalian MDCK cells, while the human and avian viruses each replicated efficiently in both PCK and MDCK cells. The PB2 single gene reassortant virus also showed restricted replication *in vivo* in the respiratory tract of squirrel monkeys and humans. Further study of this virus and of phenotypic revertants that had recovered the ability to replicate efficiently in MDCK cells allowed Subbarao *et al.* to determine that a single amino acid substitution at position 627 (Glu → Lys) was responsible for the ability of these viruses to replicate in MDCK cells, and in the respiratory tract of squirrel monkeys [47]. Interestingly, the amino acid at position 627 is a glutamic acid residue in all available sequences for avian-derived PB2 proteins, and a lysine residue in all available sequences for human-derived PB2 proteins *(Table I).* These findings clearly indicated that the PB2 gene contributes to the host range restriction of the A/Mallard/NY/6759/78 reassortant virus, but did not establish whether interactions of PB2 with cellular host factors and/or interactions of PB2 with other viral proteins are involved. This body of evidence led to the idea that specific constellations of gene segments encoding the internal proteins could be determinant for the host-range, but no such constellation has been clearly implicated for its contribution to host range restriction yet. This is mostly due to the fact that all possible constellations could generally not be isolated, which precluded unequivocal interpretation of the data.

Effect of the avian/human origin of core proteins on the activity of polymerase complexes

In order to address the question as to how efficiently the polymerase proteins derived from human and avian influenza A viruses may interact with each other within a mammalian cell, we made use of the genetic system described by Pleschka *et al.* [48] for the *in vivo* reconstitution of functional ribonucleoproteins. The ability to ensure replication of a viral-like reporter RNA in COS-1 cells was examined with heterospecific mixtures of the core proteins (PB1, PB2, PA and NP) from two strains of human viruses (A/PuertoRico/8/34 and A/Victoria/3/75) and two strains of avian viruses (A/Mallard/NY/6750/78 and A/FPV/Rostock/34) [49]. In accordance with the observations of Clements *et al.* on PB2 single gene reassortant viruses [45], PB2 amino acid 627 was identified as a major determinant of the replication of heterospecific complexes in COS-1 cells *(Table II)*. The detailed analysis of all possible constellations among the polymerase genes suggested that the mechanism by which the nature of PB2 amino acid 627 altered the efficiency of transcription/replication of the viral-like RNA relied on interactions of PB2 with both viral and cellular proteins. We observed that homospecificity between PB2 and NP appeared to enhance the functional efficiency of chimeric complexes, which suggested that PB2-NP interactions could be involved in the transcription/replication process, and could therefore impose some constraints on reassortment events involving the corresponding segments. Furthermore, replication of the viral-like reporter RNA in mammalian cells was more efficient when PB1 was derived from an avian virus whatever the origin of the other proteins *(Table II)*, suggesting that the acquisition of the PB1 segment from an avian virus may have conferred a selective advantage to the 1957 and 1968 reassortant viruses.

Using the same experimental system, the efficiency of the polymerase complexes was found to be impaired at 33 °C as compared to 37 °C in the case of the avian A/Mallard/NY/78 and A/FPV/Rostock/34 viruses, whereas it was similar at both temperatures in the case of the human A/Puerto Rico/8/34 and A/Victoria/3/75 viruses [50]. The sensitivity to cold of the avian-derived complexes was determined mostly by residue 627 of the PB2 protein, and to a lesser extent by the PA protein *(Table II)*. The abilities of human and avian viruses to replicate at the temperature of the upper respiratory tract (33 °C) were compared in order to address the question whether this observation could be related to the fact that human influenza A viruses replicate in the upper respiratory tract at a temperature of about 33 °C, whereas avian viruses replicate in the intestinal tract at a temperature close to 40 °C. Using plaque assays on MDCK cells, the virus titers and the plaque size were found to be reduced at 33 °C as compared to 37 °C in the case of avian viruses and not or only slightly reduced in the case of human viruses. The kinetics of replication of the NP-RNA segment in MDCK or COS-1 cells were similar at 33 °C and 37 °C in the case of human viruses, whereas replication was delayed at 33 °C as compared to 37 °C in the case of avian viruses [50]. These findings suggest that a reduced ability of the polymerase complex of avian viruses to ensure replication of the viral genome at the temperature of the upper respiratory tract (33 °C) could contribute to their inability to grow efficiently in humans. The role of amino acid 627 of PB2 in cold-sensitiviy of avian viruses remains to be confirmed in the context of an infectious virus produced by the reverse genetics approach, using both *in vitro* and *in vivo* assays. However, it is remarkable that this residue has alltogether been found

Table II. Effect of the origin of the polymerase protein genes on the activity of polymerase complexes reconstituted in COS-1 cells*.

	Human(1)	**HK156**(2)	**Avian**(3)
PB1	– Reduced activity as compared to PB1 proteins of avian origin at 37 °C – No PB1-mediated sensitivity at 33 °C as compared to 37 °C	– Intermediate activity with respect to PB1 proteins of human and avian origin – No PB1-mediated sensitivity at 33 °C as compared to 37 °C	– Increased activity as compared to PB1 proteins of human origin at 37 °C – No PB1-mediated sensitivity at 33 °C as compared to 37 °C
PB2 (aa 627)	– Increased activity as compared to PB2 proteins of avian origin at 37 °C – PB2-mediated increase of activity at 33 °C as compared to 37 °C	– Intermediate activity with respect to PB2 proteins of human and avian origin – PB2-mediated reduction of activity at 33 °C as compared to 37 °C	– Reduced activity as compared to PB2 proteins of human origin at 37 °C – PB2-mediated reduction of activity at 33 °C as compared to 37 °C
PA(4)	– No PA-mediated sensitivity at 33 °C as compared to 37 °C	– No PA-mediated sensitivity at 33 °C as compared to 37 °C	– PA-mediated reduction of activity at 33 °C as compared to 37 °C

* Data from Naffakh *et al.* [49] and Massin *et al.* [50].
(1) Proteins derived from the A/Puerto Rico/8/34 or A/Victoria/3/75 strains.
(2) A/Hong Kong/156/97.
(3) Proteins derived from the A/Mallard/NY/6750/78 or A/FPV/Rostock/34 strains.
(4) The effect of the human or avian origin of the PA gene on the activity of the polymerase complexes at 37 °C could not be evaluated, because the level of proteolytic activity associated with PA varied from one strain to another.

determinant for the ability of reassortant influenza A viruses to replicate in MDCK cells, the activity of heterospecific polymerase complexes reconstituted in COS-1 cells, and the cold-sensitivity of avian-derived polymerase complexes. One hypothesis could be that host-range and cold-sensitivity both rely on the same molecular interactions between PB2 and cellular proteins. In mammalian cells, these interactions would be as strong at 37 °C as at 33 °C when PB2 is derived from a human virus, while they would be weaker (at 37 °C and even more so at 33 °C) when PB2 is derived from an avian virus. There are numerous reports of PB2 being involved in the adaptation of influenza A viruses to low temperatures (25-33 °C) or in their sensitivity to high temperatures (37-40 °C). More than 20 different PB2 mutations responsible for such phenotypes have been identified using genomic sequencing [51-55] or reverse genetics methods [56-58]. A number of PA mutations have also been correlated with temperature-dependent phenotypes. The question whether natural sensitivity to temperature of human viruses, linked to some of their internal proteins, could contribute to their inability to replicate in the intestinal tract of ducks should probably be addressed. An attempt was already made by Tian *et al.* to identify the avian influenza virus genes specifying replication at 42 °C, by testing the efficiency of plaque formation at 42 °C as compared to 37 °C of A/Mallard/78 × A/Udorn/72 reassortants. Their observations suggested that although more than one gene contribute to the ability of the A/Mallard/NY/78 to replicate at 42 °C, the PB2 gene plays a major role [41].

Molecular characteristics of the core proteins involved in replication and/or pathogenicity of H5N1 viruses in humans

The experiments mentioned above have been useful to address the question of the compatibility between viral internal proteins derived from avian and human viruses and the interaction of these proteins with cellular factors. They have given some clues to the molecular basis of host range restriction and interspecies reassortment control among influenza A viruses. However, they have provided little information about the determinants of the ability of an influenza A virus to transmit and become adapted to a new host, and about the determinants of virulence for such a new host. With respect to these questions, the study of the avian influenza A (H5N1) viruses that infected humans in Hong Kong in 1997 [9-11] is of paramount interest. Alignment of the amino acid sequences from internal proteins of the H5N1 viruses isolated from human patients in Hong Kong revealed some amino acids specific for this virus subgroup and some others characteristic of the sequences derived from human strains, which could possibly be determinant in inter-species transmission *(Table I)*. In contrast, the HA and NA showed no evidence of adaptative change in humans [59]. The core proteins of one of the human H5N1 isolates (A/Hong Kong/156/97) were included in our experiments of *in vivo* reconstitution of functional ribonucleoproteins in COS-1 cells. Within heterospecific complexes, the PB1 and PB2 proteins from the A/Hong Kong/156/97 virus exhibited intermediate properties with respect to the corresponding proteins from avian or human viruses *(Table II)* [49]. Moreover, the polymerase complex from the H5N1 virus exhibited an intermediate sensitivity to cold with respect to the polymerase complexes derived from avian or human viruses, which seemed to be linked solely to the PB2 protein *(Table II)* [50]. These observations suggested that some molecular characteristics of the core proteins could at least partially account for the ability of the A/Hong Kong/156/97 virus to replicate in humans.

The BALB/c mouse has been used as a mammalian model for the evaluation of human H5N1 virus pathogenesis [60-63]. All viruses appeared to replicate efficiently in the respiratory tract of mice without prior adaptation, suggesting that all viruses shared some characteristics conferring the ability to replicate in a mammalian host. However, two groups of distinct virulence were clearly identified. Viruses exhibiting high pathogenicity (*e.g.* HK/483/97) underwent systemic replication, whereas viruses exhibiting low pathogenicity (*e.g.* HK/486/97) replicated in the respiratory tract only [60-63]. For a few viruses (HK/156/97, HK/481/97), discordant results were found, which may reflect either an intermediate level of pathogenicity, or the heterogeneity of the original isolates. Extensive sequence analysis of H5N1 viruses was performed by Katz et *al.* [63]. Substitutions at residue 223 in the NA, 15 in M1, 198 and 317 in PB1, and 355 in PB2 correlated with differences in pathogenicity in all 15 viruses analyzed. These residues did not correspond to a human/avian specificity of the sequences *(Table I)*. Interestingly, residue 627 of PB2 differed among the H5N1 viruses [60, 63]. Among the viruses with high pathogenicity, two had a Lys (typical of human strains), two had a Glu (typical of avian strains), and one was found to be a mixed population of viruses having a Lys and a Glu residue, confirming the hypothesis mentioned earlier that the H5N1 isolates could be heterogeneous. These findings suggest that the Glu627Lys substitution in PB2, in association with other molecular determinants, could contribute to an increased replicative efficiency and pathogenicity in mammals. The use of plasmid-based reverse genetics techniques will probably help to evaluate the contribution of each of the residues mentioned above, alone or in combinations, to the pathogenicity phenotype in mice, and to elucidate the corresponding mechanisms.

As a whole, the data obtained so far suggest that not one but multiple genetic features of the internal genes contribute to the potential for interspecies transmission of influenza A viruses and to their virulence. A better undestanding of this polygenic determinism is still needed in order to be able to survey the emergence of influenza A viruses with the potential to cause severe disease in humans.

References

1. Webster RG, Bean WJ Jr. Evolution and ecology of Influenza viruses: interspecies transmission. In: Nicholson KG, Webster RG, Hay AJ, eds. *Textbook of Influenza*. Ltd.: Oxford, England: Blackwell Science, 1998: 109-19.
2. Beare AS, Webster RG. Replication of avian influenza viruses in humans. *Arch Virol* 1991; 119: 37-42.
3. Murphy BR, Hinshaw VS, Sly DL, London WT, Hosier NT, Wood FT, Webster RG, Chanock RM. Virulence of avian influenza A viruses for squirrel monkeys. *Infect Immun* 1982; 37: 1119-26.
4. Scholtissek C, Rohde W, Von Hoyningen V, Rott R. On the origin of the human influenza virus subtypes H2N2 and H3N2. *Virology* 1978; 87: 13-20.
5. Scholtissek C, Hinshaw VS, Olsen CW. Influenza in pigs and their role as the intermediate host. In: Nicholson KG, Webster RG, Hay AJ, eds. *Textbook of influenza*. Oxford: Blackwell Science, 1998: 137-45.
6. Kawaoka Y, Krauss S, Webster RG. Avian-to-human transmission of the PB1 gene of influenza A viruses in the 1957 and 1968 pandemics. *J Virol* 1989; 63: 4603-8.
7. Shortridge KF. Pandemic influenza: a zoonosis? *Semin Resp Infect* 1992; 7: 11-25.
8. Kurtz J, Manvell RJ, Banks J. Avian influenza virus isolated from a woman with conjunctivitis. *Lancet* 1996; 348: 901-2.
9. Centers for Disease Control and Prevention. Update: isolation of avian influenza A (H5N1) viruses from humans-Hong Kong, 1997-1998. *MMWR* 1998; 46: 1245-7.
10. Claas EC, Osterhaus AD, van Beek R, De Jong JC, Rimmelzwaan GF, Senne DA, Krauss S, Shortridge KF, Webster RG. Human influenza A H5N1 virus related to a highly pathogenic avian influenza virus. *Lancet* 1998; 351: 472-7.
11. Subbarao K, Klimov A, Katz J, Regnery H, Lim W, Hall H, Perdue M, Swayne D, Bender C, Huang J, Hemphill M, Rowe T, Shaw M, Xu X, Fukuda K, Cox N. Characterization of an avian influenza A (H5N1) virus isolated from a child with a fatal respiratory illness. *Science* 1998; 279: 393-6.
12. Zhou NN, Shortridge KF, Class EC, Krauss SL, Webster RG. Rapid evolution of H5N1 influenza viruses in chickens in Hong Kong. *J Virol* 1999; 73: 3366-74.
13. Guan Y, Shortridge KF, Krauss S, Webster RG. Molecular characterization of H9N2 influenza viruses: were they the donors of the "internal" genes of H5N1 viruses in Hong Kong? *Proc Natl Acad Sci USA* 1999; 96: 9363-7.
14. Hoffmann E, Stech J, Leneva I, Krauss S, Scholtissek C, Chin PS, Peiris M, Shortridge KF, Webster RG. Characterization of the influenza A virus gene pool in avian species in southern China: was H6N1 a derivative or a precursor of H5N1? *J Virol* 2000; 74: 6309-15.
15. Lin YP, Shaw M, Gregory V, Cameron K, Lim W, Klimov A, Subbarao K, Guan Y, Krauss S, Shortridge K, Webster R, Cox N, Hay A. Avian-to-human transmission of H9N2 subtype influenza A viruses: relationship between H9N2 and H5N1 human isolates. *Proc Natl Acad Sci USA* 2000; 97: 9654-8.
16. Huang TS, Palese P, Krystal M. Determination of influenza virus proteins required for genome replication. *J Virol* 1990; 64: 5669-73.
17. Digard P, Block VC, Inglis SC. Complex formation between influenza virus polymerase proteins expressed in Xenopus oocytes. *Virology* 1989; 171: 162-9.
18. Toyoda T, Adyshev DM, Kobayashi M, Iwata A, Ishima A. Molecular assembly of the influenza virus RNA polymerase: determination of the subunit-subunit contact sites. *J Gen Virol* 1996; 77: 2149-57.

19. Gonzalez S, Zurcher T, Ortin J. Identification of two separate domains in the influenza virus PB1 protein involved in the interaction with the PB2 and PA subunits: a model for the viral RNA polymerase structure. *Nucleic Acids Res* 1996; 24: 4456-63.
20. Zurcher T, de la Luna S, Sanz-Ezquerro JJ, Nieto A, Ortin J. Mutational analysis of the influenza virus A/Victoria/3/75 PA protein: studies of interaction with PB1 protein and identification of a dominant negative mutant. *J Gen Virol* 1996; 77: 1745-9.
21. Braam J, Ulmanene I, Krug RM. Molecular model of a eucaryotic transcription complex: functions and movements of influenza P proteins during capped RNA-primed transcription. *Cell* 1983; 34: 609-18.
22. Biswas SK, Nayak DP. Mutational analysis of the conserved motifs of influenza A virus polymerase basic protein 1. *J Virol* 1994; 68: 1819-26.
23. Blaas D, Patzelt E, Kuechler E. Cap-recognizing protein of influenza virus. *Virology* 1982; 116: 339-48.
24. Shi L, Galarza JM, Summers DF. Recombinant-baculovirus-expressed PB2 subunit of the influenza A virus RNA polymerase binds cap groups as an isolated subunit. *Virus Res* 1996; 42: 1-9.
25. Blok V, Cianci C, Tibbles KW, Inglis SC, Krystal M, Digard P. Inhibition of the influenza virus RNA-dependent RNA polymerase by antisera directed against the carboxy-terminal region of the PB2 subunit. *J Gen Virol* 1996; 77: 1025-33.
26. Sanz-Ezquerro JJ, de la Luna S, Ortin J, Nieto A. Individual expression of influenza virus PA protein induces degradation of coexpressed proteins. *J Virol* 1995; 69: 2420-6.
27. Beaton AR, Krug RM. Transcription antitermination during influenza viral template RNA synthesis requires the nucleocapsid protein and the absence of a 5' capped end. *Proc Natl Acad Sci USA* 1986; 83: 6282-6.
28. Biswas SK, Boutz PL, Nayak DP. Influenza virus nucleoprotein interacts with influenza virus polymerase proteins. *J Virol* 1998; 72: 5493-501.
29. Lamb RA, Krug RM. Orthomyxoviridae: the viruses and their replication. In: KDM Fields BN, Howley PM, *et al.*, eds. *Virology*. Philadelphia: Lippincott-Raven, 1996: 1353-95.
30. Jin H, Leser GP, Zhang J, Lamb RA. Influenza virus hemagglutinin and neuraminidase cytoplasmic tails control particle shape. *EMBO J* 1997; 16: 1236-47.
31. Hay AJ. Functional properties of the virus ion channels. In: Nicholson KG, Webster RG, Hay AJ, eds. *Textbook of Influenza*. Oxford: Blackwell Science Ltd, 1998: 74-81.
32. Katze MG, Krug RM. Metabolism and expression of RNA polymerase II transcripts in influenza virus-infected cells. *Mol Cell Biol* 1984; 4: 2198-206.
33. Garfinkel MS, Katze MG. Translational control by influenza virus. Selective translation is mediated by sequences within the viral mRNA 5'-untranslated region. *J Biol Chem* 1993; 268: 22223-6.
34. Katze MG, DeCorato D, Krug RM. Cellular mRNA translation is blocked at both initiation and elongation after infection by influenza virus or adenovirus. *J Virol* 1986; 60: 1027-39.
35. Bergmann M, *et al.* Influenza virus NS1 protein counteracts PKR-mediated inhibition of replication. *J Virol* 2000; 74: 6203-6.
36. Talon J, Horvath CM, Polley R, Basler CF, Muster T, Palese P, Garcia-Sastre A. Activation of interferon regulatory factor 3 is inhibited by the influenza A virus NS1 protein. *J Virol* 2000; 74: 7989-96.
37. O'Neill RE, Talon J, Palese P. The influenza virus NEP (NS2 protein) mediates the nuclear export of viral nucleoproteins. *EMBO J* 1998; 17: 288-96.
38. Altmüller A, Kunerl M, Muller K, Hinshaw VS, Fitch WM, Scholtissek C. Genetic relatedness of the nucleoprotein (NP) of recent swine, turkey, and human influenza A virus (H1N1) isolates. *Virus Res* 1992; 22: 79-87.
39. Okazaki K, Kawaoka Y, Webster RG. Evolutionary pathways of the PA genes of influenza A viruses. *Virology* 1989; 172: 601-8.
40. Gorman O, Donis RO, Kawaoka Y, Webster RG. Evolution of influenza A virus PB2 genes: implications for evolution of the ribo nucleoprotein complex and origin of human influenza A virus. *J Virol* 1990; 64: 4893-902.
41. Tian SF, Buckler-White AJ, London WT, Reck LJ, Chanock RM, Murphy BR. Nucleoprotein and membrane protein genes are associated with restriction of replication of influenza A/Mallard/NY/78 virus and its reassortants in squirrel monkey respiratory tract. *J Virol* 1985; 53: 771-5.
42. Buckler-White AJ, Naeve CW, Murphy BR. Characterization of a gene coding for M proteins which is involved in host range restriction of an avian influenza A virus in monkeys. *J Virol* 1986; 57: 697-700.
43. Clements ML, Snyder MH, Buckler-White AJ, Tierney El, London WT, Murphy BR. Evaluation of avian-human reassortant influenza A/Washington/897/80 × A/Pintail/119/79 virus in monkeys and adult volunteers. *J Clin Microbiol* 1986; 24: 47-51.

44. Snyder MH, Buckler-White AJ, London WT, Tierney EL, Murphy BR. The avian influenza virus nucleoprotein gene and a specific constellation of avian and human virus polymerase genes each specify attenuation of avian-human influenza A/Pintail/79 reassortant viruses for monkeys. *J Virol* 1987; 61: 2857-63.
45. Clements ML, Subbarao EK, Fries LF, Karron RA, London WT, Murphy BR. Use of single-gene reassortant viruses to study the role of avian influenza A virus genes in attenuation of wild-type human influenza A virus for squirrel monkeys and adult human volunteers. *J Clin Microbiol* 1992; 30: 655-62.
46. Scholtissek C, Burger H, Kistner O, Shortridge KF. The nucleoprotein as a possible major factor in determining host specificity of influenza H3N2 viruses. *Virology* 1985; 147: 287-94.
47. Subbarao EK, London W, Murphy BR. A single amino acid in the PB2 gene of influenza A virus is a determinant of host range. *J Virol* 1993; 67: 1761-4.
48. Pleschka S, Jaskunas R, Engelhardt OG, Zurcher T, Palese P, Garcia-Sastre A. A plasmid-based reverse genetics system for influenza A virus. *J Virol* 1996; 70: 4188-92.
49. Naffakh N, Massin P, Escriou N, Crescenzo-Chaigne B, van der Werf S. Genetic analysis of the compatibility between polymerase proteins from human and avian strains of influenza A viruses. *J Gen Virol* 2000; 81: 1283-91.
50. Massin P, Naffakh N, van der Werf S. Cold-sensitivity of polymerase complexes from human or avian influenza A viruses. In: *Options for the control of Influenza IV*. Elsevier, 2000 (in press).
51. Cox NJ, Kitame F, Kendal AP, Maassab HF, Naeve C. Identification of sequence changes in the cold-adapted, live attenuated influenza vaccine strain, A/Ann Arbor/6/60 (H2N2). *Virology* 1988; 167: 554-67.
52. Yamanaka K, Ogasawara N, Ueda M, Yoshikawa H, Ishihama A, Nagata K. Characterization of a temperature-sensitive mutant in the RNA polymerase PB2 subunit gene of influenza A/WSN/33 virus. *Arch Virol* 1990; 114: 65-73.
53. Klimov AI, Cox NJ, Yotov WV, Rocha E, Alexandrova GI, Kendal AP. Sequence changes in the live attenuated, cold-adapted variants of influenza A/Leningrad/134/57 (H2N2) virus. *Virology* 1992; 186: 795-7.
54. Lawson CM, Subbarao EK, Murphy BR. Nucleotide sequence changes in the polymerase basic protein 2 gene of temperature-sensitive mutants of influenza A virus. *Virology* 1992; 191: 506-10.
55. Herlocher ML, Clavo AC, Maassab HF. Sequence comparisons of A/AA/6/60 influenza viruses: mutations which may contribute to attenuation. *Virus Res* 1996; 42: 11-25.
56. Subbarao EK, Park EJ, Lawson CM, Chen AY, Murphy BR. Sequential addition of temperature-sensitive missense mutations into the PB2 gene of influenza A transfectant viruses can effect an increase in temperature sensitivity and attenuation and permits the rational design of a genetically engineered live influenza A virus vaccine. *J Virol* 1995; 69: 5969-77.
57. Murphy BR, Park EJ, Gottlieb P, Subbarao K. An influenza A live attenuated reassortant virus possessing three temperature-sensitive mutations in the PB2 polymerase gene rapidly loses temperature sensitivity following replication in hamsters. *Vaccine* 1997; 15: 1372-8.
58. Parkin NT, Chiu P, Coelingh K. Genetically engineered live atenuated influenza A virus vaccine candidates. *J Virol* 1997; 71: 2772-8.
59. Bender C, Hall H, Huang J, Klimov A, Cox N, Hay A, Gregory V, Cameron K, Lim W, Subbarao K. Characterization of the surface proteins of influenza A (H5N1) viruses isolated from humans in 1997-1998. *Virology* 1999; 254: 115-23.
60. Gao P, Watanabe S, Ito T, Goto H, Wells K, McGregor M, Cooley AJ, Kawaoka Y. Biological heterogeneity, including systemic replication in mice, of H5N1 influenza A virus isolates from humans in Hong Kong. *J Virol* 1999; 73: 3184-9.
61. Lu X, Tumpey TM, Morken T, Zaki SR, Cox NJ, Katz JM. A mouse model for the evaluation of pathogenesis and immunity to influenza A (H5N1) viruses isolated from humans. *J Virol* 1999; 73: 5903-11.
62. Tumpey TM, Lu X, Morken T, Zaki SR, Katz JM. Depletion of lymphocytes and diminished cytokine production in mice infected with a highly virulent influenza A (H5N1) virus isolated from humans. *J Virol* 2000; 74: 6105-16.
63. Katz JM, Lu X, Tumpey TM, Smith CB, Shaw MW, Subbarao K. Molecular correlates of influenza A H5N1 pathogenesis in mice. *J Virol* 2000; 74: 10807-10.
64. Suarez DL, Perdue ML, Cox N, Rowe T, Bender C, Huang J, Swayne DE. Comparisons of highly virulent H5N1 influenza A viruses isolated from humans and chickens from Hong Kong. *J Virol* 1998; 72: 6678-88.

Emergence and Control of Zoonotic Ortho- and Paramyxovirus Diseases
B. Dodet, M. Vicari, eds.

H5N1 virus: beaten, but is it vanquished?

Kennedy F. Shortridge[1], Malik Peiris[1], Yi Guan[1], Kitman Dyrting[2], Trevor Ellis[2], Leslie Sims[2]

[1] *Department of Microbiology, The University of Hong Kong, University Pathology Building, Queen Mary Hospital, Hong Kong SAR, China*
[2] *Department of Agriculture, Fisheries and Conservation, Government of the Hong Kong SAR, China*

Abstract – This commentary takes stock of the background of the H5N1 virus's crossing the species barrier from chicken to humans consequent upon its amplification in chicken in the live poultry markets in Hong Kong in the "bird flu" incident of 1997. Retrospective studies indicate the involvement of a precursor H5N1 virus from the goose and H9N2 and H6N1 viruses from quail in the genesis of the pathogenic H5N1/97 virus. The genetic homology of their internal genes and the continued presence of all three subtypes in the region raises the possibility of the re-emergence of the pathogenic H5N1/97 virus there. Thus, in spite of the eradication of this virus in late 1997 through the slaughter of chicken and other poultry across the SAR, it may not be vanquished. It also raises the stakes for the potential for pandemicity of H9N2 and H6N1 viruses. In particular, the H9N2 virus has been isolated from humans and pigs in Hong Kong and has spread across Eurasia and to southern Africa. Good surveillance of humans and animals in the region and beyond is the key to anticipation and critical for baseline pandemic preparedness. One of the lessons from the H5N1 incident was that the state of preparedness was far from satisfactory. While we are aware of the potential importance of the H5N1 virus, are we really prepared for it?

In 1997 the Hong Kong SAR found itself in a public health crisis with an H5N1 outbreak in humans. Eighteen patients were diagnosed and six succumbed [1, 2]. The situation posed a potential pandemic threat. Save for minimal genetic differences, the same totally avian H5N1 virus that had claimed high mortality on chicken farms in the rural New Territories [3] was present in retail and wholesale markets across the SAR to the extent that around 20% of chicken were infected [4] providing an unprecedented opportunity for those entering the markets to be exposed to the virus.

Why the H5 subtype?

Fifteen H subtypes of influenza virus have been recognized in nature to date; there may be more. There is no reason to suppose that all H subtypes would not occur in southern China, a region recognized as a hypothetical epicentre for the emergence of pandemic influenza viruses in part due to its abundance and diversity of avian influenza viruses

[5]. What special advantages did the H5 subtype have over other avian H subtypes in leading to interspecies transmission in humans and causing disease? Indeed, it might be reasoned that pandemics might arise in the epicentre as frequently as interpandemic variants of H3N2 arise. After all, humans in the rural areas of Southern China show evidence of antibodies directed against all the H subtypes examined, indicating that exposure to a miscellany of avian influenza viruses is not uncommon [6]. If there were an opportunity for H5 subtype viruses to cause human disease, a cue might be taken from the H5N2 viruses that had claimed high mortality in chickens in Pennsylvania and Mexico some 12-14 years earlier following introduction into chicken [7, 8]. In both these incidents, human exposure, although considerable, was limited to a relatively small number of persons working directly in the poultry industry. It did not lead to significant human infection and did not pose a pandemic threat. This proved to be cold comfort to Hong Kong when an H5N1 virus was isolated from the index human case in May, 1997.

Why was the H5N1/97 in particular able to cross the species barrier and infect humans in the Hong Kong SAR?

It is now known that this virus still showed a preference for binding to the avian sialic acid receptor containing the N acetylneuramic acid -α2,3 gal linkage and was not ideally adapted to the human receptor containing the -α2,6 gal linkage [9]. This probably was a reason why transmission of infection to humans was so inefficient and why, fortunately for mankind, human-to-human transmission was so poor. Given the high prevalence of the virus in the live poultry markets of Hong Kong, a large number of persons in Hong Kong were exposed. A key difference from the situation in Pennsylvania and Mexico was that in Hong Kong, human exposure was not restricted to poultry workers but extended to the many people who shopped in the almost 1000 retail live poultry markets across the SAR.

Those few who got the disease were the exception rather than the rule and were presumably unusually "susceptible" to infection by the virus. This susceptibility was not due to immuno-suppression or to any of the known risk factors for influenza [2]. It may be speculated that genetic host differences in receptors available for virus attachment were contributory or that there were other host factors. A key difference contributing to human disease following the H5 outbreaks in poultry in Hong Kong and the USA may simply be the much larger number of humans exposed to the virus in Hong Kong through the live poultry retail market system prevalent there.

A second notable feature of the H5N1 infections was the severe disease associated with human infections, especially in adults. In the course of the incident, pathogenicity for chicken was often equated with pathogenicity for humans. The H5N1/97 virus had multiple basic amino acids at the cleavage site of the haemagglutinin and a readily cleavable haemagglutinin [4] which is characteristic of highly pathogenic avian influenza viruses. The virus grew readily in MDCK cells without the need for exogenous trypsin in the culture medium. However, though there was indication of multiple organ dysfunction in human patients with severe H5N1 disease, there was no direct evidence that the virus had disseminated beyond the respiratory tract [10]. The post-mortem data was limited and in some patients, death occurred many weeks after the acute infection and a definitive answer to this question is not available. Clearly, pathogenicity is a polygenic characteristic dependent on the gene constellation of a virus [11]. In another mammalian system, *i.e.* the mouse model, H9N2 viruses of the G1 lineage, which share internal genes with H5N1/97, also have unusually high pathogenicity for mice [12]. Furthermore, evidence presented at this meeting suggests that the PB2 gene of H5N1/97 virus is a key factor in mouse virulence [13].

It is to be noted that the previous pandemic viruses of 1957 (H2N2) and 1968 (H3N2) did not have multiple basic amino acid motifs at the haemagglutinin cleavage site. Data from the molecular archaeology carried out on the pandemic H1N1 virus of 1917 also suggests that this virus also lacked a highly cleavable haemagglutinin [14]. It remains to be seen what ancestral genetic information toward this will emerge from the current investigations being carried out on its fragments. Experimental studies involving reverse genetics on the H5N1/97 virus may point to a way forward in understanding the basis of pathogenicity in humans, one that is central to influenza pandemic preparedness should a virus in the epicentre or elsewhere be recognized in a non-human host.

Pandemicity and virulence are not necessarily the same thing! The H5N1/97 virus in Hong Kong had high virulence but limited pandemic potential because of its poor human-to-human transmissibility. The concern was that the virus may have acquired greater transmissibility through mutation or reassortment with current human influenza viruses. What effect such "human adaptation" as has been suggested might have occurred with the 1918 pandemic virus [15] would have had on the virulence of the H5N1 virus is unknown.

The slaughter of chicken and other poultry across the SAR in late December 1997 eliminated the source of the H5N1 virus for humans and a seemingly averted pandemic. This is a cue toward control of a pandemic at source but would it really be practicable to slaughter poultry selectively over a wide region, economic factors notwithstanding? And was the slaughter of poultry in Hong Kong in 1997 nothing more than a short term respite from the H5N1 virus?

Tracing the source of the H5N1 virus

It had never been possible to trace the precursor viruses or their source in past pandemics. Any information that might be gathered from the H5N1 incident might prove useful in pandemic preparedness should the H5N1 virus re-emerge or another H subtype emerge. This was approached by genetically examining influenza viruses that were present in poultry in the SAR's markets in 1997, *i.e.* H9N2 and an H6N1 isolate in addition to H5N1 [3], and viruses found in a range of poultry in post-1997 surveillance. Two important sets of information arose.

Firstly, the H5N1/97 virus shared its internal genes with H9N2 viruses of the G1 lineage and H6N1 viruses of the W321 lineage and its neuraminidase gene with these H6N1 viruses [16, 17]. The haemagglutinin was derived from an H5N1 virus isolated previously from geese, *i.e.* A/Goose/Guangdong/96-like virus [18]. Secondly, the H9N2 and H6N1 viruses carrying the internal gene complex of H5N1/97 still continue to circulate in this region with quail being a major host for both of them. In contrast, the H5 haemagglutinin is so far confined to geese (unpublished data). Could the quail be the "mixing vessel" in which reassortment takes place? Might the chicken also be involved? Are the live retail markets the "site" in which this reassortment takes place? And could chicken, by virtue of their numerical strength in the retail markets, be the amplifying host that transmits these viruses to humans? Good surveillance will be important in resolving this issue.

Can the pathogenic H5N1/97 virus re-emerge?

While the highly pathogenic H5N1/97 virus had been eradicated from the live poultry markets in the poultry slaughter, the precursor viruses are still present in the wider region. In so far as Hong Kong is concerned, the opportunity for reassortment to occur in its live poultry retail system has been minimized since geese (which carry the donor of the H5 haemagglutinin) are now centrally slaughtered and not allowed into the retail markets which sell live land-based poultry only. The donors of the internal genes and the neuraminidase gene are still present in live land-based poultry imported into the SAR. However, this does not preclude opportunity for such a mixing occurring elsewhere in the wider region.

In addition to its recognition in East Asia in the mid-1990's [19, 20], the H9N2 virus has also been recognized in Pakistan, the Middle East, Europe and Southern Africa [21]. This takes the H9N2 precursor virus beyond the hypothetical epicentre providing the opportunity for it or a reassortant of it to give rise to a possible pandemic virus. This view is taken on the grounds that H9N2 viruses of the G1 lineage have been isolated from two children in Hong Kong with influenza-like illness [22, 23] and of the Y280 lineage from pigs also in Hong Kong (Peiris *et al.* in preparation). There is an unconfirmed report of the isolation of H9N2 viruses from humans in Guangdong Province adjacent to Hong Kong.

However, both H5N1 and H6N1 precursor viruses have so far only been isolated from poultry imported from Guangdong Province, implying, at least for the present, that an H5N1 virus similar to the highly pathogenic 1997 viruses could still arise in the epicentre. In other words, while the H5N1 virus may have been beaten in 1997, there is every possibility that it has not been vanquished and it could re-emerge should the opportunity for reassortment arise in the future. Good surveillance must be maintained. In Hong Kong, there are 62 out-patient clinics and over 40 sentinel physicians regularly providing samples from cases of influenza-like illness to the Department of Health. The Departments of Agriculture, Fisheries and Conservation, and Food and Environmental Hygiene as well as The University of Hong Kong monitor poultry and pigs upon entry into Hong Kong, and poultry on farms and in the wholesale and retail poultry markets.

It was during routine sampling in September 2000 that haemagglutination inhibiting activity to the H5 virus was detected in three sets of chicken on a farm in the New Territories. Further studies confirmed the H5 specificity in virus infectivity neutralization tests and N1 specific antibody in neuraminidase inhibition on representative sera (unpublished data). However the virus could not be isolated and subsequent sentinel birds exposed to the flock failed to seroconvert. It is clear that the farm chicken had been exposed to H5N1 virus or antigens but it is not possible to say whether it was similar to the pathogenic H5N1/97 or not. However, exposure in whatever form, is worrying enough. The details of this investigation will be reported elsewhere (Sims *et al.*, in preparation). Failure to isolate the virus may have been due to the fact that about half the chicken had antibody to H9N2 virus raising the possibility that cell mediated immunity arising from shared non-surface antigens [24] modulated the H5N1 infection and reduced virus shedding.

Pandemic preparedness

In the light of the H5N1 incident in Hong Kong in 1997, the isolation of H9N2 viruses from pigs and humans in Hong Kong in 1998 and 1999, respectively, and the additional recognition in 1998 of the involvement of H6N1 virus in the genesis of the highly pathogenic H5N1/97 virus [17], have led to an initial issuance of supplementary diagnostic kits for H5, H9 and H6 subtypes through the Centre for Diseases Control and Prevention, Atlanta, under the auspices of the World Health Organization, Geneva, for evaluation and distribution. Experimental vaccines are under study. This is the first time such a venture in preparedness has been possible. Yet again, each year brings us closer to a pandemic, influenza being such an unpredictable virus; it remains to be seen whether the information currently being accumulated about the H5, H9 and H6 candidate H subtypes will enable us to get ahead of a pandemic caused by any of these H subtypes. The scientific evidence about the possible involvement of the avian H subtypes is accumulating but will it really be enhanced for the common good? In this respect, influenza is more a political problem that might only be dealt with by political means.

What if the H5N1 virus were to re-emerge as a pandemic virus?

Given that current information indicates that the precursor H5N1 virus is found in Southern China, it is essential that surveillance for the highly pathogenic reassortant of it be stepped-up for it there. How it would behave as a pandemic virus can only be a matter of speculation. The high case fatality rate of the H5N1/97 virus poses sobering questions. Given that the UK did not have enough hospital beds to cope with the Sydney variant of H3N2 in 1999 and that there is inadequate vaccine available for the 2000-01 influenza season in the US largely because of problems encountered with the H3N2 Moscow variant, it does raise the question how the industrialized countries, let alone other countries, could cope in the face of a full-blooded H5N1 pandemic. A satisfactory H5N1 vaccine has not yet been prepared three years after the incident, H5 antigens from surrogate viruses possibly offering a way out. While vaccination must be the front-line of defence, antiviral agents may be useful but would sufficient quantities be available and at an affordable price? This raises questions of the usefulness of the antineuraminidase compounds.

Interestingly, amantadine is available over the counter in China and might well find application if, as seems likely, a pandemic H5 virus might arise there. In the Hong Kong SAR, it is available only by prescription. Unfortunately, the circumstances under which it was used in the SAR in the H5N1 incident in 1997 did not allow evaluation of its therapeutic usefulness [2]. Whatever the scenario, good virus surveillance is important to get ahead of the virus. The 1918 and 1968 pandemics were recognized Hong Kong in June [25] and the index H5N1 case occurred in May in 1997. Early summer or summer is a time when surveillance in Hong Kong and China should be keenest. In this sense, Hong Kong is an important sentinel influenza post for the region.

Acknowledgements

Thanks are due to The Wellcome Trust grant 057476/Z/99/Z and the National Institute of Allergy and Infectious Diseases grant AI 95357.

References

1. Shortridge KF, Gao P, Guan Y, Ito T, Kawaoka Y, Markwell DD, Takada A, Webster RG. Interspecies transmission of influenza viruses: H5N1 virus and a Hong Kong SAR perspective. *Vet Microbiol* 2000; 74: 141-7.
2. Yuen KY, Chan PKS, Peiris JSM, Tsang DNC, Que TL, Shortridge KF, Cheung PT, To WK, Ho ETF, Sung R, Cheng AFG and members of the H5N1 Study Group. Clinical features and rapid viral diagnosis of human disease associated with avian influenza A H5N1 virus. *Lancet* 1998; 351: 467-71.
3. Shortridge KF. Poultry and the influenza H5N1 outbreak in Hong Kong, 1997: abridged chronology and virus isolation. *Vaccine* 1999; 17 (Suppl 1): S26-9.
4. Claas ECJ, Osterhaus ADME, van Beek R, De Jong JC, Rimmelzwaan FG, Senne AD, Shortridge KF, Webster RG. Human influenza A (H5N1) virus related to a highly pathogenic avian influenza virus. *Lancet* 1998; 351: 472-7.
5. Shortridge KF, Stuart-Harris CH. An influenza epicentre? *Lancet* 1982; ii: 812-3.
6. Shortridge KF. Pandemic influenza: a zoonosis? *Semin Respir Infect* 1992; 7: 11-25.
7. Kawaoka Y, Webster RG. Evolution of the A/Chicken/Pennsylvania/83 (H5N2) influenza viruses. *Virology* 1985; 146: 130-7.
8. Horimoto T, Rivera E, Pearson J, Senne D, Krauss S, Kawaoka Y, Webster RG. Origin and molecular changes associated with emergence of a highly pathogenic H5N2 influenza virus in Mexico. *Virology* 1995; 213: 223-30.
9. Matrosovich M, Zhou N, Kawaoka Y, Webster RG. The surface glycoproteins of H5 influenza viruses isolated from humans, chickens and wild aquatic birds have distinguishable properties. *J Virol* 1999; 73: 1146-55.
10. To KF, Chan PKS, Chan KF, Lee WK, Lam PWY, Wong KF, Tang NLS, Tsang DNC, Sung R, Buckley T, Tam JS, Cheng AFB, Lee JCK. Pathology of fatal human disease associated with avian influenza A H5N1 virus. *J Med Virol* 2001; 63: 242-6.
11. Scholtissek C. Virus genes involved in host range and pathogenicity. In: *Molecular basis of viral and microbial pathogenesis*, no. 38: Colloquium Mosbach. Berlin, Germany, Springer-Verlag, 1987: 39-50.
12. Guo YJ, Krauss S, Senne DA, Mo IP, Lo KS, Xiong XP, Norwood M, Shortridge KF, Webster RG, Guan Y. Characterization of the pathogenicity of members of the newly established H9N2 influenza virus lineages in Asia. *Virology* 2000; 267: 279-88.
13. Naffakh N, Massin P, Van Der Werf S. Internal genes as determinants of interspecies transmission and host specificity of influenza A viruses. In: Dodet B, Vicari M, eds. Emergence and control of zoonotic ortho- and paramyxovirus diseases. Paris: John Libbey Eurotext, 2001: 79-89.
14. Reid AH, Fanning TG, Hultin JV, Taubenberger JK. Origin and evolution of the 1918 "Spanish" influenza hemagglutinin gene. *Proc Natl Acad Sci USA* 1999; 96: 1615-56.
15. Shortridge KF. The 1918 "Spanish" flu: pearls from swine? *Nature Med* 1999; 5: 384-5.
16. Guan Y, Shortridge KF, Krauss S, Webster RG. Molecular characterization of H9N2 influenza viruses: were they the donors of the "internal" genes of H5N1 viruses in Hong Kong? *Proc Natl Acad Sci USA* 1999; 96: 9363-7.

17. Hoffmann E, Stech J, Chin PS, Leneva I, Krauss S, Scholtissek C, Peiris M, Shortridge KF, Webster RG. Characterization of the influenza A virus gene pool in avian species in southern China: was H6N1 a derivative or precursor of H5N1? *J Virol* 2000; 74: 6309-15.
18. Xu X, Subbarao K, Cox NJ, Guo Y. Genetic characterization of the pathogenic influenza A/Goose/ Guangdong/1/96 (H5N1) virus: similarity of its hemagglutinin gene to those of H5N1 viruses from the 1997 outbreaks in Hong Kong. *Virology* 1999; 261: 15-9.
19. Mo IP, Song CS, Kim KS, Rhee JC. An occurrence of non-highly pathogenic avian influenza in Korea. In: Swayne D, Slemons R, eds. *Proc 4th Intl Symp Avian Influenza.* United States Animal Health Association, Rose Printing Company, Tallahassee, FL, 1997: 379-83.
20. Shortridge KF. The next pandemic influenza virus? *Lancet* 1995; 346: 1210-2.
21. Alexander DJ. Ecology of avian influenza in domestic birds. In: Dodet B, Vicari M, eds. *Emergence and control of zoonotic ortho- and paramyxovirus diseases.* Paris : John Libbey Eurotext, 2001: 25-33.
22. Peiris M, Yuen KY, Leung CW, Chan KH, Ip PL, Lai WM, Orr WK, Shortridge KF. Human infection with influenza H9N2. *Lancet* 1999; 354: 916-7.
23. Lin YP, Shaw M, Gregory V, Cameron K, Lim W, Klimov A, Subbarao K, Guan Y, Krauss S, Shortridge KF, Webster RG, Cox N, Hay A. Avian-to-human transmission of H9N2 subtype influenza A viruses: relationship between H9N2 and H5N1 human isolates. *Proc Natl Acad Sci USA* 2000; 97: 9654-8.
24. O'Neil E, Krauss S, Riberdy JM, Webster RG. *Heterosubtypic immunity against H5N1 influenza A virus infection. Options for the Control of Influenza IV.* September 2000. Hersonissos, Crete, Greece, 2001: 104 and 106.
25. Shortridge KF. Pandemic influenza; application of epidemiology and ecology in the region of southern China to prospective studies. In: Laver WG, ed. *The Origin of Pandemic Influenza Viruses.* New York: Elsevier Science Publishing Co., Inc. 1983: 191-200.

Emergence and Control of Zoonotic Ortho- and Paramyxovirus Diseases
B. Dodet, M. Vicari, eds.

The significance of antigenic evolution for swine influenza vaccine efficacy: learning from vaccination-challenge studies in pigs

Kristien Van Reeth, Sophie De Clercq, Maurice Pensaert
Laboratory of Virology, Faculty of Veterinary Medicine, Ghent University, Merelbeke, Belgium

Abstract – The current swine influenza vaccines for use in Europe are inactivated bivalent vaccines containing A/Port Chalmers/1/73 (H3N2) and either A/New Jersey/8/76 or Sw/Netherlands/80 (H1N1), and an oil adjuvant. To examine whether antigenic drift within H1N1 or H3N2 subtypes may require substitution of these strains with more recent strains, we have performed vaccination-challenge studies in pigs. Pigs were vaccinated twice intramuscularly with a 4 week interval. Two or three weeks after the second vaccination, they were challenged intratracheally with H1N1 or H3N2 swine influenza viruses isolated in 98. Pre-challenge haemagglutination inhibition (HI) antibody titres against the challenge virus, and clinical signs and lung virus titres after challenge were examined. In a first series of studies, pigs were vaccinated with experimental monovalent vaccines based on New Jersey, Port Chalmers or recent swine influenza virus strains. In a second series of studies, a commercial swine influenza vaccine containing New Jersey and Port Chalmers strains was used. Antibody titres against the H1N1 challenge virus were at least 5-fold lower for the experimental New Jersey-based vaccine than for vaccines based on more recent strains, and virological protection was significantly better for the latter vaccines. However, the New Jersey-derived commercial vaccine induced a more than 10-fold higher serological response against the challenge virus than the experimental vaccine, and an outstanding virological protection. Similarly, complete protection against the H3N2 challenge virus was obtained in all vaccinates with HI antibody titres ≥ 160-320 against this virus, irrespective of the vaccine strain. Furthermore, all vaccinates in this study were protected from disease. In conclusion, there is insufficient argument to replace the current New Jersey (H1N1) and Port Chalmers (H3N2) swine influenza vaccine strains. The different potencies of experimental and commercial New Jersey-derived vaccines in this study suggest that the antigenic dose and adjuvant may be of critical importance.

The swine influenza situation in Europe

The epidemiology of swine influenza in Europe is complex, and three different swine influenza virus subtypes are currently circulating. The major subtypes, H1N1 and H3N2, have been enzootic in a number of European countries for at least 20 years. Most H1N1 viruses closely resemble H1N1 viruses from wild waterfowl, and they appear to have spread from birds into the pig population in 1979 when continental Europe was hit by a series of swine flu epizootics [1, 2]. These "avian-like" H1N1 viruses differ antigenically from "classical" swine H1N1 viruses [1, 3], which are the primary strains in the USA and in Asia. The H3N2 virus originates from variants of the human influenza virus that caused the "Hong Kong flu" pandemic in 1968 [4]. These "human-like" H3N2 viruses have established a stable lineage in swine populations in Europe and Asia and continue to circulate long after their disappearance from the human population. Genetic analyses of swine H3N2 viruses isolated in Italy between 1985 and 1989 have provided evidence of reassortment between the surface glycoprotein genes from human-like H3N2 viruses and the internal protein genes from avian-like H1N1 viruses [5]. In areas of high pig density, H1N1 and H3N2 viruses are implicated in up to 50% of acute respiratory disease outbreaks [6]. The third and most recent virus subtype, H1N2, appears to be a double reassortant with the haemagglutinin (HA) of a human H1N1 virus from the early 1980's and the neuraminidase (NA) of a swine H3N2 virus [7]. H1N2 has been associated increasingly with swine flu outbreaks throughout Great Britain since 1994 [8] and it was recently diagnosed in a few outbreaks on the European mainland.

Swine influenza vaccines became commercially available in some European countries in the mid 1980's. These vaccines are inactivated whole virus or split virus preparations for intramuscular administration. They contain one representative of the H1N1 and H3N2 subtype in combination with an oil adjuvant. Unlike influenza vaccines for humans, swine flu vaccines have never been updated. Indeed, all vaccines include A/Port Chalmers/1/73 (H3N2) and either A/New Jersey/8/76 (H1N1) or Sw/Netherlands/25/80 (H1N1). The Port Chalmers strain is representative of the human H3N2 virus that crossed the species barrier into pigs in Asia in the early 1970's. The New Jersey strain was isolated from recruits at Fort Dix, New Jersey, in 1976 and probably had been transferred from pigs to humans [9]. This strain resembles classical swine H1N1 viruses more closely than avian-like H1N1 viruses. Both A/Port Chalmers/1/73 and A/New Jersey/8/76 protected sufficiently against swine influenza viruses circulating in the mid 1980's [10, 11]. More than 15 years later, however, there is uncertainty as to whether these vaccines provide comprehensive protection against the current field viruses. On the one hand, antigenic drift in pigs is relatively minor when compared to that in humans. On the other hand, some degree of antigenic variation has been reported, and it was recently suggested that drift of the H3N2 subtype necessitates vaccine strain updating [12].

Vaccination-challenge studies in pigs

For swine influenza vaccines in particular, it is difficult to recommend vaccine strains based on the results of antigenic analysis alone. Unlike for human viruses, there is only limited surveillance of swine influenza viruses. Furthermore, the available antigenic data are difficult to interpret, because there is no standardization of the reagents and methods used in different laboratories. Most important, the significance of observed antigenic differences for vaccine efficacy is uncertain. Therefore, *in vivo* vaccination-challenge studies in pigs are most reliable to evaluate vaccine strain performance. A challenge method for swine influenza vaccine efficacy studies was developed at the Laboratory of Virology, Ghent University, some 15 years ago [10]. In this type of challenge study, pigs are inoculated intratracheally with as much as $10^{7.5}$ EID50 virus, so as to obtain reproducible lower respiratory tract illness and massive virus replication in the lungs. Within 24 hours after such a severe challenge, unvaccinated control pigs develop clinical signs typical of influenza such as fever, anorexia, depression, tachypnoea, dyspnoea and abdominal breathing. Also, virus titres in their lungs reach up to $10^{7.0-9.0}$ EID_{50}/g lung. In vaccinated pigs, the reduction of clinical signs and of virus titres are indicative of vaccine efficacy. Using this model, two administrations of a commercial vaccine containing A/New Jersey/8/76 (H1N1) and A/Port Chalmers/1/73 (H3N2) were shown to provide complete virological and clinical protection against challenge with swine influenza viruses from the mid 1980's [10, 11]. A single vaccination conferred only partial virological protection, but was still sufficient to prevent disease. This same intratracheal challenge model was used here to answer questions about the protective efficacy of swine influenza vaccines against more recent virus strains. In all experiments below, pigs were vaccinated twice at the age of 4 and 8 weeks, challenged 2 or 3 weeks after the second vaccination, and euthanatized 24 or 72 hours after the challenge. The serum haemagglutination inhibiting (HI) antibody profile before challenge, virus titres in the lungs and clinical signs after challenge were used to evaluate vaccine efficacy.

The effects of antigenic variation on vaccine efficacy

To examine whether antigenic drift between vaccine and circulating strains may compromise swine influenza vaccine efficacy, we prepared experimental monovalent vaccines based on older or more recent virus strains. Vaccines were prepared from egg allantoic fluid, inactivated with beta-propiolactone and diluted in phosphate-buffered saline to give 320 haemagglutinating units (HAU) per vaccine dose. Immediately before use, an oil-in-water adjuvant with vitamin E (Microsol Diluvac Forte®, Intervet NV) was mixed with the vaccines.

In a first experiment, vaccines based on three different H1N1 strains - the current A/New Jersey/8/76 vaccine strain, and the avian-like Sw/Belgium/1/83 and Sw/Belgium/1/98 viruses - were compared for their efficacy against Sw/Belgium/1/98 (H1N1) challenge. This experiment has been described in detail elsewhere [13]. After two vaccinations, mean serum HI antibody titres against the homologous vaccine virus were similar for the three vaccines. Antibody titres against the challenge virus were significantly lower for the New Jersey/76 vaccine group (mean HI titre 16) than for the Belgium/83 (mean HI titre 91) or Belgium/98 (mean HI titre 197) groups. Both of the most recent strains induced a significantly better virological protection. Only 2 of 8 New Jersey-vaccinated pigs were completely protected against virus replication, compared to 6 and 7 out of 8 pigs in the Belgium/83 and Belgium/98 groups respectively. Clinical signs after challenge were negligible in all vaccinates. Thus, in this experiment, protection against H1N1 swine influenza virus infection was directly correlated to the antigenic relatedness of the vaccine strain to the challenge strain.

Two preliminary experiments were designed to compare H3N2 strains for their protection against Sw/Flanders/1/98 (H3N2) challenge. The vaccines used were derived from the current vaccine strain A/Port Chalmers/1/73, or from Sw/Gent/1/84 or Sw/Flanders/1/98 viruses. As shown in *Table I*, the serological response to vaccination and protection against challenge were dependent on the vaccine dose. In the first experiment, primary and booster vaccinations were performed with 320 HAU of each vaccine.

Table I. Serological profile and protection against Sw/Flanders/1/98 (H3N2) infection after 2 vaccinations of pigs with different experimental H3N2 vaccines.

			Vaccine dose (HAU)		Mean HI antibody titre against			No. of pigs/total with virus in lungs	
Experiment	**Vaccine**	*n*	1st vacc.	2nd vacc.	A/PC 1/73	Sw/G 1/84	Sw/Fl 1/98	24h PC	72h PC
1	A/ P Chalmers/1/73	4	320	320	2153	538	640	0/2	0/2
	Sw/Gent/1/84	4	320	320	226	380	260	1/2	0/2
	Sw/Flanders/1/98	4	320	320	40	80	269	2/2	0/2
	None	4	–	–	< 20	< 20	< 20	2/2	2/2
2	A/P Chalmers/1/73	4	320	254	905	160	160	1/2	1/2
	Sw/Gent/1/84	4	320	640	160	190	226	1/2	1/2
	Sw/Flanders/1/98	4	320	1280	113	226	761	0/2	0/2
	None	4	–	–	< 20	< 20	< 20	2/2	2/2

HAU: haemagglutinating units; h PC: hours post challenge; –: not applicable.

The mean homologous antibody titre was several times higher with the A/Port Chalmers/1/73 (mean HI titre 2153) vaccine than with Sw/Gent/1/84 (mean HI titre 380) or Sw/Flanders/1/98 (mean HI titre 269) vaccines. The mean HI antibody titre against the challenge virus was 640 in the Port Chalmers/73 group, but only 260 and 269 in the Gent/84 and Flanders/98 groups respectively. Moreover, the Port Chalmers vaccine protected better against Sw/Flanders/1/98 challenge than the Sw/Gent/1/84 or homologous vaccines.

In the second experiment, we tried to obtain comparable homologous antibody titres for the different vaccines. To this purpose, booster vaccinations were performed with only 254 HAU of the A/Port Chalmers/1/73 vaccine, compared to 640 and 1280 HAU of the Sw/Gent/1/84 and Sw/Flanders/1/98 vaccines respectively. Homologous antibody titres were still highest in the Port Chalmers group, but the differences between the groups were smaller than in the first experiment. This time, challenge virus antibody titres were lower in the Port Chalmers/73 (mean HI titre 160) and in the Gent/84 groups (mean HI titre 226) than in the Flanders/98 group (mean HI titre 761). Consequently, the A/Port Chalmers/1/73 and Sw/Gent/1/84 vaccination provided poorer protection than the Sw/Flanders/1/98 vaccination. All pigs in both experiments were protected from clinical disease. Despite the discordance between experiments 1 and 2, both experiments revealed an identical correlation between challenge virus antibody titres and virological protection. All vaccinates with HI antibody titres ≥ 160-320 against Sw/Flanders/1/98 showed complete protection against challenge *(Figure 1)*. Unfortunately, these H3N2 experiments failed to compare the protective efficacy of the virus strains as such. It remains unknown why the Port Chalmers strain induced higher antibody titres than the other strains. We wonder whether Port Chalmers is just more immunogenic. Another possibility is that the Port Chalmers vaccine was administered at relatively higher doses than both other vaccines in experiment 1. The haemagglutination assay is not the most reliable method to standardize the HA content in influenza vaccines, but there are few alternatives for swine influenza viruses. It would be most useful to develop assays to measure vaccine potency in micrograms of haemagglutinin. Such assays are needed for an objective comparison of vaccine strains and to establish the relationship between HA content and protective levels of immunity.

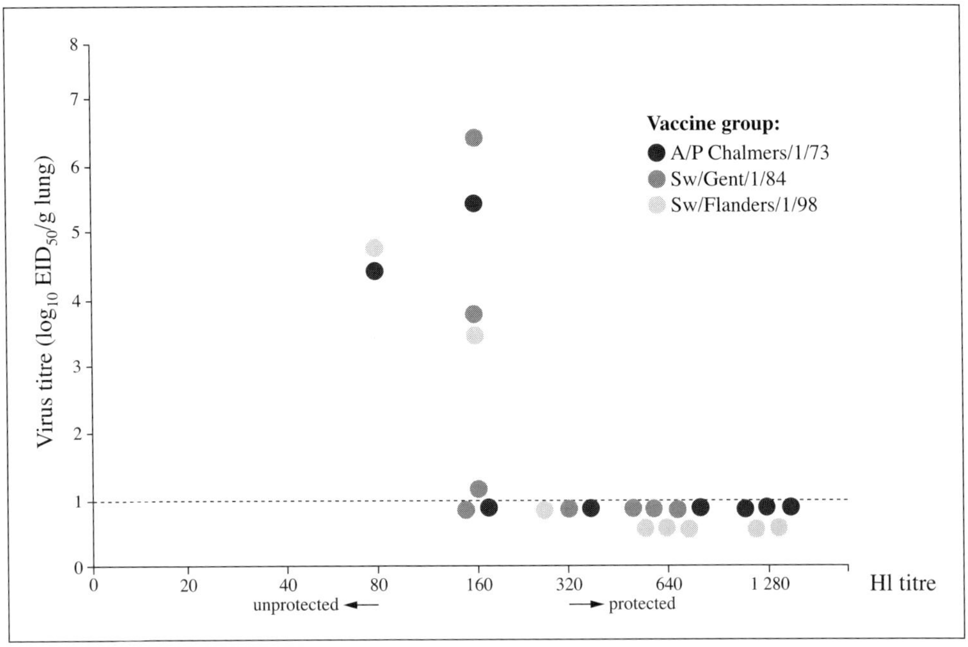

Figure 1. Correlation between serum HI antibody titres against the Sw/Flanders/1/98 (H3N2) challenge strain and protection against infection in pigs vaccinated with different experimental H3N2 vaccines. Each dot represents the results of an individual pig.

Efficacy of the current commercial swine influenza vaccines

The experimental vaccines used in our studies differ in several respects from the existing commercial vaccines. To examine whether these commercial vaccines need to be updated, pigs vaccinated with such a vaccine were challenged with the Sw/Belgium/1/98 (H1N1) or Sw/Flanders/1/98 (H3N2) viruses. The commercial vaccine was a bivalent split-virus product containing A/New Jersey/8/76 (H1N1) and A/Port Chalmers/1/73 (H3N2) in an oil-in-water adjuvant (Gripovac®, Merial SA, Lyon, France). The manufacturer uses a serological method to determine the minimal antigenic content. Each vaccine dose contains at least 1.7 HI units (HIU) of the New Jersey strain and 2.2 HIU of the Port Chalmers strain. One HIU is the amount needed to obtain an HI antibody titre of 1 log_{10} after two vaccinations of pigs.

Remarkably, the commercial New Jersey-derived vaccine protected far better against Sw/Belgium/1/98 (H1N1) challenge than the experimental New Jersey vaccine used in the previous experiments. The mean challenge virus antibody titre after 2 vaccinations was 197. Also, six of eight vaccinated pigs showed complete virological protection.

In an H3N2 challenge experiment, the mean antibody titre against Sw/Flanders/1/98 (H3N2) was 174. Six out of eight individual pigs had HI titres $\geq$ 160, and four of these pigs were fully protected against Sw/Flanders/1/98 infection *(Figure 2)*.

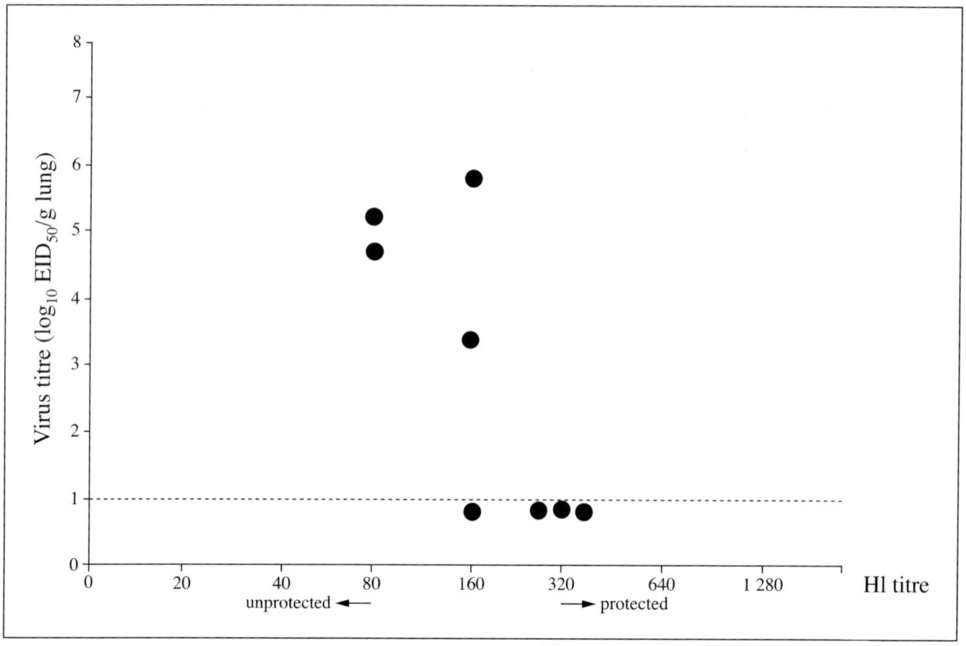

Figure 2. Correlation between serum HI antibody titres against the Sw/Flanders/1/98 (H3N2) challenge strain and protection against infection in pigs vaccinated with a commercial vaccine. Each dot represents the results of an individual pig.

Thus, most vaccinated pigs were fully protected against a severe challenge with a current H1N1 or H3N2 swine influenza virus. In addition, all vaccinates remained clinically healthy.

Final comments

Antigenic differences between vaccine and challenge strain can have a significant impact on swine influenza vaccine efficacy. The experimental A/New Jersey/8/76 vaccine, for example, protected less efficiently against challenge with Sw/Belgium/1/98 (H1N1) virus than the homologous or an avian-like swine H1N1 virus. Paradoxically, an antigenically distant strain can afford a very solid protection if antibody titres against the challenge virus are at sufficient levels. As an illustration, the New Jersey-derived commercial vaccine elicited a more than 10-fold higher serological response against Sw/Belgium/1/98 than the experimental vaccine, and an outstanding virological protection. Similarly, complete protection against Sw/Flanders/1/98 (H3N2) challenge was obtained in all vaccinates with HI antibody titres ≥ 160-320 against this virus, irrespective of the vaccine strain. Thus, like in humans and horses [14], there appears to be a tight correlation between serum antibody levels and protection against a given swine influenza virus. We will try to further establish this relationship, because postvaccination antibody levels to the current field viruses may predict susceptibility very accurately.

Factors other than the suitability of the vaccinal strain may also play important roles in swine influenza vaccine efficacy. The vaccine dose, for example, can have a tremendous impact on vaccine potency, as seen in the studies with experimental H3N2 vaccines. Differences in the antigenic dose may also explain the different potencies of commercial and experimental New Jersey vaccines. The lack of rigid techniques to measure HA content is an important problem with swine influenza vaccines. Another factor which has been shown to play a crucial role in protection against heterologous challenge is the adjuvant [15, 16]. Differences in the adjuvant formulation of commercial and experimental New Jersey vaccines may also contribute to their different potencies. It is noteworthy that human influenza vaccines generally do not contain an adjuvant, while most equine influenza vaccines have aluminium hydroxide, carbomer or ISCOM adjuvants. Because all the available swine influenza vaccines contain highly immunogenic oil adjuvants, criteria for the replacement of swine influenza vaccine strains should differ from those for human or equine strains.

Overall, there is insufficient argument at present to replace the current H1N1 and H3N2 swine influenza vaccine strains. We feel, however, that addition of an H1N2 component may be required. The H1N2 subtype is similarly pathogenic as H1N1 and H3N2 subtypes and appears to have become increasingly widespread on the European continent [17, 18]. There is no cross-protection between HI antibodies to H1N2 and H1N1 or H3N2. Interestingly, pigs immune against infection with H1N1 or H3N2 were still susceptible to H1N2 challenge [19]. Therefore, it is unlikely that the current swine influenza vaccines will protect against H1N2 and this issue is currently under study.

Acknowledgements

This work was financially supported by the Belgian Ministry of Agriculture and by the Fund for Scientific Research – Flanders (fellowships of Kristien Van Reeth and Sophie De Clercq). The authors thank Lieve Sys and Fernand De Backer for excellent technical assistance, Merial Inc. for providing vaccine and Intervet Inc. for help with preparation of the experimental vaccines.

References

1. Pensaert M, Ottis K, Vandeputte J, Kaplan MM, Bachmann PA. Evidence for the natural transmission of influenza A virus from wild ducks to swine and its potential importance for man. *Bull WHO* 1981; 59: 75-8.
2. Scholtissek C, Burger H, Bachmann PA, Hannoun C. Genetic relatedness of hemagglutinins of the H1 subtype of influenza A viruses isolated from swine and birds. *Virology* 1983; 129: 521-3.
3. Brown IH, Ludwig S, Olsen CW, *et al.* Antigenic and genetic analyses of H1N1 influenza A viruses from European pigs. *J Gen Virol* 1997; 78: 553-62.
4. Haesebrouck F, Biront P, Pensaert MB, Leunen J. Epizootics of respiratory tract disease in swine in Belgium due to H3N2 influenza virus and experimental reproduction of disease. *Am J Vet Res* 1985; 46: 1926-8.
5. Castrucci MR, Donatelli I, Sidoli L, Barigazzi G, Kawaoka Y, Webster RG. Genetic reassortment between avian and human influenza A viruses in Italian pigs. *Virology* 1993; 193: 503-6.
6. Loeffen WLA, Kamp EM, Stockhofe-Zurwieden, *et al.* Survey of infectious disease agents involved in acute respiratory disease in finishing pigs. *Vet Rec* 1999; 145: 175-80.

7. Brown IH, Harris PA, McCauley JM, Alexander DJ. Multiple genetic reassortment of avian and human influenza A viruses in European pigs, resulting in the emergence of an H1N2 virus of novel genotype. *J Gen Virol* 1998; 79: 2947-55.
8. Brown IH, Chakraverty P, Harris PA, Alexander DJ. Disease outbreaks in pigs in Great Britain due to an influenza A virus of H1N2 subtype. *Vet Rec* 1995; 136: 328-9.
9. Hodder RA, Gaydos JC, Allen RG, Top Jr FH, Nowosiwsky T, Russel PK. Swine influenza A at Fort-Dix New Jersey January-February 1976. Extent of spread and duration of outbreak. *J Infect Dis* 1977; 136: S369-S75.
10. Haesebrouck F, Pensaert M. Effect of intratracheal challenge of fattening pigs previously immunized with an inactivated influenza H1N1 vaccine. *Vet Microbiol* 1986; 11: 239-49.
11. Vandeputte J, Brun A, Duret C, Haesebrouck F, Devaux B. Vaccination of swine against H3N2 influenza using a Port Chalmers/1/73 vaccine. *Proc Int Pig Vet Soc*, Barcelona, Spain, 1986, p. 219.
12. De Jong JC, van Nieuwstadt AP, Kimman TG, *et al.* Antigenic drift in swine influenza H3 haemagglutinins with implications for vaccination policy. *Vaccine* 1999; 17: 1321-8.
13. Van Reeth K, Labarque G, De Clercq S, Pensaert M. Efficacy of vaccination of pigs with different H1N1 swine influenza viruses using a recent challenge strain and different parameters of protection. *Vaccine* 2001; 19: 4479-86.
14. Mumford JA, Chambers TM. Equine influenza. In: Nicholson KG, Webster RG, Hay AJ, eds. *Textbook of influenza.* Oxford: Blackwell Science, 1998: 146-62.
15. Webster RG, Thomas TL. Efficacy of equine influenza vaccines for protection against A/Equine/Jilin/89 (H3N8) – a new equine influenza virus. *Vaccine* 1993; 11: 987-93.
16. Mumford JA, Jesset DM, Rollinson EA, Hannant D, Draper MA. Duration of protective efficacy of equine influenza immunostimulating complex/tetanus vaccines. *Vet Rec* 1994; 143: 158-62.
17. Marozin S, Gregory V, Cameron K, *et al.* Antigenic and genetic diversity among swine influenza viruses in Europe. Abstracts Options for the Control of Influenza IV, Hersonissos, Crete, 2000: 70.
18. Van Reeth K, Brown IH, Pensaert M. Isolations of H1N2 influenza A virus from pigs in Belgium. *Vet Rec* 2000; 146: 588-9.
19. Van Reeth K, De Clercq S, Pensaert M. Lack of cross-protection between European H1N1 and H1N2 swine influenza viruses. In: Osterhaus A, *et al.*, eds. *Options for the Control of Influenza IV.* New York: Elsevier, 2001, in press.

Emergence and Control of Zoonotic Ortho- and Paramyxovirus Diseases
B. Dodet, M. Vicari, eds.

Equine influenza: epidemiology, surveillance and vaccine performance

Jenny A. Mumford
Animal Health Trust, Lanwades Park, Newmarket, Suffolk, UK

The ever increasing international movement of equidae for competition and breeding purposes presents a complex challenge for control of equine influenza. Explosive epizootics have been described during the last 20 years which have been attributed to the introduction of infected animals into susceptible indigenous populations [1]. In the last 10 years, all such outbreaks described have been caused by the A/equine-2 (H3N8) subtype of equine influenza and there is a clear need to develop control measures for this infection on a global basis. Successful measures require knowledge of the epidemiology of the disease, rapid diagnostic techniques and effective vaccines of adequate potency.

Although inactivated vaccines against equine influenza have been available since the 1960's [2], there has been little effort to develop international standardisation of their potency and efficacy. Nevertheless, the value of vaccination is recognised in many countries and is mandatory among some groups of horses such as the European thoroughbred racing population and non thoroughbreds competing under Federation Equestre Internationale rules. The effectiveness of such policies is undermined by the poor efficacy of some products which result in vaccinated animals shedding virus, often in the absence of clinical signs. Thus, when horses travel on temporary import permits, which are based on a system of health certification and a compulsory vaccination scheme agreed between importing and exporting countries, the risk of transmission cannot be eliminated. Recognising the short-lived immunity provided by some vaccines, the Code Commission of the Office International des Epizooties (OIE) recommends that importing countries which are free of influenza should require that all horses travelling from endemic areas are fully vaccinated and should have received their last booster dose within the 2-8 weeks prior to travel.

In spite of these efforts, outbreaks associated with infected imported animals still occur and a number of reasons have been proposed for the failure of vaccines to eliminate viral shedding. While it is recognised that products vary in their potency and inadequate antigenic content is likely to be the major factor, responses to vaccination can also be highly variable between individuals. Poor responders to vaccination are likely to be high risk animals in terms of virus shedding. Of much wider concern is the accumulating evidence that out of date strains in vaccines are likely to result in ineffective control of virus excretion [1]. Since there has been no formal procedure for updating vaccine viruses, many products remain with outdated viruses which are unlikely to eliminate virus shedding.

In recent years a number of steps have been taken to improve our ability to control equine influenza on an international level which include improved surveillance of equine influenza in the field [3], development of rapid diagnostic techniques [4], development of methods to standardise the potency of influenza vaccines [5] and the introduction of a vaccine strain selection system under the auspices of OIE [6].

This scientific progress has been applied and implemented at a practical level in Europe through the development of a fast-track licensing system for vaccines containing updated strains [7], and the adoption of more rigorous potency standards among licensing authorities [8]. The development of regulations relating to movement of animals which utilise improved diagnostic techniques and adoption of vaccination policies which recognise the limitations of current products [9] has also contributed to improved control.

Epidemiology

During the last 10 years, repeated influenza outbreaks in Europe and the Americas have been reported to the International Thoroughbred Breeders International Collating Centre on an annual basis with some countries such as Sweden, being particularly badly affected [10, 11]. During this period there have also been some serious outbreaks associated with the importation of infected animals [1]. In 1992, influenza A/equine-2 was imported into Hong Kong from the United Kingdom and the outbreak which subsequently occurred in the vaccinated population in Hong Kong seriously disrupted racing and affected the majority of horses in Hong Kong [12]. In 1995, an outbreak occurred in Dubai as a result of the importation of polo ponies from America. While this outbreak was restricted to immediate in-contacts, it nevertheless presented a risk to international thoroughbred racing which was in progress in the Emirates at that time [13]. Outbreaks have also occurred in Puerto Rico, in the Caribbean in 1997 (Chambers, personal communication) and in the Philippines in 1997 as a result of the importation of horses from America.

Since economic and competitive issues dictate that it is desirable for horses to move through lengthy quarantine procedures with the minimum of disruption to their training programmes, there is a reliance on surveillance of influenza in the population from which animals are leaving and on the effectiveness of vaccines to prevent viral shedding. When disease screening is ineffective, subclinically infected horses shedding virus are transported, and the short quarantine periods often in place fail to prevent introduction of infection [12, 13].

Diagnosis

Our ability to diagnose influenza infections in a field situation has been substantially improved with the advent of ELISAs capable of detecting viral antigen (nucleoprotein) directly in nasopharyngeal secretions [4, 13, 14]. This test can provide a same day diagnosis if influenza is suspected. It is particularly valuable in differentiating influenza from other respiratory pathogens when classical signs of influenza such as coughing and pyrexia are absent in vaccinated animals [15].

A more challenging objective is to maintain an awareness of influenza activity in vaccinated populations in which few clinical signs are evident, or in circumstances where nasopharyngeal swabs cannot be taken or processed easily. In heavily vaccinated populations mild infections may fail to stimulate significant serological responses to the haemagglutinin (HA). The introduction of a serological test able to differentiate antibody responses to infection and vaccination with inactivated whole virus vaccines [16] has improved surveillance. This ELISA test is based on the detection of antibody to a non-structural protein (NS1) which is produced during infection but is not incorporated into inactivated whole virus vaccines. The test is useful for both confirmation of infection in vaccinated animals which have been sampled after the acute period of disease, or in animals vaccinated in the face of infection [17].

Used together, these tests provide valuable information about the risks associated with horses travelling from particular populations and provide a means by which animals can be rapidly screened for viral shedding whilst still in quarantine at their destination before being released into potentially susceptible local populations.

Vaccines

Variable potency of vaccines

Most current equine influenza vaccines contain inactivated whole virus with and without adjuvants including oil, alhydrogel, carbomer, and subunit vaccines such as ISCOMs or micelles combined with Quil A. More recently a cold adapted virus vaccine has been launched in North America [18, 19]. Historically antigenic content in inactivated vaccines has been measured in terms of chick cell agglutinating (CCA) units of HA and potency in terms of haemagglutinin inhibition (HI) antibody responses induced in guinea pigs and horses. However some manufacturers have now adopted the Single Radial Diffusion (SRD) test for in process testing of antigenic content [20].

An international collaborative study to examine the reproducibility of the HI test between laboratories revealed that differences in titre between laboratories could be as much as 1,000 fold. This has highlighted the need to establish international reference preparations to standardise serological tests for potency evaluation of final products. The historical lack of standardisation of vaccines from different sources and the undemanding standards of some licensing authorities has resulted in the use of products with variable potency in terms of their ability to stimulate antibody to the HA. In studies in which antibody responses to 5 European vaccines available in the early 1990's were evaluated following three doses, the peak levels and duration of antibody were shown to vary widely [17]. Only two vaccines induced protective levels of SRH antibody (150 mm^2) after the second dose, and three products did so following the third dose only. Given that SRH antibody is closely correlated with protection against infection both in experimental [21] and field studies [15], this data indicated that many vaccinated horses would have had insufficient antibody to prevent infection and virus shedding. Increased efforts by manufacturers in recent years has resulted in European products of greater potency which maintain clinically protective levels of antibody for up to one year following the third vaccination [22].

Serological studies in North America have revealed that several American vaccines fail to stimulate protective levels of antibody even in previously vaccinated animals [23] and that in immunologically naïve animals 3 to 4 doses were required to stimulate detectable SRH antibody and in some instances the levels achieved were not protective even after 4 doses [24].

This data indicates there is an urgent need to harmonise standards for inactivated equine influenza vaccines through provision of reagents to standardise measurement of antigenic content and serological responses used in potency testing. More extensive use of challenge studies would also assist in the evaluation of vaccine efficacy particularly for live vaccines. In recent studies the level of protection provided by a single dose of live cold adapted vaccine has been demonstrated at one, six and twelve months post-vaccination using challenge infections. From these studies it was demonstrated that, although significant protection could be achieved six months after a single dose, immunity was not reliant on the presence of circulating SRH antibody.

Poor responders

In a series of trials undertaken to examine the serological responses to influenza vaccines in ponies, it has been observed that peak antibody levels induced in individual animals can be highly variable and that some individuals respond poorly [17]. The number of poor responders appears to relate to the type and potency of vaccine (whole virus or subunit) and the adjuvant used, with poor responders being more common, among animals receiving subunit vaccines. Field studies have also shown that poor responders to vaccination occur among thoroughbred horses and in the 1989 epidemic of influenza in the UK, it was noted that poor responders which had antibody levels of less than 50 mm^2 were 15 times more likely to be the index case of influenza within premises than horses with antibody levels greater than 50 mm^2 [25].

Vaccine strains

Antigenic drift over time

Vaccines developed in the 1960's contained the prototype strains A/equine/1/Prague/56 (H7N7) or A/equine/2/Miami/63 (H3N8) or similar viruses isolated at those times. In the early years there was little information about antigenic variation among isolates or how closely strains selected for vaccines reflected the most prevalent viruses circulating in the population. Subsequently it was shown that significant antigenic differences existed among isolates from 1963 [26-29], highlighting the importance of having a co-ordinated surveillance programme capable of monitoring antigenic drift and providing the information from which to select the vaccine viruses most appropriate for control of the prevalent viruses circulating. However, there has been no regular and formal review of vaccine strains and their relevance to viruses causing field outbreaks, thus the same vaccine strains were used over a 20-30 year period. In response to ad hoc studies on genetic and antigenic drift in A/equine 1 and A/equine 2 isolates [28-30], some vaccines were updated to include more recent isolates of A/equine 2 such as Fontainebleau/79, Brentwood/79 and Kentucky/81.

The first compelling field evidence for the importance of antigenic drift for vaccine efficacy was collected during the 1989 epidemic of influenza in the UK [31]. Firstly, the disease was initially identified in annually vaccinated horses with high levels of vaccine-induced antibody at the time of exposure. In spite of this programme of vaccination, they succumbed to infection and disease. The infection spread rapidly in the vaccinated population; however, severe clinical signs of classical influenza were only seen in unvaccinated animals. When antibody levels in horses affected by influenza during the outbreak were examined, it was found that although a correlation between antibody level and severity of disease could be identified, as has been shown from data collected under experimental conditions, only horses with very high levels of antibody, *i.e.* greater than 190 mm^2, were protected against infection [25]. This represented only 12% of animals which had received vaccine in the previous 3 months. These observations suggested that vaccine induced SRH antibody raised against viruses from 1963 or the 1979-1981 period, although cross-reacting in SRH and to a lesser extent HI tests, was ineffective in suppressing replication of the recent 1989 virus probably as a result of antigenic drift.

This hypothesis was subsequently confirmed experimentally [17]. Although vaccines containing outdated strains provided clinical protection, vaccine efficacy in terms of ability to eliminate virus excretion was directly correlated with the degree of antigenic relatedness between vaccine and challenge strain This study provided valuable evidence that regular updating of vaccine strains with viruses representative of those predominantly circulating in the field was important for vaccine efficacy over time.

Geographical diversity

An increased effort in surveillance and virus characterisation since 1989 has also revealed that A/equine 2 viruses which had previously been described as evolving as a single lineage [29], appeared to diverge into two families. Daly *et al.* [32] compared the HA sequences of A/equine 2 strains isolated between 1963 and 1994 and noted that from about 1987 viruses evolved as two lines, one family of strains isolated from horses in Europe, China and Mongolia (the Eurasian family) and the other strains isolated in the USA and Argentina (the American family). This phylogenetic tree has subsequently been extended to include viruses isolated as recently as 2000 *(Figure 1)*.

Although the geographical clustering of these two families was initially strong, one isolate from Canada Saskatoon/90 [33] belongs to the Eurasian family, identified in 1996, and a series of viruses isolated from European horses have been identified as American-like viruses. These include viruses from the UK (Newmarket/1/93,

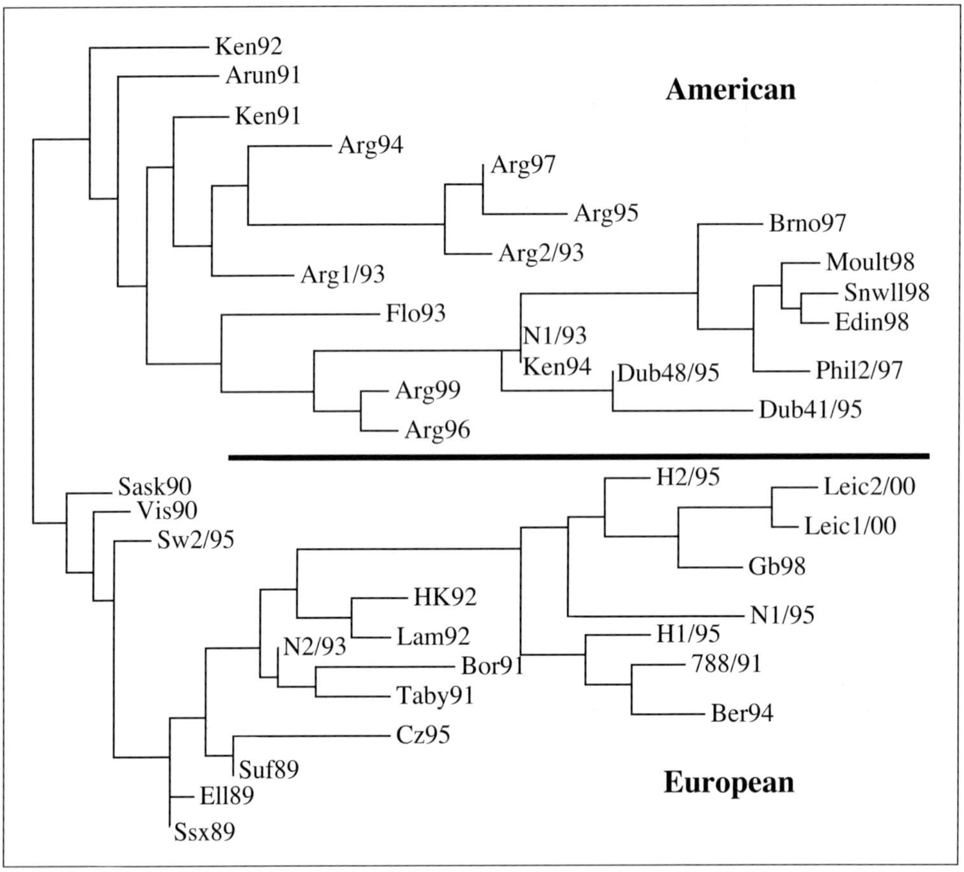

Figure 1. Philogenetic tree (amino acid) of HA1 (H3N8) viruses.

Newmarket/98, Edinburgh/98), Sweden (Soderala/94, Bollnas/96, Alvdalen/96), Switzerland (Switzerland/2/95) and Czech Republic [11, 32]. American-like viruses have also been recovered from horses in the Philippines in 1997 and in Dubai in 1995 [13] after the importation of influenza with horses from the Americas.

The divergence in HA sequence of the two families was also reflected by a difference in antigenic character detectable in HI tests using post-infection ferret sera. Six antigenic groups have been identified dating back to 1963. A dendrogram of antigenic resemblance coefficients among pairs of recent isolates grouped them into 3 clusters *(Figure 2)*. These observations raised the question of the potential importance of geographical variations in antigenic character for vaccine efficacy. Since many horses travel internationally and could expect exposure to both American and Eurasian viruses, vaccination with only one antigenic type may provide less than optimal protection against the other.

To investigate this possibility a series of vaccine and challenge studies have been performed in ponies to examine the cross protective activity of antibody stimulated by American-like viruses for infection with Newmarket/2/93, a European strain, and *vice*

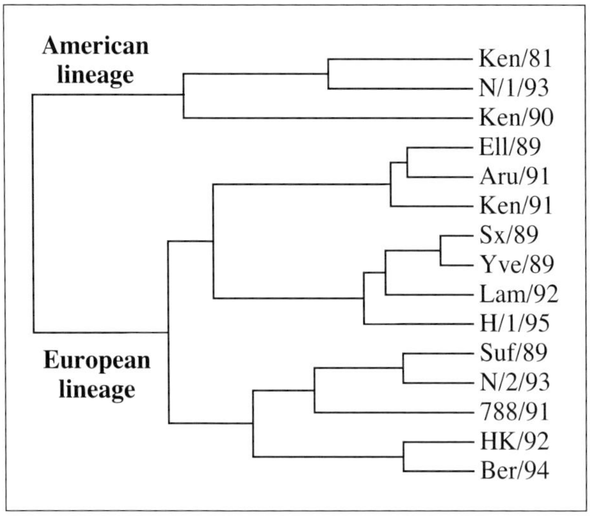

Figure 2. Antigenic dendrogram.

versa. In the first study, vaccines prepared against Arundel/91 (American-like) and Newmarket/2 (European-like) were compared and found to be similar in their ability to protect against Newmarket/2/93 taking into account the levels of prechallenge antibody [17]. These findings correlated with the cross reactivity of post-infection ferret and post vaccination horse sera in HI tests. Similarly monovalent vaccines containing either Newmarket/1/93 (American-like) or Newmarket/2/93 (European-like) were not significantly different in their ability to protect against Newmarket/2/93 [34]. These observations also correlated with the cross reactivity observed with post-infection ferret and horse sera [17].

However, reciprocal HI tests using post-infection ferret sera and post infection and post-vaccination horse sera revealed that Newmarket/1/93 virus reacted poorly with post-infection ferret and horse sera raised against Newmarket/2/93, raising the possibility that vaccines containing European viruses may protect less well against American-like viruses. A study to test this hypothesis has demonstrated that ponies vaccinated with Newmarket/2/93 virus are less well protected against Newmarket/1/93 virus than ponies vaccinated with the homologous virus and this data reflects the specificity of antibody in post-infection ferret and horse sera (Yates, unpublished observation).

Similar results have been obtained in cross protection studies using hamsters as a small animal model and provides the opportunity to investigate further the significance of antigenic differences observed between viruses isolated in the field *e.g.* Czech/95, Grosbois/98, and current vaccine strains Suffolk/89 and Newmarket/2/93 *(Table I)*.

Although experimental studies in horses are few, the data accumulating suggests that the antigenic differences between viruses on the American and European lineages may effect vaccine efficacy, and recent field observations would support this conclusion [35].

Table I. Antigenic analysis of equine influenza viruses with ferret sera.

		Ferret sera raised against:											
Virus	**Origin**	**N1/93**	**N2/93**	**Czech/3/95**	**Holl1/95**	**Swit/2/95**	**Dub/48/95**	**Phil/2/97**	**Brno/97**	**Edin/1/98**	**Mab 7.4A1/2**	**Lineage by antigenicity**	**Lineage by phylogeny**
Fontainebleau/79	France	32	< 8	16	< 8	16	6	< 8	20	< 8	< 8		
Grosbois/93	France	10	< 8	8	< 8	6	5	< 8	6	< 8	< 8		Font-like*
Grosbois/98	France	< 8	< 8	< 8	< 8	< 8	< 8	< 8	< 8	< 8	< 8		European
Cagnes-Mer/06/00	France	256	128	512	256	128	64	64	128	32	< 8	European	Unknown
Drome/26/00	France	256	256	256	512	128	128	64	128	32	< 8	European	Unknown
Seine-et-Marne/77/99	France	256	256	256	512	64	64	64	128	32	< 8	European	American
Isere/00	France	256	256	256	512	128	128	64	128	32	< 8	European	Unknown
Newmarket/1/93	UK	642	5	256	40	321	161	512	512	321	> 1,024	American	American
Newmarket/2/93	UK	101	64	51	642	20	10	< 8	32	< 8	< 8	European	European
Czechoslovakia/3/95	Czech	4	4	79	6	4	4	< 8	< 8	< 8	< 8	European	European
Holland/1/95	Holland	5	16	45	362	4	4	< 8	< 8	< 8	< 8	European	European
Switerland/2/95	Switzerland	891	45	256	114	256	256	> 1,024	32	1,024	8,192	American	Unclear
Dubai/48/95	UAE	1,450	64	725	512	512	256	nd	nd	nd	8,192	American	American
Philippines/2/97	Philippines	512	16	256	32	384	256	> 1,024	1,024	512	4,096	American	American
Brno/97	Czech	1,024	16	256	32	256	256	> 1,024	1,024	1,024	12,288	American	American
Edinburgh/1/98	UK	256	16	512	64	256	256	> 1,024	1,024	512	4,096	American	American

* Fontainebleau-like

Implementation of research findings for improved control

Influenza surveillance programme

Over the past 15 years persuasive evidence has accumulated indicating that equine influenza vaccine viruses need regular updating. As with human influenza, the challenge is to predict important changes and update vaccines to contain newly emerging viruses before major epidemics occur. This requires constant surveillance of influenza worldwide and rapid identification of new variants which may replace old established strains. There is also a requirement for a rapid licensing system for vaccines containing updated strains to enable vaccine manufacturers to respond effectively to changing epidemiological conditions.

Using the human influenza surveillance and vaccine strain selection scheme as a model, scientists, reference laboratories, regulators and vaccine manufacturers have been working together through a series of meetings co-ordinated by WHO and OIE experts to establish a framework for rapidly updating equine influenza vaccine strains *(Table II)*.

Table II. Four WHO/OIE meetings on equine influenza.

1983	Informal workshop on vaccination against equine influenza
1992	Consultation on newly emerging strains of equine influenza
1995	Consultation of OIE and WHO experts on progress in surveillance of equine influenza and application to vaccine strain selection
1999	Fourth International Meeting of OIE and WHO Experts on control of equine influenza. Surveillance and vaccine efficacy: the American perspective

This has required establishing an acceptable level of surveillance internationally, with supporting genetic and antigenic characterisation of viruses isolated, the development of criteria on which to base the decision to change vaccine strains, the establishment of annual reporting mechanisms by an expert surveillance panel on the need to update vaccine strains, the introduction of a fast track licensing system in which vaccine evaluation is based largely on *in vitro* potency testing rather than clinical trials and the provision of reference reagents for vaccine potency and serological testing.

Annual review of vaccine strains by the expert surveillance panel

Following the report of the Conclusions and Recommendations of the 1995 meeting to the Standards Commission of the OIE, the OIE supported the initiative to establish a formal vaccine strain review system through the establishment of an Expert Surveillance Panel [17] and agreed to publish their findings on an annual basis in the OIE Bulletin [36-39]. At the 1995 meeting, the Expert Surveillance Panel concluded that for horses to be adequately protected against H3N8 viruses, vaccines should contain representative strains of American and European-like viruses, similar to Kentucky/94 and Suffolk/89 respectively. It was further recommended that ancient viruses, such as Miami/63, should be removed from current vaccines. Review of information arising between 1995 and 2000 has provided no evidence to indicate that these recommendations require modification, although occasional antigenic variant viruses have been isolated, *e.g.* in Czech Republic (Czech M2/95) and France (Grosbois /1998) *(Table I).*

Criteria for recommending a change in vaccine strain

Based on experience with human influenza vaccines, recommendations to change vaccine strains are dependent on a number of criteria. These include field information on vaccine breakdown in the presence of vaccinal antibody, recognition of antigenic differences between vaccine and field isolates by equine post-vaccinal antibody, antigenic analysis of new isolates using post-infection ferret and horse sera, cross protection studies in horses and hamsters and sequence analysis of the HA gene. Currently all these features are taken into consideration and a conservative approach adopted. Only when the majority of these tests demonstrate significant differences between the majority of field isolates and vaccine strains would a change be recommended. Studies to date indicate that a relationship is emerging between virus antigenicity as characterised in HI tests with ferret and horse sera, and protection in hamsters and horses. Viruses identified as antigenically different using ferret and horse sera in HI tests are subsequently examined in cross protection studies in hamsters and, if shown to overcome immunity to current vaccine strains such viruses would become candidates for cross protection studies in horses. For example viruses such as Czech/95 and Grosbois/98 are candidates for further study in hamsters on the basis that they react poorly with ferret sera to the majority of recent isolates and with post-infection horse sera raised against current vaccine strains *(Tables III and IV).*

It is well recognised that post-vaccinal antibody from repeatedly vaccinated horses is likely to be highly cross-reactive [40]. It has been argued that any antigenic difference detected by such cross reactive sera are likely to be important for immunity in the

Table III. Summary of HI data with post-infection equine sera.

	European		**American**	
Virus	**Sussex/89**	**N/2/93**	**N/1/93**	**Lineage**
Grosbois/93	10	20	40	?
Grosbois/98	4	4	4	?
Cagnes-Mer/06/00	256	1,024	110	European
Drome/26/00	64	128	64	European
Seine-et-Marne/77/99	256	512	40	European
Isere/00	128	420	80	European
Sussex/89	205	420	26	European
Newmarket/1/93	80	512	630	American
Newmarket/2/93	160	256	26	European

Table IV. Summary of HI data from sero-surveys.

	Geometric mean titres			
Antigen	**Jan. 1999**	**June 1999**	**Dec. 1999**	**Jun. 2000**
Miami/63	11	57	22	34
Fontainebleau/79	–	42	17	15
Kentucky/81	6	40	17	18
Suffolk/89 (Sf89)	10	60	26	27
Newmarket/1/93	12	65	24	43
Newmarket/2/93	11	73	32	57
Newmarket/1/95	10	61	24	38
Holland/1/95	9	53	15	38
Switzerland/2/95	30	77	32	171
Czechoslovakia/M2/95 (C95)	6	38	25	19
Brno/97	29	56	35	46
Grosbois/98 (GB98)	4	4	nd	nd
Balaton/98	21	81	55	143
Fold difference of C95:Sf89	1.67	1.58	1.04	1.42
Fold difference of GB98:Sf89	2.5	15	nd	nd
No. of sera analysed	36	36	15	19

horse. Most virus strains so far isolated react strongly in HI tests with post-vaccinal antibody to the prototype European virus Suffolk/89 with the exception of Czech/95 and Grosbois/98, which react less well with antibody stimulated against current vaccines *(Table IV)*. This observation demonstrates the need for careful surveillance to monitor emerging variants, which may overcome vaccine-induced immunity. It is therefore essential that intensive efforts are made to isolate influenza viruses rather than relying solely on rapid techniques such as ELISAs and PCR for the diagnosis.

Fast track licensing system

Following the introduction of a vaccine strain selection system and recognition of the need to use epidemiologically relevant viruses [41], it was necessary to develop a fast track licensing system for vaccines incorporating new strains in order to facilitate the rapid introduction of updated vaccines. Guidelines for "Harmonisation of Requirements for Equine Influenza Vaccines, Specific Requirements for Substitution or Addition of a Strain or Strains" have been developed by the Committee for Veterinary Medicinal Products (CVMP) which are based on the premise that the performance of equine influenza vaccines is well understood and that the substitution or addition of a strain is unlikely to materially alter the composition of the product.

The Guidelines are based on manufacturers selecting a virus antigenically similar to that recommended by the Expert Surveillance Panel. Control tests required during production include in process testing of immunologically active antigen by Single Radial Diffusion (SRD) or a similarly validated *in vitro* test [20]. Specific reagents for use with an A/equine/1 (H7N7) virus (Prague/56) and American and European-like H3N8 viruses have been prepared by the National Institute for Biological Standards and Control.

Potency testing of adjuvanted final product is performed in guinea pigs and horses using SRH or a similarly validated serological test to measure antibody responses following two doses of vaccine. Since the correlation between SRH antibody and protection is so well established [15, 21] challenge studies to demonstrate efficacy are not required; however, it has been recognised that reference antisera are essential for evaluation of the sensitivity of the serological assays used to demonstrate potency. Post-infection antisera have been prepared against representative strains of the European (Newmarket/2/93) and American (Newmarket/1/93) families of the H3N8 virus and against Newmarket/77 (H7N7) virus and freeze dried by the European Pharmacopoeia to provide the necessary reagents for standardisation of serological assessment of vaccine potency. Values have been assigned based on an international collaborative study and these sera are currently now available [41].

Thus, based on the relationships demonstrated between antigenic content measured by SRD, antibody responses in horses measured by SRH and protection against challenge infection [21], it has been possible to develop a fast track licensing system which does not require challenge studies or duration data before market authorisation.

Conclusions

Many of the activities are now in place to provide vaccine manufacturers with the necessary information for production of effective vaccines containing epidemiologically relevant viruses. The steps taken should result in vaccines better able to eliminate virus shedding, a requirement identified by the equine industry, and vaccine manufacturers should be encouraged to adopt them. There is now an urgent need to work towards international harmonisation of standards for licensing vaccines. At the meeting of OIE and WHO experts held in Miami in 1999 it was recommended that a group be established to progress this objective under the auspices of the Veterinary International Committee for Harmonisation.

Although the provision of a broader range of diagnostic assays has further increased our ability to monitor influenza activity world-wide and avoid transmission of infection with movement of horses from areas where the infection is active, there are still important goals to be met. These include increased surveillance and virus recovery and characterisation from large equine populations in the Americas and Far East, where relatively little is known about the viruses circulating.

References

1. Mumford JA, Chambers TM. Equine Influenza. In: *Textbook of Influenza*. Nicholson, Hay, Webster. Blackwell Healthcare Communications Ltd. 1998: 146-62.
2. Bryans JT, Doll ER, Wilson JC, McCollum WH. Immunisation for equine influenza. *J Am Vet Med Assoc* 1966; 148: 413-7.
3. Mumford JA, Wood J. Conference report on WHO/OIE meeting: Consultation on newly emerging strains of equine influenza. *Vaccine* 1993; 11: 1172-5.
4. Cook RF, Sinclair R, Mumford JA. Detection of influenza nucleoprotein antigen in nasal secretions from horses infected with A/equine influenza (H3N8) viruses. *J Virol Meth* 1988; 20: 41-12.
5. Wood JM, Mumford JA, Dunleavy U, Seagroatt V, Newman RW, Thornton D, Schild GC. Single radial immunodiffusion potency tests for inactivated equine influenza vaccines. In: Powell DG, ed. *Proc 5th Intl Conf Equine Infectious Diseases*. Lexington: Kentucky University Press, 1988: 74-9.
6. OIE. Manual of Standards for Diagnostic Tests and Vaccines. Third Edition, 1996, 412-414. Eds OIE, Paris, France.
7. EMEA/CVMP/112/98 (1998) "Notes for Guidance: Harmonisation of Requirements for Equine Influenza Vaccines – Specific Requirements for substitution or addition of a strain or strains" (EMEA/CVMP/112/98 Consultation).
8. European Pharmacopoeia. Monograph on Equine Influenza Vaccines, 3RD Edition 1998.
9. OIE. International Animal Health Code, Seventh Edition. Office International des Epizooties, Paris, France, 1998.
10. Oxburgh L, Berg M, Klingeborn B, Emmoth E, Linne T. Evolution of H3N8 equine influenza virus from 1963 to 1991. *Virus Res* 1994; 34: 153-65.
11. Oxburgh L, Akerblom L, Fridberger T, Klingeborne B, Linné T. Identification of two antigenically and genetically distinct lineages of H3N8 equine influenza virus in Sweden. In: Wernery U, Wade JF, Mumford JA, Kaaden OR, eds. *Proc 8th Intl Conf Equine Infectious Diseases*. Newmarket: Publishers R & W Ltd, 1999: 471.
12. Powell DG, Watkins KL, Li PH, Shortridge KF. Outbreak of equine influenza among horses in Hong Kong during 1992. *Vet Rec* 1995; 136 (21): 531-6.
13. Wernery R, Yates PJ, Wernery U, Mumford JA. Equine influenza outbreak in a polo club in Dubai, United Arab Emirates in 1995/96. *Proc 8th Intl Conf Equine Infectious Diseases*. Newmarket: Publishers R & W Ltd, 1999: 342-6.
14. Chambers TM, Shortridge KF, Li PH, Powell DG, Watkins KL. Rapid diagnosis of equine influenza by the Directigen FLU-A enzyme immunoassay. *Vet Rec* 1994; 135 (12): 275-9.
15. Newton JR, Townsend HGG, Wood JLN, Sinclair R, Hannant D, Mumford JA. Immunity to equine influenza: relationship of vaccine induced antibody in young thoroughbred racehorses to protection against field infection with influenza A/equine-2 viruses (H3N8). *Equine Vet J* 1999; 32: 65-74.
16. Birch-Machin I, Rowan A, Pick J, Mumford JA, Binns MM. Expression of the nonstructural protein NS1 of equine influenza A virus: detection of anti-NS1 antibody in post infection equine sera. *J Virol Meth* 1996; 65: 255-63.
17. Mumford JA. Control of Influenza from an international perspective. In: Wernery U, Wade JF, Mumford JA, Kaaden OR, eds. *Proc 8th Intl Conf Equine Infectious Diseases*. Newmarket: Publishers R & W Ltd, 1999: 11-24.
18. Holland RE, Chambers TM, Townsend HGG, *et al.* New modified live equine influenza virus vaccine: safety and efficacy studies in young equids. In: *Proc 45th Annu Conv Am Assoc Equine Practnr* 1999: 38-40.
19. Townsend HGG, Cook A, Watts TC, *et al.* Efficacy of a cold-adapted, modified-live virus influenza vaccine. a double-blind challenge trial. In: *Proceedings 45th Annu Conv Am Assoc Equine Practnr* 1999; 43-4.
20. Wood JM, Schild GC, Folkers C, Mumford J, Newman RW. The standardisation of inactivated equine influenza vaccines by single-radial immunodiffusion. *J Biol Stand* 1983; 11: 133-6.
21. Mumford JA, Wood J. Establishing an acceptable threshold for equine influenza vaccines. *Dev Biol Stand* 1992; 79: 137-46.
22. Klein N, *et al.* Presented in Fourth International Meeting of OIE and WHO Experts on Control of Equine Influenza: Surveillance and vaccine efficacy: the American perspective. Unpublished 2000.
23. Townsend HGG, Moore S, Bogdan J, Haines D. Antibody response of horses to vaccination against influenza. In: *Proc IBC's 4th Intl Symp Veterinary Vaccines* 1999.

24. Townsend HGG. The role of vaccines and their efficacy in the control of infectious respiratory disease of the horse. Presented in *Proc 46th Annu Conv Am Assoc Equine Practnr* 2000: 21-6.
25. Wood JLN. *Equine Influenza: history and epidemiology and a description of a recent outbreak.* MSc Dissertation, London School of Hygiene and Tropical Medicine, University of London, 1991.
26. Pereira H, Takimoto S, Piegas N, Valle L. Antigenic variation of equine (Heq2Neq2) influenza virus. *Bull WHO* 1972; 47: 465-9.
27. Van Oirschot J, Masurel N, Huffels A, Anker W. Equine influenza in the Netherlands during the winter of 1978-1979; antigenic drift of the A-equi 2 virus. *Tijdschrift Voor Diergeneeskunde* 1981; 106: 80-4.
28. Hinshaw V, Naeve C, Webster R, Douglas A, Skehel J, Bryans J. Analysis of antigenic variation in equine 2 influenza A viruses. *Bull WHO* 1983; 61: 153-8.
29. Kawaoka Y, Bean W, Webster R. Evolution of the haemagglutinin of equine H3 influenza viruses. *Virology* 1989; 169: 283-92.
30. Gibson C, Daniels R, McCauley J, Schild G. Haemagglutinin gene sequencing studies of equine-1 influenza A viruses. In: Powel DG, ed. *Equine Infectious Diseases V.* Lexington: University Press of Kentucky, 1988: 51-9.
31. Livesay G, O'Neill T, Hannant D, Yadav MP, Mumford JA. The outbreak of equine influenza (H3N8) in the United Kingdom in 1989: diagnostic use of an antigen capture ELISA. *Vet Rec* (1993; 133: 515-9.
32. Daly J, Lai A, Binns M, Chambers T, Barrandeguy M, Mumford J. Recent worldwide antigenic and genetic evolution of equine H3N8 influenza A viruses. *J Gen Virol* 1996; 77: 661-71.
33. Bogdan JR, Morley PS, Townsend HGG, Haines DM. Effect of influenza A/equine/H3N8 virus isolate varation on the measurement of equine antibody responses. *Can J Vet Res* 1993; 57: 126-30.
34. Yates P, Mumford JA. Equine influenza vaccine efficacy: the significance of antigenic variation. *Vet Microbiol* 2000; 74: 173-7.
35. Newton JR, Verheyen K, Wood JLN, Yates PJ, Mumford JA. Equine influenza in the United Kingdom in 1998. *Vet Rec* 1999; 145: 449-52.
36. OIE. Conclusions and recommendations from the consultation meeting of OIE and WHO experts on equine influenza, Newmarket, United Kingdom, 18-19 September 1995. *OIE Bull* 1996; 6 (96): 482-4.
37. OIE. Report of the Expert Surveillance Panel on Equine Influenza Vaccine Strain Selection. *OIE Bull* 1997; 3 (97): 265.
38. OIE. Report of the Expert Surveillance Panel on Equine Influenza Vaccine Strain Selection. *OIE Bull* 1998; 4 (98): 365.
39. OIE. *Report of the Expert Surveillance Panel on Equine Influenza Vaccine Strain Selection*, 1999.
40. Burrows R, Denyer M. Antigenic properties of some equine influenza viruses. *Arch Virol* 1982; 73: 15-24.
41. European Pharmacopoeia. European Pharmacopoeia forum special issue biologicals. Bio2000-1, 5-22. ISSN 10135294.

Emergence and Control of Zoonotic Ortho- and Paramyxovirus Diseases
B. Dodet, M. Vicari, eds.

Anti-influenza drugs: implications of resistance

Larisa V. Gubareva[1], Frederick G. Hayden[1, 2]
[1] *Department of Internal Medicine School of Medicine, University of Virginia, Charlottesville, VA, USA*
[2] *Department of Pathology School of Medicine, University of Virginia, Charlottesville, VA, USA*

Amantadine and rimantadine target the ion channel formed by the M2 protein of influenza A viruses. They are effective for prevention and treatment of influenza A infections in humans, experimentally infected mammals and in birds. Because influenza B viruses lack the M2 protein, they are not susceptible to these drugs. The development of resistance to M2 inhibitors is rapid in animals and humans and is caused by a single amino acid substitution at one of five residues in the transmembrane domain of the M2 protein. The resistant mutants are cross-resistant and appear to be as infectious and virulent as wild-type viruses [1].

One of the advances in the treatment of influenza during the past decade has been the development of potent inhibitors of the influenza virus neuraminidase (NA). Recently, two NA inhibitors, zanamivir and oseltamivir, have been approved for use in humans [2]; and the third inhibitor, RWJ-270201, is currently undergoing clinical evaluation [3]. Despite the difference in their structure, all three drugs are potent and specific inhibitors of both influenza A and B NAs. There are two recognized mechanisms of resistance to NA inhibitors: reduced virus binding to receptors and NA enzyme resistance. Reduced binding may result from substitutions in the hemagglutinin (HA) receptor-binding site, which aids virus release from infected cells by reducing virus dependence on NA activity. Resistant enzymes acquire substitutions at one of four identified positions 119, 152, 274, and 292 (N2 numbering) of NA active site. Some NA inhibitor-resistant viruses have changes in both viral proteins HA and NA [4].

Emergence of NA resistance in immunocompetent adults is a relatively rare event (< 2%) [5]. NA-resistant mutants demonstrate attenuation in the animal models, although the level of attenuation varies depending on a particular substitution. Monitoring of virus resistance to NA inhibitors is based on NA enzyme activity inhibition assay and sequence analysis of the HA and NA genes [6]. In contrast to results of the studies involving amantadine/rimantadine, there was no apparent emergence or transmission of resistance in the families treated with zanamivir [7]. Escalation in the use of NA inhibitors would require a reliable and relatively simple assay for routine monitoring of drug-resistance in clinical isolates.

Materials and methods

Neuraminidase enzyme assay

Virus in cell culture supernatants was used as a source of NA activity. A fluorometric assay developed by Potier *et al.* [8] was used to measure influenza NA activity and its inhibition by antiviral drugs. The assay measures 4-methylumbelliferone released from the fluorogenic substrate 2'-(4-methylumbelliferyl)-α-D-*N*-acetylneuraminic acid (MU-NANA) by the enzymatic activity of influenza virus enzyme.

Measurement of neuraminidase activity

Neuraminidase activity for virus was determined prior to testing for NA inhibition, due to variation between viruses. Titration of NA activity was performed through serial dilutions of each virus. Virus and substrate were mixed in 96-well black plates and incubated at 37 °C for 30 minutes. Reactions were stopped with the addition of 150 µl of 0.1M glycine buffer, pH 10.7, containing 25% ethanol. Fluorescence was read using an HTS 7000 Bio Assay Reader (Perkin Elmer) with an excitation wavelength of 365 nm and an emission wavelength of 460 nm. In the present study we have utilized two modifications of the assay for measurement of influenza virus NA activity.

Neuraminidase inhibition assay

The concentration of NA inhibitor required to inhibit enzyme activity by 50% (IC_{50} value) was determined by serial half-log dilutions (from 10 µM to 0.00001 µM) of the NA inhibitor against a standard amount of virus. Equal volumes of the virus and inhibitor were mixed and incubated at room temperature for 30 min. After addition of the substrate, the reaction mixture was incubated for 1 hour at 37 °C. Reaction was stopped by addition of stop solution and the fluorescence of each combination of compound and virus was measured. These data were plotted as log inhibitor concentration against percent fluorescence inhibition. The IC_{50} values were obtained from the resulting graph by extrapolation.

NA inhibition assay A

The working virus dilution was made in saline containing 6.8 mM $CaCl_2$. Five µl of the virus dilution were mixed with 5 µl of the inhibitor diluted in 0.4 M sodium phosphate buffer, pH 5.9. The mixture was incubated at room temperature for 30 min. Ten µl of the substrate diluted in distilled water was added yielding a final concentration of 1 mM.

To evaluate the effect of the substrate concentration on the IC_{50} value readings, assay A was also performed with the final concentrations of the substrate of 10 and 100 µM.

NA inhibition assay B

The working virus dilution was made in 33 mM MES containing 4 mM $CaCl_2$, pH 6.5. Twenty µl of the virus dilution were mixed with 20 µl of the inhibitor diluted in the same buffer and incubated 30 min at room temperature. The substrate diluted in the same buffer was added yielding a final concentration of 75 µM.

Effect of EDTA on measurement of NA activity

The NA activities of the wild type virus and their zanamivir-resistant variants were normalized by diluting viruses in 33 mM MES buffer, pH 6.5. Twenty µl of the working dilution of each virus were mixed with 20 µl of the same buffer containing 0 mM, 0.6 mM, and 0.8 mM of EDTA. Mixtures were incubated for 30 min at room temperature and then the substrate diluted in the same buffer (containing corresponding concentrations of EDTA) was added and reactions were incubated for 1 hour at 37 °C.

Results and discussion

The enzyme sensitivities of the influenza viruses and their NA-inhibitor-resistant counterparts *(Table I)* were tested in two NA inhibition assays *(Tables II and III)*. Based on the IC_{50} values, there was no significant difference in zanamivir-sensitivity of the wild type enzymes of type A (N1 and N2) and type B between the assays. Similarly to wild type enzymes, the oseltamivir-selected mutant carrying substitution (His → Tyr) at position 274 was sensitive to zanamivir *(Table II)*. The zanamivir-selected mutant with Lys at position 292 exhibited a low level of zanamivir-resistance (8-12-fold), while mutants with the substitution at position 119 were zanamivir-resistant, although the level of resistance varied substantially between the assays. Thus, there was an approximately 10-fold increase in the IC_{50} values determined for the mutant Gly119 and an approximately 20-fold increase for the mutant Ala119. The mutant Lys152 exhibited the highest level of resistance in assay A with a greater than 3,000-fold increase in IC_{50}, whereas the resistance estimated in assay B was substantially lower. Thus, assay A was more sensitive in detection of substitution at position 152 than assay B.

Table I. Influenza viruses with drug-resistant enzymes selected in the presence of NA inhibitors and used in the present study.

Residue in NA active site	Function	Substitution	NA type and subtype	Reference
119 Glu	Framework	Gly and Ala	A/N2	[11, 14]
292 Arg	Catalytic	Lys	A/N2	[11]
274 His	Framework	Tyr	A/N1	[15]
152 Arg	Catalytic	Lys	B	[16]

Table II. Assessment of zanamivir-resistance of mutant variants selected in the presence of neuraminidase inhibitors.

NA type and subtype	Amino acid substitution	Inhibition of NA activity by zanamivir			
		Assay A		Assay B	
		IC_{50}, nM	Fold[a]	IC_{50}, nM	Fold
A/N2	Wild type	3.0	1	2.5	1
	Gly 119	1,000	333	100	40
	Ala 119	1,250	417	50	20
	Lys 292	35	12	20	8
A/N1	Wild type	2.0	1	1.5	1
	Tyr 274	2.5	1.3	1.8	1.2
B	Wild type	3.2	1	3.3	1
	Lys 152	10,000	3,125	100	30

[a] The ratio of the mean IC_{50} value for the mutant *versus* the IC_{50} for the wild-type enzyme.

Table III. Assessment of oseltamivir carboxylate-resistance of mutant variants selected in the presence of neuraminidase inhibitors.

NA type and subtype	Amino acid substitution	Inhibition of NA activity by oseltamivir carboxylate			
		Assay A		Assay B	
		IC_{50}, nM	Fold[a]	IC_{50}, nM	Fold
A/N2	Wild type	0.9	1	0.4	1
	Gly119	1.0	1.1	0.5	1.3
	Ala119	24	27	1.1	2.8
	Lys292	> 1,000	> 1,000	3,750	9,375
A/N1	Wild type	2.0	1	2.0	1
	Tyr274	> 1,000	>500	450	225
B	Wild type	40	1	4.3	1
	Lys152	> 1,000	> 25	750	174

[a] The ratio of the mean IC_{50} value for the mutant *versus* the IC_{50} for the wild-type enzyme.

The substitution at position 119 (Glu → Val) in the N2 enzyme was detected in the virus recovered from a patient treated with oseltamivir [9]. This mutant enzyme exhibited an approximately 20-fold decrease in the sensitivity to oseltamivir carboxylate. This finding prompted us to test oseltamivir carboxylate-sensitivity of the mutants with substitution at position 119 (Glu → Gly or Ala) which were selected in the presence of zanamivir. The wild type N2 and the mutant Gly119 were sensitive to oseltamivir carboxylate *(Table II)*. Peculiarly, the other mutant with the substitution at position 119 (Glu → Ala) exhibited an approximately 27-fold decrease in oseltamivir carboxylate-sensitivity in assay A but not in assay B. The zanamivir-selected mutant Lys292 was highly resistant (> 1,000 nM) to oseltamivir carboxylate which is in accordance with results reported by other groups [4] *(Table III)*. The oseltamivir-selected mutant Tyr274 demonstrated resistance to this inhibitor. Again, the wild type N1 was drug-sensitive in both assays. In contrast, the sensitivity of the wild type B enzyme to oseltamivir carboxylate was much lower based on the results of assay A in comparison to assay B (10-fold difference). The mutant Lys152 was highly resistant to oseltamivir carboxylate in both assays.

The behavior of the mutants with substitution at functional residues was different from those of the framework. Thus, the substitutions of arginines by lysines at positions 152 or 292 resulted in drug-resistance in both assays against both NA inhibitors.

Because the zanamivir-resistance of the mutant Lys 152 was substantially higher (100-fold) in assay A, we wanted to test whether it was due to the difference in the concentration of the substrate. However, when the concentration of MUNANA was reduced by 10-fold in assay A, the IC_{50} values were still higher than those in the assay B (results are not shown). The drug-sensitivity of the mutant Ala119 was also lower in assay A than in assay B.

Ca^{2+} is known to effect interactions of the influenza NA with the substrate and inhibitor [10]. To ascertain the effect of Ca^{2+} depletion on activity of the viral enzymes, we added EDTA to 33 mM MES buffer, pH 6.5, and compared the effect of EDTA on the activity of the wild type enzymes *versus* the mutants under such conditions. The depletion of Ca^{2+} by EDTA (concentration of EDTA in the buffer added to viruses was 0.6 mM, or 0.8 mM) had no or little effect on N2 and B virus enzymatic activity. In contrast, the addition of EDTA had a profound effect on the activity of the enzyme with the substitution Arg152 → Lys *(Table IV)*. The activity of the mutant carrying the same mutation at residue 292 was not reduced but enhanced under similar conditions.

The presence of EDTA in the reaction buffer resulted in a substantial reduction of the NA activity of the mutant with the substitution at position 119 *(Table IV)*. Therefore, the interactions of the mutants carrying substitutions at positions 119 and 152 with the substrate and inhibitors are more sensitive to conditions of the experiment than the wild type enzymes. The mutant Lys292 exhibited an enhanced activity after addition of

Table IV. EDTA effect on measurement of neuraminidase activity of wild type viruses and drug-resistant variants.

NA	Change (%) in NA activity[a]	
	+ 0.6 mM EDTA	+ 0.8 mM EDTA
Wild type N2 NA	+ 4	- 4
Ala119	- 39	- 41
Lys292	+ 60	+ 36
Wild type B NA	+ 14	+ 1
Lys152	- 20	- 100

[a] 100% – enzyme activity of the virus in 33mM MES, pH 6.5.

EDTA in the present study. We have previously reported that Lys292 has reduced enzymatic activity at physiological pH [11].

Two distinct Ca^{2+} binding sites have been found in the NA tetramer [12]. One site of weak affinity is located on the 4-fold axis (central Ca^{2+}) and the other site of high affinity is located in each subunit close to the active site (in vicinity of Arg292). This central Ca^{2+} may be important in holding together the tetramer [12]. NA is enzymatically active only in a tetrameric form, and each monomer has an enzyme active site. It was suggested that central Ca^{2+} binds at the subunit interface transmitting a conformational change to the enzyme active site [10]. Chong *et al.* speculated that the binding of Ca^{2+} at the subunit interface orientates the three active-site residues Glu119, Asp151, and Arg152 *via* movement of the two loops, to optimize the binding of substrates and inhibitors. It was demonstrated previously that the central Ca^{2+} can easily be removed by EDTA [13]. Our results support the hypothesis [10] about the essential role of central Ca^{2+} in enzyme interaction with the substrate and inhibitor.

The practical consideration is that detection of the mutant enzymes with substitutions at positions 119 or 152 could be more efficient in the NA inhibition assay performed in the phosphate buffer and at high concentration of substrate. Although the mutant Lys292 used in our study was selected in the presence of zanamivir, it exhibited the high level of resistance to oseltamivir carboxylate. This result suggests that the detection of some mutants could be done more effectively with a panel of NA inhibitors.

The oseltamivir carboxylate-sensitivity of NA in influenza B virus was reduced (up to approximately 10-fold) in assay A in comparison to assay B. This result indicates that the buffer and substrate concentration could effect not only interactions of the mutant enzymes with inhibitor but also interaction of certain wild type enzymes with a particular NA inhibitor.

Monitoring of virus resistance to NA inhibitors is based on the NA inhibition assay where the estimated IC_{50} values of viruses isolated before and after treatment are compared. The accumulated experience and knowledge in detection of the mutants with altered NA sensitivity to the drugs provides a good foundation for monitoring of resistance in clinical settings. However, the development of the assay detecting the mutant viruses which confer resistance to NA inhibitors by other mechanisms is desirable.

Acknowledgements

This work was supported by a grant R01 AI45782 from National Institute of Allergy and Infectious Diseases and in part by a grant from the R.W. Johnson Pharmaceutical Research Institute.

We thank Douglas W. Schallon for excellent technical assistance.

References

1. Hayden FG. Amantadine and rimantadine – Clinical Aspects. In: Richman DD, ed. *Antiviral drug resistance*. John Wiley & Sons Ltd., 1996: 59-77.
2. Gubareva LV, Kaiser L, Hayden FG. Influenza virus neuraminidase inhibitors. *Lancet* 2000; 355: 827-35.
3. Hayden FG, Treanor JJ, Qu R, Fowler C. Safety and efficacy of an oral neuraminidase inhibitor RWJ-270201 in treating experimental influenza A and B in healthy adult volunteers. *40th Interscience Conf Antimicrobial Agents and Chemotherapy*, Toronto, Ontario, Canada, September 17-20. 2000. (Abstract.)
4. McKimm-Breschkin JL. Resistance of influenza viruses to neuraminidase inhibitors. [Review]. *Antivir Res* 2000; 47: 1-17.
5. Covington E, Mendel DB, Escarpe PA, Tai CY, Soberbarg K, Roberts NA. Phenotypic and genotypic assay of influenza virus neuraminidase indicates a low incidence of viral drug resistance during treatment with oseltamivir. *2nd Int Symp Influenza and Other Respiratory Viruses*, December 10-12, Grand Cayman. 1999. (Abstract.)
6. Tisdale M. Monitoring of viral susceptibility: new challenges with the development of influenza NA inhibitors. *Rev Med Virol* 2000; 10: 45-55.
7. Hayden FG, Gubareva LV, Monto AS *et al.* Inhaled zanamivir for the prevention of influenza in families. *N Engl J Med* 2000; 343: 1282-9.
8. Potier M, Mameli L, Belisle M, Dallaire L, Melancon SB. Fluorometric assay of neuraminidase with a sodium (4-methylumbelliferyl-alpha-D-N-acetylneuraminate) substrate. *Anal Biochem* 1979; 94: 287-96.
9. Carr J, Ives J, Roberts NA *et al.* An oseltamivir treatment-selected influenza A/Wuhan/359/95 virus with an E119V mutation in the neuraminidase gene has reduced infectivity *in vivo*. *2nd Intl Symp Influenza and other Respiratory Viruses*, Grand Cayman, Cayman Islands, December 10-12, 1999. (Abstract.)
10. Chong AK, Pegg MS, von Itzstein M. Influenza virus sialidase: effect of calcium on steady-state kinetic parameters. *Biochim Biophys Acta* 1991; 1077: 65-71.
11. Gubareva LV, Robinson MJ, Bethell RC, Webster RG. Catalytic and framework mutations in the neuraminidase active site of influenza viruses that are resistant to 4-guanidino-Neu5Ac2en. *J Virol* 1997; 71: 3385-90.
12. Burmeister WP, Ruigrok RW, Cusack S. The 2.2 A resolution crystal structure of influenza B neuraminidase and its complex with sialic acid. *EMBO J* 1992; 11: 49-56.
13. Burmeister WP, Cusack S, Ruigrok RW. Calcium is needed for the thermostability of influenza B virus neuraminidase. *J Gen Virol* 1994; 75: 381-8.
14. Gubareva LV, Bethell R, Hart GJ, Murti KG, Penn CR, Webster RG. Characterization of mutants of influenza A virus selected with the neuraminidase inhibitor 4-guanidino-Neu5Ac2en. *J Virol* 1996; 70: 1818-27.
15. Gubareva LV, Kaiser L, Matrosovich MN, Soo-Hoo Y, Hayden FG. Selection of influenza virus mutants in experimentally infected volunteers treated with oseltamivir. *J Infect Dis* 2001; 183: 523-31.
16. Gubareva LV, Matrosovich MN, Brenner MK, Bethell RC, Webster RG. Evidence for zanamivir resistance in an immunocompromised child infected with influenza B virus. *J Infect Dis* 1998; 178: 1257-62.

Emergence and Control of Zoonotic Ortho- and Paramyxovirus Diseases
B. Dodet, M. Vicari, eds.

Developing vaccines against potential pandemic influenza viruses

John M. Wood
National Institute for Biological Standards and Control, Hertfordshire, United Kingdom

Abstract – In the event of an influenza pandemic, there will be urgent need for a vaccine. The human infections with influenza A (H5N1) and A (H9N2) viruses served as pandemic warnings and initiated world-wide efforts to develop suitable vaccines. This was not straightforward, however, due to safety considerations and many practical problems that were encountered. This is primarily an account of the three main strategies for H5 vaccine development: attenuation of the pathogenic A/Hong Kong/97 (H5N1) virus; expression of H5 haemagglutinin in baculovirus vectors; and use of avirulent H5 avian viruses. Progress with H9 vaccine development is also reviewed.

Over the past two and a half years, we have learnt a great deal about our ability to respond to an influenza pandemic. Some of the improvements that could be made for the future are summarised.

During the period May to December 1997, an outbreak of human influenza A (H5N1) infections in Hong Kong SAR gave serious cause for concern [1]. At the time, there was no indication whether human infection would remain linked to poultry infections, or whether the H5N1 virus would acquire the ability to transmit from person-to-person. A few months later, human infections caused by a further avian influenza virus subtype, H9N2, were detected in China and Hong Kong SAR [2, 3]. In response to these events, there was an urgent need to develop H5N1 and H9N2 vaccines, which could be used to combat possible pandemic activity. Several laboratories throughout the world were involved with vaccine development and at the time of writing, two such vaccines have been clinically evaluated and a third is under testing. Although neither an H5N1 nor an H9N2 pandemic actually materialised, the process of vaccine development was extremely useful nonetheless. Different development strategies were adopted, some more successful than others and most laboratories encountered problems at some stage of vaccine development. There are important lessons to be learned from our experiences, which should help us to respond more effectively in future. The following is an account of vaccine development.

Safety issues

Ideally an influenza vaccine should be safe for man and the environment both during vaccine development and also during clinical use. The H5N1 virus was highly pathogenic for man and several species of animals [4] and the H9N2 virus caused clinical illness in man, and was capable of infecting chickens and ducks without symptoms, but was pathogenic in mice [5]. It was important therefore to review safety procedures, before vaccine development could begin. By common consent among WHO influenza laboratories, a high level of containment (*e.g.* BSL 3 or 4) was necessary for the H5N1 virus, whereas the H9N2 virus was less of a hazard and could be handled at lower levels of containment (BSL 2 + or BSL 3). There were also important public health and veterinary regulations to observe and permits to be obtained before work could begin. The first stages of H5N1 vaccine development were directed at producing a safe vaccine virus and this work, together with the initial preparation for safe handling of the pathogenic H5N1 virus, meant that some delays were experienced.

One of the general safety issues that emerged was the safe handling of novel viruses within vaccine production areas. Most production areas are designed to protect the product from extraneous agents, but not to protect staff. Thus in order to avoid accelerating a possible pandemic by infecting staff, a containment facility would be needed for vaccine production. This is an important consideration during the time when a novel virus is not circulating widely (*e.g.* WHO pandemic plan phases 0 and possibly 1 [6]). It may however be considered appropriate to relax such precautions if vaccine production is based on an attenuated virus or indeed if a pandemic is imminent.

Strategies for vaccine production

In considering which strategy to adopt for H5N1 or H9N2 vaccine production, choices had to be made between developing a vaccine by a licensed process and using alternative approaches which offered advantages but were as yet unlicensed processes. Thus for H5N1, three main strategies were adopted:

- attenuate the pathogenic A/Hong Kong/97 virus so that it was no longer lethal for poultry and other animal species;
- produce purified H5 haemagglutinin (HA) by recombinant technology using genetically-modified baculovirus vectors;
- produce a conventional inactivated virus vaccine from an apathogenic H5N1.

Attenuation of A/Hong Kong/97 virus

Three laboratories pursued this approach. In the USA [7], the HA gene of A/Hong Kong/97 virus was genetically modified by deleting the stretch of basic amino acids at the cleavage site. Then by reverse genetics, the modified H5 HA gene and the NI NA gene from HK/97 virus were rescued into the attenuated cold-adapted A/Ann Arbor/60 virus background. The resulting 6:2 reassortant had trypsin-dependant replication in mammalian cells, was apathogenic in chickens and ferrets, possessed the cold-adapted phenotype and grew well in eggs. A second laboratory in the USA attempted to rescue a modified H5 HA gene and the N1 gene into either A/PR/8/34 (H1N1) or A/Mal/New York/78 (H2N2) viruses, but this approach appeared to be less successful (Subbarao, personal communication). In Japan, similar modifications to A/HK/97 HA were made and a reassortant was prepared using an avirulent strain A/Duck/Hong Kong/836/80 (H3N1) [8]. The reassortant was avirulent in a variety of animal species and grew well in eggs (Tashiro, personal communication).

As yet, safety for man for such genetically attenuated viruses is unknown, but there is clearly considerable potential for this approach to quickly develop safe and productive seed viruses for use in inactivated vaccines. Furthermore, the use of cold-adapted parental strains provides a basis for development of live attenuated vaccines for use in a pandemic.

Recombinant proteins

The first H5 vaccine to be available anywhere in the world was a recombinant HA protein expressed in recombinant baculovirus-infected *S. frugiperda* cells. At present only small amounts of vaccine can be produced using this technology, but there is potential for scale-up to meet future demands.

Vaccines derived from apathogenic avian H5 viruses

An avirulent H5N3 strain, A/Duck/Singapore-Q/F119-2/97, was selected for vaccine development due to the antigenic and genetic similarity of the HA with that of the HK/97 HA. Furthermore, the DK/Sing virus did not have the polybasic amino acids at the HA cleavage site and it was not pathogenic in poultry (Alexander, personal communication). Unfortunately the virus grew poorly in hens' eggs and had an N3, not an N1 NA. Attempts were made to improve the situation by producing high growth reassortants. However, despite repeated attempts in several laboratories to produce reassortants by conventional means in eggs, there has been only limited success. Virus growth has been improved by selecting variants of DK/Sing, NIB-40 and ARIV-1, but it was not possible to substitute the NA. It is significant that the only complete success to produce a high growth H5N1 virus from DK/Sing virus was in MDCK cells using plaquing techniques [9]. An avirulent H5N1 vaccine virus has also been developed in Japan [8], by producing an H5N1 reassortant, R513 between A/Duck/Hokkaido/67/96 (H5N4) and A/Duck/Hong Kong/301/78 (H7N1). The HA of DK/Hok virus was antigenically related to that of A/HK/97 virus. Experimental lots of NIB-40 and R513 have been produced for animal studies, but only NIB-40 has been used on a larger scale to produce clinical trial lots of purified surface antigen vaccine [10]. Here the greatest problem was that of poor virus growth, which created difficulties in downstream processing (Colegate, personal communication). Another significant issue was the availability of eggs. It was fortunate that only small amounts of vaccine were needed for clinical trials and this could be accommodated during a normal vaccine production season. If an H5N1 pandemic had materialised, it would have been difficult to mass-produce an egg-grown NIB-40 vaccine.

H9N2 vaccines

In Europe, clinical trial lots of conventional whole virus and surface antigen vaccines have been made from the A/Hong Kong/99 (H9N2) virus. The virus grew well in eggs and vaccine processing was not a problem. Again the availability of eggs was an issue and, as mentioned earlier, containment facilities were needed for the early stages of vaccine production.

A recombinant H9 HA protein has also been produced for experimental use (Lambert, personal communication).

General production issues

In 1998, plans were developed in the UK to produce pilot lots (approx. 1,000 doses) of an inactivated vaccine from the pathogenic HK/97 virus, for subsequent clinical comparison with NIB-40 vaccines. The first stages of vaccine production took place at BSL4 containment and this was very successful. However, during downstream processing at another site, there were severe problems, which led to complete loss of the vaccine. Such losses were due to processing small amounts of experimental vaccine in a normal vaccine production facility. It is likely that if a small scale production facility had been available, the losses would have been avoided. This was extremely unfortunate but the experience does illustrate that it should be possible to produce pilot lots of vaccine from un-modified novel viruses and this could be a first response while attempts are being made to seek safer alternatives.

Immunogenicity and efficacy

Attenuated A/Hong Kong/97 vaccines

Pre-clinical assessment of the attenuated viruses was performed in the USA and Japan. Cold adapted reassortants were administered to chickens by the intravenous route and they stimulated serum haemagglutination-inhibition (HI) responses against wild type HK/97 virus. When the chickens were challenged with lethal HK/97 viruses, 11 out of 16 survived [7]. Studies with inactivated vaccines prepared from attenuated HK/97 virus were performed in Japan. Mice were immunised by the intraperitoneal route and one dose stimulated HI and virus neutralising (VN) antibody responses. When vaccine was administered by the intra-nasal route, mucosal and systemic antibody was produced and approximately 90% of mice survived a lethal HK/97 challenge [8].

These experiments illustrate the potential of vaccines prepared from attenuated influenza viruses and plans are in place to assess their safety and immunogenicity in man.

Recombinant proteins

Immunogenicity and protective efficacy of baculovirus-expressed avian H5 and H7 HA's in animals has been demonstrated [11] and there are ample results to show immunogenicity of human influenza HA's in man. The first lots of recombinant H5 HA were available for clinical use early in 1998 and they were administered as two, 10 or 20 μg doses, to 56 subjects in a phase I trial. Somewhat surprisingly, only 2 of 28 subjects receiving the 10 μg dose and only 6 of 28 subjects receiving the 20 μg dose, developed significant VN antibody titres (≥ 80) [12]. This was a weaker immune response than expected, in view of earlier trials of HA derived from conventional human influenza viruses. In a subsequent phase II dose escalating study, even two 90 μg doses could only stimulate significant VN antibody in 40% of recipients [13]. Thus although the recombinant H5 protein was well tolerated, it was only modestly immunogenic.

Vaccines derived from apathogenic avian H5 viruses

In order to assess the protective efficacy of DK/Sing vaccines, mouse challenge studies were performed. For comparative purposes, four experimental inactivated whole virus vaccines were prepared: 1) DK/Sing virus, 2) A/Hong Kong/156/97 virus, 3) A/Hong Kong/489/97 virus, 4) A human H3N2 virus, A/Shanghai/24/90. Balb/C mice were immunised with two intramuscular doses of 15 μg HA, given 21 days apart. High levels of HI antibody to HK/156 virus HA were induced by HK/156 and HK/489 vaccines, whereas the HI titres induced by DK/Sing vaccine were somewhat lower. This reflected the small antigenic differences between the DK/Sing vaccine and the HK/156 virus used for serological tests. The Shg/90 vaccine was as immunogenic as the H5 vaccines (high H3 antibody titres). The mice were subsequently challenged in a BSL4 laboratory with a lethal infection of HK/156 virus. All the mice died within a seven-day period in an unvaccinated control group and in the H3N2 vaccine group, but there was complete survival of mice in all three H5 vaccine groups [14].

Similar results have been obtained in other laboratories using inactivated vaccine prepared from DK/Sing virus [15] or from A/Hokkaido/67/96 (H5N4) or an H5N1 reassortant R513 described earlier [8]. In each case, the avirulent H5 avian virus provided an effective inactivated vaccine against lethal HK/97 virus challenge.

As was described earlier, pilot lots of NIB-40 vaccine have been produced for clinical evaluation. In a phase I dose escalating trial, a conventional surface antigen vaccine was compared with an MF59 – adjuvanted surface antigen vaccine. Subjects received one or two doses of 7.5, 15 or 30 μg HA. Although both types of vaccine were well tolerated, there were significant differences in immunogenicity. Two doses of the non-adjuvanted vaccine produced seroconversion in only 22% of individuals (VN data), whereas 94% of individuals seroconverted after receiving two doses of the adjuvanted vaccine (Nicholson *et al.*, unpublished data). The conclusion from this study is that a conventional surface antigen vaccine prepared from DK/Sing is poorly immunogenic and normal doses are unlikely to protect against the pathogenic HK/97 viruses.

H9N2 vaccines

Pre-clinical evaluation of inactivated vaccines prepared from HK/99 virus have been performed in mice. A whole virus vaccine stimulated good HI responses in all mice and gave complete protection against challenge with HK/99 virus, whereas a surface antigen vaccine was poorly immunogenic even after two doses and gave incomplete protection [16]. This is further evidence that surface antigen vaccines may not make good pandemic vaccines. Clinical trial evaluation of the H9N2 vaccines is currently underway.

Other H5N1 vaccines

H5 DNA vaccines have been shown to protect mice against the lethal effects of HK/97 virus challenge (Robertson, unpublished data), even when the encoded H5 DNA (A/Turkey/Ireland/1/83) differed by 12% in the HA1 region from the HK/156 challenge virus [17]. However neither the H5 nor an H9 DNA vaccine appeared to be capable of preventing virus replication after challenge. Thus a DNA vaccine may offer adequate protection, even if a homologous vaccine is not available. At present, the most likely use of a DNA vaccine in the context of a pandemic is to protect chickens and to prevent an initial focus of infection. The safety and efficacy of DNA vaccines in man is, as yet, unproven.

The efficacy of ISCOM's as adjuvants for H5N1 vaccines has been investigated in chickens. Purified surface antigens of HK/97 virus induced no antibody responses and no protection against lethal H5N1 challenge, whereas the same surface antigens prepared as ISCOM's were highly immunogenic and gave complete protection [18]. ISCOM's are at present undergoing evaluation for use in normal human influenza vaccines and they offer potential to augment immune responses to pandemic vaccines.

Vaccine serology

It was extremely difficult to detect antibody to H5N1 human infections in Hong Kong, using the conventional HI test and it was necessary to use alternative tests such as VN [19]. The inadequacies of the HI test were further revealed when immune responses to baculovirus HA vaccines [12] and NIB-40 inactivated vaccines (Nicholson, unpublished data) were examined. It was only by the use of VN, ELISA or single-radial haemolysis techniques that vaccine immunogenicity could be evaluated. If HI insensitivity is a general phenomenon among avian subtypes, it is important that alternative safe and reliable techniques are developed.

Reagents for vaccine potency testing

The internationally accepted test for measurement of influenza vaccine potency is single-radial-diffusion (SRD). It was therefore important to develop SRD reagents (calibrated antigen and specific anti-HA sera) for H5 and H9 vaccines prior to evaluation of their immunogenicity. Normally it takes about two months to develop SRD reagents, but much longer was needed for H5 (4 months) and H9 (10 months) reagents. The delays were due to a variety of reasons such as poor virus growth, need for containment facilities, difficulties in purifying H9 HA and availability of recombinant HA. Although the reagents were available in time for the animal and human vaccine studies there may have been problems if the H5N1 or H9N2 viruses had become pandemic.

Conclusions

Over the past two and a half years, we have learnt a great deal about our ability to respond to an influenza pandemic. We cannot ignore the fact that it took 8 months (dating from the second human H5N1 case) to produce the first lots of H5 vaccine by conventional means, that the vaccine virus grew so poorly that mass-vaccination would have been virtually impossible and that conventional surface antigen vaccines probably would not have afforded adequate protection. The H5N1 and H9N2 outbreaks have served as warnings that improvements are needed, before we can effectively combat an influenza pandemic by vaccination.

The following are some lessons that can be learnt:

– develop and maintain dialogue between veterinary and public health authorities to reduce administrative barriers and to obtain appropriate permits and containment facilities;

– develop and rehearse contingency plans for production of pandemic vaccines. Such plans should involve the use of containment laboratories;

– develop methods to attenuate pathogenic viruses by reverse genetics;

– develop alternative technologies (*e.g.* plaquing in cell cultures; reverse genetics) for production of high growth reassortants;

– produce libraries of vaccine viruses from a range of avian subtypes, beginning with those considered most likely to transmit to mammals (*e.g.* H2, H5, H7, H9);

– develop new vaccine technologies that do not depend upon the availability of hens' eggs; produce vaccine quicker than conventional methods and/or present vaccine more efficiently to the immune system (*e.g.* mammalian cell culture vaccine, recombinant proteins, DNA vaccines, adjuvants);

– reach a consensus on the role of live attenuated vaccines in a pandemic;

– prepare contingency plans for fast-track licensing and official testing of pandemic vaccines. Such plans should allow novel vaccines to be used;

– evaluate dose requirements and immunogenicity for conventional vaccines, adjuvanted vaccines and novel vaccines prepared from novel subtypes;

– develop antiserum reagents to standardise the potency of vaccines made from novel subtypes;

– strengthen and maintain pandemic response teams to develop vaccines. The teams could include Directors of WHO Influenza Centres, public health officials, national control authorities, clinicians, academic institutions and vaccine manufacturers.

Acknowledgements

I am grateful for helpful discussion and permission to use unpublished information from Dr's J. Katz, A. Klimov, K. Subbarao, CDC, USA; L. Lambert NIAID, USA; R. Levandowski CBER, USA; M. Tashiro, NIID, Japan; A. Osterhaus, Erasmus University, The Netherlands and A. Colegate, Chiron Vaccines, Italy.

References

1. Bender C, Hall H, Huang J, Klimov A, Cox N, Hay A, Gregory V, Cameron K, Lim W, Subbarao K. Characterisation of the surface proteins of influenza A (H5N1) viruses isolated from humans in 1997-1998. *Virology* 1999; 254: 115-23.
2. Peiris M, Yuen KY, Leung CW, Chan KH, Ip PLS, Lai RWM, Orr WK, Shortridge KF. Human infection with influenza H9N2. *Lancet* 1999; 354: 916-7.
3. Guo Y, Li JW, Cheng I. Discovery of humans infected by avian influenza A (H9N2) virus. *Chin J Exp Clin Virol* 1999; 15: 105-8.
4. Shortride KF, Zhou NN, Guan Y, Gao P, Ito T, Kawaoka Y, Kodihalli S, Krauss S, Markwell D, Murti KG, Norwood M, Senne D, Sims L, Takada A, Webster RG. Characterisation of avian H5N1 influenza viruses from poultry in Hong Kong. *Virology* 1998; 252: 331-42.
5. Guo YJ, Krauss S, Senne DA, Mo IP, Lo KS, Xiong XP, Norwood M, Shortridge KF, Webster RG, Guan Y. Characterisation of the pathogenicity of members of the newly established H9N2 influenza virus lineages in Asia. *Virology* 2000; 267: 279-88.
6. Influenza pandemic preparedness plan. WHO Geneva Switzerland, 1999.
7. Li S, Liu C, Klimov A, Subbarao K, Perdue M, Mo D, Ji Y, Woods L, Hietala S, Bryant M. Recombinant influenza A virus vaccines for the pathogenic human A/Hong Kong/97 (H5N1) viruses. *J Infect Dis*; 179: 1132-8.
8. Takada A, Kuboki N, Okazaki K, Ninomiya A, Tanaka H, Ozaki H, Itamura S, Nishimura H, Enami M, Tashiro M, Shortridge KF, Kida H. Avirulent avian influenza virus as a vaccine strain against a potential human pandemic. *J Virol* 1999; 73: 8303-7.
9. Mabrouk T. Vaccines and related biological products advisory committee meeting regarding influenza vaccine formulation for 1999-2000. 1999. www.fda.gov/ohrms/dockets/ac/99/transcpt/3494t1
10. Wood JM. Vaccines and related biological products advisory committee meeting regarding influenza vaccine formulation for 1999-2000. 1999. www.fda.gov/ohrms/dockets/ac/99/transcpt/3494t1
11. Crawford J, Wilkinson B, Vosnesensky A, Smith G, Garcia M, Stone H, Perdue ML. Baculovirus-derived haemagglutinin vaccines protect against lethal influenza infections by avian H5 and H7 sub-types. *Vaccine* 1999; 17: 2265-74.
12. Katz J, Treanor J. Vaccines and related biological products advisory committee meeting regarding influenza vaccine formulation for 1999-2000. 1999. www.fda.gov/ohrms/dockets/ac/99/transcpt/3494tl
13. Treanor JJ, Wilkinson B, Blackwelder W, Katz JM. Evaluation of the haemagglutinin (HA) of the H5N1 influenza A/Hong Kong/156/97 virus expressed in insect cells by recombinant baculovirus (rH5) as an influenza vaccine in healthy adults [Abstract No. 682]. *39th Intl Conf Antimicrobial Agents and Chemotherapy*, San Francisco, 1999.
14. Wood JM, Major D, Daly J, Newman RW, Dunleavy U, Nicholson C, Robertson JS, Schild GC. Vaccines against H5N1 influenza. Letter to *Vaccine* 2000; 19: 579-80.
15. Lu X, Tumpey TM, Morken T, Zaki SR, Cox NJ, Katz JM. A mouse model for the evaluation of pathogenesis and immunity to influenza A (H5N1) viruses isolated from humans. *J Virol* 1999; 73: 5903-11.
16. Major D, Newman RW, Dunleavy U, Heath A, Ploss K, Wood JM. Evaluation of candidate H9N2 influenza vaccine strains in Balb C mice. In: Osterhaus ADME, *et al.*, eds. *Options for the control of influenza IV.* Exerpta Medica International Congress Series. Elsevier Science, 2000.
17. Kodihalli S, Goto H, Kobasa DL, Krauss S, Kawaoka Y, Webster RG. DNA vaccine encoding haemagglutinin provides protective immunity against H5N1 influenza virus infection in mice. *J Virol* 1999; 73: 2094-8.
18. Rimmelzwaan GF, Claas ECJ, Van Amerongen G, de Jong JC, Osterhaus ADME. ISCOM vaccine induced protection against a lethal challenge with a human H5N1 influenza virus. *Vaccine* 1999; 17: 1355-8.
19. Rowe T, Abernathy RA, Hu-Primmer J, Thompson WW, Lu X, Lin W, Fukuda K, Cox NJ, Katz JM. Detection of antibody to avian influenza A (H5N1) virus in human serum by using a combination of serological assays. *J Clin Microbiol* 1999; 37: 937-43.

Emergence and Control of Zoonotic Ortho- and Paramyxovirus Diseases
B. Dodet, M. Vicari, eds.

Neuraminidase in the development of an anti-influenza vaccine

Lionel Gérentes, Michèle Aymard, Olivier Ferraris, Jeanine Jolly, Nicole Kessler
National Influenza Center, Laboratory of Virology, Lyon, France

Two glycoproteins of the influenza virus participate in its infectious ability: hemagglutinin antigen (HA) mediates the binding of influenza virus to host receptors *via* terminal sialic acid moieties and subsequent penetration of the virus by a fusion procedure, while neuraminidase antigen (NA), by removing sialic acid residues, mainly participates in the virus release from the cells and the destruction of aggregates of new progeny virions.

On the viral envelope, there are 4 to 5 times more HA than NA spikes and both glycoproteins are antigens primarily involved in induction of specific humoral immunity; nevertheless, due to their relative abundance, and to their interference with early stages of viral infection, neutralising anti-HA antibodies are thought to play a predominantly prophylactic role in preventing infection. On the contrary, anti-NA antibodies are considered as non-neutralising and inefficient for preventing infection but are responsible for significant reduction in virus replication and in the occurrence and severity of illness. As a consequence NA is considered as a minor antigen. Nevertheless, decades ago, Schulmann *et al.* [1] described the protective effect of specific anti-NA immunity against influenza infection in mice and Monto *et al.* [2] reported that persons who did not show clinical influenza during the Hong Kong 1968-69 pandemic carried anti-N2 antibodies.

NA properties as reviewed by Coleman [3] confer pathogenicity to influenza virus: (i) the cleavage of sialic acid bonds with the penultimate sugar and destroys viral receptors and fluidifies the mucus, allowing for virus release and diffusion in the respiratory tract; (ii) the cleavage of the sialic acid from the viral HA might facilitate the cleavage of the HA0 precursor by cellular proteases; (iii) NA, as a glycoprotein, stimulates the production of numerous cytokines (IFN, IL1, IL6, TNFα) and so plays an important role in feverish and systemic reactions. As it has been shown recently that NA inhibitors are effective in reducing the influenza disease and virus excretion, it could be assumed that anti-NA antibodies induced by vaccination could also protect against influenza as do the antibodies produced during natural infection.

We report here the two different approaches we have chosen to demonstrate *in vivo* the protecting efficacy of anti-NA neutralising antibodies, *i.e.* the passive transfer in mice of anti-NA N2 specific monoclonal antibodies and the vaccination of mice with pure NA N2 proteins. In both series of experiments, the animals were challenged with 1 to 10 lethal doses of homologous virus. In order to evaluate protection, a biological (lung virus titre, pathology of lung) or clinical (mortality) monitoring of the infection was performed in mice as a function of the dose of virus we used for the challenge.

In vitro functional characteristics of anti-NA MAbs

Monoclonal antibodies (MAbs) directed against the NA of X117 (A/Beij/32/92 H3N2 reassortant) virus were produced, which divided into 3 different groups, whose functional properties were as follows:

- **Group 1 anti-NA MAbs** presented a high ELISA titre, an important capacity to inhibit NA activity on both macromolecular (fetuin) and micromolecular (NANL) substrates, and a moderate neutralising capacity due to their interaction with the late stages of the viral cycle.
- **Group 2 anti-NA MAbs** presented a high ELISA titre, an important capacity to inhibit NA activity on the sole macromolecular substrates (fetuin) and high neutralising capacity due to their interaction with the early stage of viral cycle.
- **Group 3 anti-NA MAb** presented a high ELISA titre, but was devoid of NA inhibiting activity and exhibited a very weak virus neutralising potency *in vitro*. Its hemagglutination inhibition property was due to steric hindrance.

Considering the different profiles of these anti-NA MAbs *in vitro*, we deemed interesting to evaluate their protective potency *in vivo*. As a control we introduced into our experiments an anti-HA H3 MAb which was shown to exhibit a very high ELISA titre, a high capacity to inhibit HA activity and to neutralise virus infectivity *in vitro* by interacting with the early stages of the viral cycle.

In vivo protection conferred by passive transfer of anti-NA MAbs

In order to analyse the role of anti-NA antibodies in protection against influenza infection, we examined the ability of passively transferred anti-NA N2 MAbs to protect BALB/c mice from an intranasal challenge with A/Lyon/2286/93 (H3N2) virus (A/Beijing/32/92-like).

Two different models of passive transfer and virus challenge were developed. In model A, the mice received an intramuscular injection of MAb two days prior to viral challenge, while in model B the mice received an intranasal inoculation of MAb six hours after viral infection. Both models were performed using two different infection conditions: in "**standardised infection**", mice were challenged with 50 MID_{50} per mouse (equivalent to 1LD_{50} per mouse) of virus so that 100% of animals had developed an infection in the respiratory tract with a $10^{7,7 \pm 0,24}$ $TCID_{50}$ of virus per lung (n = 35), when sacrificed 2 days post-infection.

In "**lethal infection**", mice were challenged with 2 to 10 lethal doses (LD_{50}) and were monitored for mortality over a 21 days period following infection. Mortality of infected controls was consistently observed 5 to 8 days post-infection.

Protection against standardised infection

Table I summarizes the results regarding the protection conferred by the different anti-NA MAbs when passively transferred, according to either model A or model B, to mice challenged under standard infection conditions. All three groups of anti-NA MAbs were capable of protecting mice efficiently against influenza infection. In agreement with *in vitro* Nt tests, group 2 and group 3 anti-NA MAbs were shown to protect mice by interacting with the early stages of the virus cycle exclusively, while group 1 anti-NA MAbs interacted only with the late stages of the virus cycle; indeed in model A, MAbs were present in the lung from the beginning of infection so that they were potentially capable of interacting with early and late stages of viral cycle.

In additional sets of experiments, we tested *in vitro* and *in vivo* the synergistic effects of two or more MAbs in combination. MAbs were mixed under their protective neutralising limiting dilutions and the mixture was then submitted to serial log2 dilutions. Results were expressed in percentage of inhibition of viral multiplication in lung/MDCK cells. *Figure 1 (a, b, c)* shows the synergistic effects with the different anti-NA MAb pairs. The largest synergistic effects (2 dilutions *in vivo*/4 dilutions *in vitro*) were observed when associating two anti-NA MAbs interacting with early (group 2) and late (group 1) stages of the viral cycle respectively. In a similar manner optimal gain in protective (2 dilutions)/neutralising (3 dilutions) titre was observed when anti-HA MAb interacting with the early stages of the viral cycle was mixed with group 1 anti-NA MAb interacting with the late stages of the viral cycle. When testing multi-MAb associations (2 to 5 MAbs), the synergistic effect ranged between 1 to 4 dilutions *in vivo* and 2 to 7 dilutions *in vitro*. It is interesting to notice that one protective dose of anti-NA MAb was shown to correspond to 40 (group 1) to 80 (group 2) neutralising doses, while one protective dose of anti-HA MAb corresponded to 3,200 neutralising doses.

Table I. Protection conferred by the passive transfer of anti-NA MAbs.

	Protective titre /ml		Deduced interaction with viral cycle
Anti-NA MAbs	**Model A**	**Model B**	
Group 1	50	50	Late
Group 2	50,000	< 8	Early
Group 3	20	< 8	Early
Anti-HA MAb			
Anti-H3 (HA_1)	100	< 8	Early

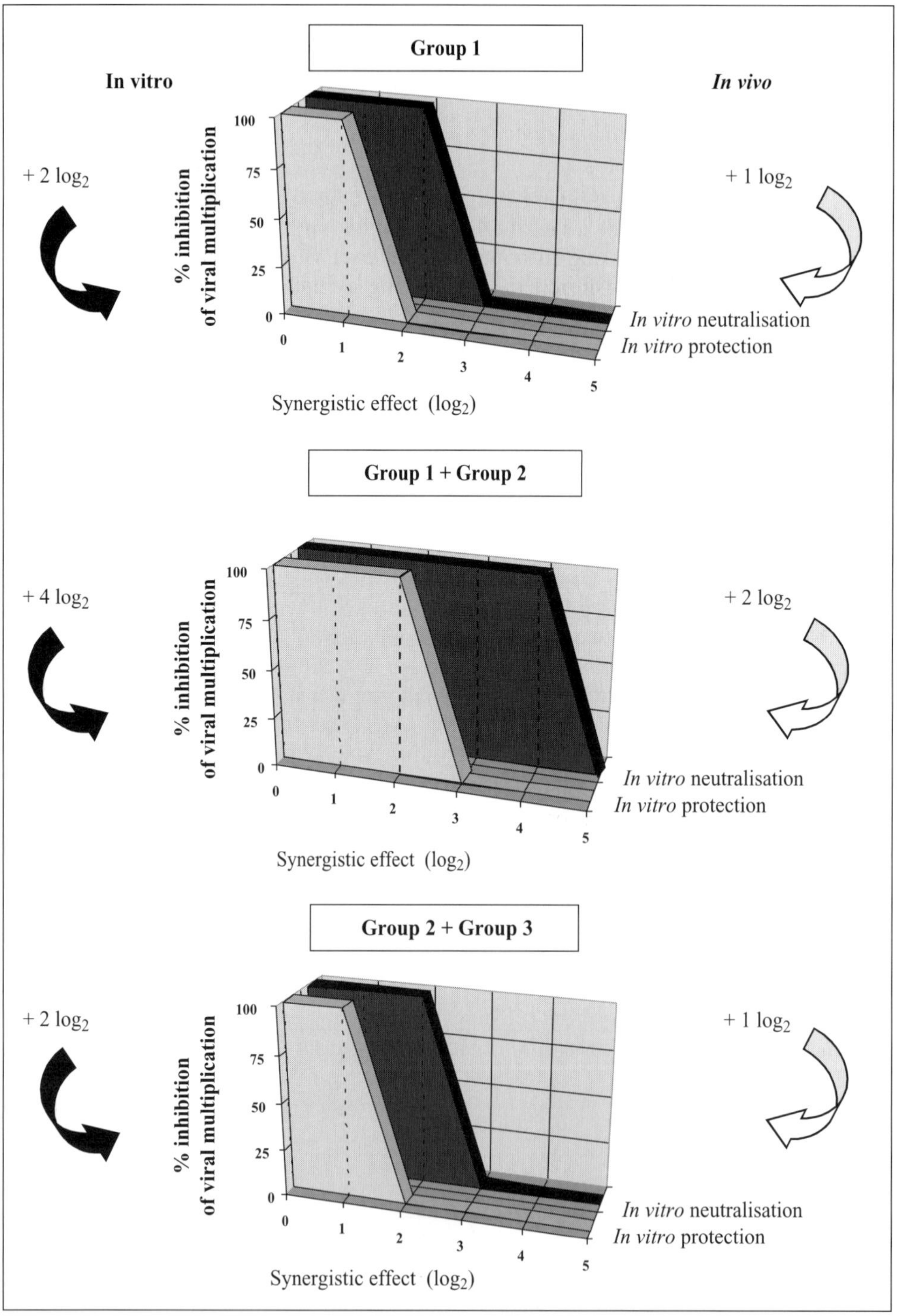

Figure 1. Protection against standardized infection: synergistic effects with different anti-NA MAb pairs.

Protection against lethal infection

The results presented above were obtained in mice challenged under standardised infection conditions, corresponding to one lethal dose. In order to confirm our results regarding the protective efficacy of anti-NA MAbs, mice passively transferred with MAbs were challenged with higher doses of influenza virus ranging from 2 to 10 lethal doses. Group 1 and group 2 anti-NA MAbs were capable of efficiently protecting all mice (6/6) against 5 lethal doses of virus while only 4/6 mice were protected by group 3 anti-NA MAb. It is interesting to notice the presence of histo-pathological lesions in the lungs of passively transferred mice surviving a challenge with 5 lethal doses of virus; such lesions signal viral multiplication in the lungs. None of the different groups of anti-NA MAbs were capable of conferring complete protection to mice when challenged with 10 lethal doses of influenza virus. Nevertheless, pooling MAbs generated a synergistic effect, so that mice could be efficiently protected against 10 lethal doses of virus. As previously mentioned for mice challenged under standardised infection conditions, such a synergistic effect was optimal when MAbs interacting with early stages for the one and late stages of viral cycle for the other(s) were added to the mixture.

Protection against influenza by vaccination of mice with purified NA and/or HA proteins

NA and HA proteins of the X117 reassortant virus were purified by immunochromatography according to Gérentes *et al.* [4]. Groups of 21 mice were vaccinated with one unique intraperitoneal injection (200 µl) of purified protein: NA, HA or NA + HA mixture in presence of complete Freund adjuvant, in order to mimic the situation in human vaccinees. Various antigen doses were tested ranging from 0.25 µg to 4 µg per mouse. Control mice received adjuvant in PBS.

Fifteen days after vaccination, 3 mice per group were sacrificed in order to analyse the immune response and the remaining mice were challenged under either standardised infection conditions (50 MID_{50}/mouse) or lethal infection conditions (2 to 10 LD_{50}/mouse). The protection was evaluated by either MDCK titration of infectious virus in the lung (standardised infection) or monitoring of mice mortality (lethal infection).

Primary immune response of vaccinated mice

In order to study the primary immune response of mice vaccinated with either single or pooled NA/HA glycoproteins, sera were introduced in a series of immunological tests such as NA and HA ELISA on purified protein, hemagglutination inhibition (HI) and neuraminidase inhibition (NI) tests, neutralisation tests and competition ELISA with anti-NA MAbs. The results are summarised in *Table II*.

When vaccinated with purified NA or HA proteins, the ELISA titre of anti-NA/anti-HA antibodies increased linearly with the amount of injected proteins and the titre

Table II. Characterisation of the immune response.

Vaccine doses		ELISA/ml	NI/ml	HI/ml	Standard Nt	Early Nt	Late Nt
Control PBS		< 10	< 10	< 10	< 10	< 10	< 10
NA	≤ 1 µg	40,000	800	< 10	200	< 10	400
	2 µg	80,000	1,600	< 10	400	< 10	800
	4 µg	320,000	3,200	< 10	800	50	1,600
HA	≤ 1 µg	20,000	< 10	400	200	200	< 10
	2 µg	40,000	< 10	800	200	400	< 10
	4 µg	80,000	< 10	1,600	800	800	< 10
NA + *HA*	≤ 3 µg	20,000/*20,000*	400	400	800	200	200
	3 < 4 µg	40,000/*40,000*	800	800	3,200	400	400
	4 µg (2 + 2)	80,000/*40,000*	2,400	800	3,200	400	800

of anti-NA antibodies was twice that of anti-HA antibodies in mice immunised with equal amounts of antigen.

Mice immunised with purified NA did not produce HI antibodies, as expected from the purity of NA preparations, whereas the NI antibodies titres increased from 800 to 3,200 according to the amount of antigen. Mice immunised with purified HA did not produce any NI antibodies, whereas the HI antibodies titres increased from 400 to 1,600 according the amount of antigen.

Depending on the antigen used for immunisation (NA or HA), differences were observed in terms of Nt antibodies. These differences did not appear when introducing immune sera in the "standard" Nt test allowing antigen/antibody contact prior to seeding on cells, since similar amounts of Nt antibody were raised in mice primed with similar HA or NA vaccine doses. In contrast, significant differences were detected when using the Nt tests, which we modified in order to allow the interaction of antibodies with either the early or the late stages of the viral cycle. Depending on the vaccine dose, the NA antigen was shown to generate one unique category of Nt antibodies interacting with the late stages of the viral cycle or two different categories of Nt antibodies interacting with early and late stages of the viral cycle, respectively. On the contrary, irrespective of the vaccine dose, the HA was shown to induce the generation of a unique category of Nt antibodies reacting with the early stages of the viral cycle in mice.

When vaccinated with NA + HA mixtures, mice exhibited serum NA-ELISA and HA-ELISA titres similar to those of mice vaccinated with an equal single dose of HA or NA. In addition, our results showed that there was no antigenic competition between purified NA and HA protein antigens when injected together in mice. Regarding Nt antibodies, a synergistic effect was observed when mice received 4 µg of NA + HA (1:1) instead of 4 µg of HA or NA protein. As expected from the presence of HA in the different pooled vaccine doses, immune sera exhibited both categories of Nt antibodies, irrespective of the amount of total antigen used for vaccinating the mice: early viral stage reacting Nt antibodies were mainly induced by HA while late viral stage reacting Nt antibodies were induced by NA.

In order to monitor the different anti-NA antibody epitope specificities generated in mice vaccinated with pure NA or pooled NA + HA antigen doses, immune sera were introduced in competition-ELISA tests with anti-NA MAbs from the three different groups previously used. The results summarised in *Table III* show that differences in terms of anti-NA antibody specificities were observed as a function of the vaccine dose: while group 1 and group 3 antibodies were found in immune sera independently of the NA vaccine dose, those group 2 antibodies exhibiting the highest neutralising potency were found exclusively in mice having received a ≥ 2 µg dose of NA. When considering the different NA antibodies specificities, which were generated by NA or NA + HA vaccination they ranged as following: group 1 > group 2 ≥ group 3.

Table III. Distribution of anti-NA antibody specificities in post-vaccinal mouse sera.

Vaccine doses	Group 1	Group 2	Group 3	Protection (standardised infection)
NA 1 µg/mouse	++	–	±	–
NA 2 µg/mouse	+++	±	±	Reduction of infection
NA 4 µg/mouse	+++	+	±	+
HA 4 µg/mouse	–	–	–	+
NA + HA 2 + 2 µg/mouse	+++	±	±	+

The last approach we used to characterise the humoral response of mice to NA and/or HA vaccination was the quantification of antibody secreting cells (ASC) in lungs. For this, groups of six mice were immunised with every vaccine formulation and then sacrificed fifteen days later. Pulmonary leukocytes were collected and then introduced into ELISPOT test (adapted from [5]). The mean results were calculated from quadruplicate samples. Similar profiles of ASC distribution were obtained, *i.e.* 78% IgG, 17% IgM, 5% IgA, irrespective of both the vaccine antigen (NA or HA) and the amount of antigen. Nevertheless, the number of ASC for 10^6 leukocytes varied with the amount of antigen, with 100 ASC induced by a 2 µg vaccine dose and 190 ASC induced by a 4 µg vaccine dose; in addition, the number of NA specific ASC was always 5 to 25% lower than that of HA specific ASC. The very low percentage of IgA secreting cells could be related to the intraperitoneal route we used for vaccinating the mice.

Protection of mice conferred by vaccination with NA or HA protein

Mice challenged under standardised infection conditions

The results obtained when using the different antigens and vaccine doses are summarised in *Table IV*. A 4 µg dose of purified NA, HA or HA + NA protein was shown to be necessary for inducing complete protection, due to the prevention of infection in mice challenged under standardised infection conditions. Lower doses of NA or HA antigen did not confer protection to the vaccinated mice, but it is interesting to note that contrary to HA, the 2 µg dose of NA was shown capable of reducing the infection in the lungs to 0.01% of infected controls. Results of virus titration in the lungs were confirmed by histo-pathological observations; under standardised infection, a consolidation of the lungs was observed in infected controls and in NA/HA vaccinated animals in which the immune response was too low to prevent infection.

Table IV. Protection conferred by vaccination (NA/HA) against standardised infection (50 MID_{50}/mouse).

Vaccine doses		Lung infectious titre	Interpretation
Control PBS		$10^{7.3 \pm 0.17}$ $TCID_{50}$/lung	Infection
NA	≤ 1 µg	$10^{7.3 \pm 0.19}$ $TCID_{50}$/lung	Infection
	2 µg	$10^{3.3 \pm 0.26}$ $TCID_{50}$/lung	Reduction of infection
	4 µg	< 10 $TCID_{50}$/lung	Protection
HA	≤ 1 µg	$10^{6.9 \pm 0.14}$ $TCID_{50}$/lung	Infection
	2 µg	$10^{6.6 \pm 0.17}$ $TCID_{50}$/lung	Infection
	4 µg	< 10 $TCID_{50}$/lung	Protection
NA + HA	≤ 3 µg	$10^{6.9 \pm 0.18}$ $TCID_{50}$/lung	Infection
	3 < 4 µg	$10^{4 \pm 0.12}$ $TCID_{50}$/lung	Reduction of infection
	4 µg (2 + 2)	< 10 $TCID_{50}$/lung	Protection

Mice challenged under lethal infection conditions

As shown in *Table V* similar results were obtained when using equivalent amounts of NA, HA or NA + HA proteins. All mice receiving a ≥ 2 µg dose of purified protein were capable of surviving to 2 LD_{50} of virus while a 4 µg protein dose of antigen was required to protect 100% of mice receiving 5 lethal doses. Such a 4 µg protein dose of NA, HA or NA + HA was unable to protect all the animals challenged with 10 lethal doses, since, according to the antigen used for vaccination, 33% to 66% of the vaccinated mice did not survive the infection.

Table V. Protection conferred by vaccination (NA/HA) against lethal infection (% of survivor).

Vaccine doses		Lethal doses		
		2 LD_{50}	5 LD_{50}	10 LD_{50}
Control PBS		0%	0%	0%
NA	2 µg	100%	33%	0%
	4 µg	100%	100%	66%
HA	2 µg	100%	33%	0%
	4 µg	100%	100%	33%
NA + HA	4 µg (2 + 2)	100%	100%	66%

Conclusion

Control of influenza through vaccination is especially difficult due to the fact that the two influenza virus surface glycoproteins, NA and HA, exhibit continual antigenic variations. The currently licensed split inactivated influenza vaccines target chiefly the anti-HA antibody response which is considered as the sole one capable of preventing infection.

In spite of the fact that (i) the immune response to NA lasts longer than the response to HA and (ii) the variations of NA antigen are independent from the HA variations,

NA is still considered as a minor antigen due to earlier evidence that NA-specific immunity is infection permissive over a broad range of antibody levels [6-9].

In the present study, by using two different approaches, the passive transfer of NA specific monoclonal antibodies and the vaccination with NA as purified protein, we have been able to show that NA specific immunity is capable of preventing infection in mice.

Regarding passive immunisation, all different groups of NA specific MAbs protected mice from standardised infection as efficiently as did the HA specific MAb we used as a control and, to our knowledge, it is the first time that anti-NA antibodies were shown to be capable of preventing infection. Nevertheless, significant differences were observed between anti-NA MAbs in terms of their capability to prevent infection when considering their NI activity, as is usually done. Indeed a high NI antibody titre in serum ($\geq$ 100) was necessary for group 1 MAbs to prevent infection while group 2 MAbs diluted to undetectable levels in serum were capable of completely inhibiting viral multiplication in the lungs. When we consider the respective neutralising activity of anti-NA MAbs, group 1 and group 2 antibodies exhibited a similar protection potency with a protective threshold in serum equivalent to a 2-6 Nt titre. In addition, a very interesting and novel observation was that group 1 and group 2 anti-NA MAbs used two different mechanisms to neutralise virus infectivity, interaction with the late stages of the viral cycle, as usually described for the former, and interaction with the early stages of the viral cycle for the latter. These two different pathways of virus neutralisation are responsible for the optimal synergistic effect observed *in vitro* as well as *in vivo* when pooling group 1 and group 2 anti-NA MAbs. Group 1 and group 2 anti-NA MAbs protected mice from lethality when the animals were challenged with five LD_{50} per mouse. These data confirmed the observation of Deroo *et al.* [10] who underlined the important mediator role of circulating anti-NA antibodies in the mechanism by which NA vaccination confers viral resistance.

NA and HA appeared as equivalent immunogens in primary immune response when equal amounts of antigen were given to mice but in addition to the observation of Johansson *et al.* [8] regarding the synthesis of ELISA reacting antibodies we showed that NA and HA induced identical levels of Nt antibodies.

When compared with the anti-HA immune response, the original feature in the anti-NA immune response is the capability of sera from vaccinated mice to neutralise infection as well *in vitro* as *in vivo* by interacting with both the early and late stages of the viral cycle. As expected from the data we obtained with anti-NA MAbs, such a particularity was shown to be due to the fact that group 2 antibodies are one of many anti-NA antibody specificities. Challenging the mice immunised with either purified NA, HA or NA + HA proteins confirmed the evidence obtained from passive immunisation studies, that immunity to NA is capable of protecting mice as efficiently as immunity to HA, by preventing infection of the lungs or mortality of animals in proportion to the number of lethal doses administered to the vaccinees.

In conclusion, our dual approach for analysing the role of anti-NA antibodies in protecting against influenza infection and consequently for determining the right place of NA in influenza vaccines gave us sound arguments for the rehabilitation of the neuraminidase antigen as a full partner in vaccine formulations. The present study clearly shows that (i) NA and HA are equivalent in stimulating antibody response,

(ii) anti-NA antibodies are neutralising and capable of preventing infection, (iii) equivalent monovalent NA/HA vaccine doses are capable to confer similar protection level and (iv) a balanced NA plus HA formulation produced an optimal immune response without antigenic competition and conferred an optimal protection.

Our data confirm and complete those of Johansson *et al.* [11] who reported on the supplementation of conventional influenza A vaccine with purified NA. Therefore we can conclude that a significant improvement in influenza vaccine would probably depend on the readjustment of their NA content by either supplementating split vaccine with purified NA or developing balanced influenza glycoproteins formulations.

References

1. Schulmann JL, Khakpour M, Kilbourne ED. Protective effects of specific immunity to viral neuraminidase on influenza virus infection of mice. *J Virol* 1968; 2: 778-86.
2. Monto AS, Kendal AP. Effect of neuraminidase antibody on Hong Kong influenza. *Lancet* 1973; 24: 623-5.
3. Coleman PM. Neuraminidase. Enzyme and Antigen. In: Krug RM, ed. *The influenza viruses*. New York: Plenum Press, 1989: 175-218.
4. Gérentes L, Kessler N, Thomas G, Aymard M. Simultaneous purification of influenza hemagglutinin and neuraminidase proteins using immunochromatography. *J Virol Meth* 1996; 58: 155-65.
5. Sedgwick JD, Holt PG. A solid-phase immunoenzymatic technique for enumeration of specific antibody secreting-cells. *J Immunol Meth* 1983; 57: 301.
6. Ogra P, Chow T, Beutner K, Rubi E, Demello S, Rizzone C. Clinical and immunologic evaluation of neuraminidase-specific Influenza A vaccine in humans. *J Infect Dis* 1977; 134: 499.
7. Schulman JL, Kilbourne ED. Independent variation in nature of hemagglutinin and neuraminidase antigens of influenza virus: distinctiveness of hemagglutinin antigen of Hong Kong/68 virus. *Proc Natl Acad Sci USA* 1969; 63: 326-33.
8. Johansson BE, Bucher DJ, Kilbourne ED. Purified influenza virus hemagglutinin and neuraminidase are equivalent in stimulation of antibody response but induce contrasting types of immunity to infection. *J Virol* 1989; 63: 1239-46.
9. Schulman JL. The role of anti-neuraminidase antibody in immunity to influenza virus infection. *Bull WHO* 1969; 41: 647-50.
10. Deroo T, Min Jou W, Fiers W. Recombinant neuraminidase vaccine protection against lethal influenza. *Vaccine* 1996; 14: 561-9.
11. Johansson BE, Matthews JT, Kilbourne ED. Supplementation of conventional influenza A vaccine with purified viral neuraminidase results in a balanced and broadened immune response. *Vaccine* 1998; 16: 1009-15.

Paramyxoviruses

Emergence and Control of Zoonotic Ortho- and Paramyxovirus Diseases
B. Dodet, M. Vicari, eds.

Canine distemper virus infections in terrestrial carnivores

Max J. G. Appel[1], Brian A. Summers[2], Richard J. Montali[3]

[1] *James A. Baker Institute for Animal Health*
[2] *Department of Biomedical Sciences, College of Veterinary Medicine, Cornell University, Ithaca, NY, USA*
[3] *Smithsonian National Zoological Park, Washington, DC, USA*

Abstract – Canine distemper virus (CDV) is a member of the *Paramyxoviridae* and has been classified as a morbillivirus together with measles virus, rinderpest virus, peste de petits ruminants virus and now phocine distemper virus, and dolphin and porpoise morbilliviruses. The classification of the newly discovered and related Hendra, Nipah, Tioman, and Menangle viruses is still debated.

Epidemiology

Canine distemper (CD) is an acute or subacute contagious febrile, often fatal disease of dogs and other carnivores with a worldwide distribution that has been known for centuries. The mortality rate in dogs is approximately 50% but it varies greatly between species from subclinical infection to 100% mortality. During the acute phase of the infection virus is shed in all body secretions, most abundant in respiratory exudates. Virus shedding begins approximately seven days post infection. Transmission occurs by aerosol. Virus transmission is also possible during the subacute phase of the disease up to three months after infection. However, fully recovered animals are not persistently infected, do not shed virus and are immune for life [1].

Canine distemper virus affects susceptible dogs and other carnivores of all ages, but puppies are most susceptible when maternal antibody is lost. With a half-life of maternal antibody in puppies of 9 1/2 days [2], they become susceptible between six and 12 weeks of age. Transplacental infection has been reported [3].

Since modified live (ML) virus vaccines for CD became available in the 1960s, the disease in dogs has been under control. However, because of widespread CD outbreaks in wildlife carnivores [4], eradication seems not to be possible. In addition, insufficient vaccination and/or vaccines with low efficacy in certain areas can cause severe disease outbreaks in dog populations. Such examples were reported from Finland [5], Denmark

[6], Greenland [7], Alaska (Preslar, 1997, personal communication), and Indiana, USA [8]. Tens of thousands of mink died from CD in Minnesota and Wisconsin in 1998 after use of a faulty vaccine (unpublished).

Canine distemper virus has a wide host range, which appears to be increasing. Most terrestrial carnivores are susceptible to natural CDV infection *(Table I)*. The morbidity and mortality rate ranges greatly from up to 100% mortality in *Mustelidae* to approximately 25% to 75% mortality in *Canidae* to predominantly subclinical infections in *Hyaenidae* and bears.

Epizootic outbreaks of CD in large cats are a recent phenomenon. The first reported outbreak occurred at the Wildlife Waystation in San Fernando, California in 1992, where 17 lions, tigers, and leopards died from CD. Most animals died after episodes of anorexia, and gastrointestinal and/or respiratory disease followed by seizures. Canine distemper virus was isolated from 3 lions, 3 tigers, and 3 leopards that died or were euthanized when moribund [9]. Virus isolations were also made from 2 raccoons with signs of CD that were trapped at the Waystation.

Table I. Host range of canine distemper in terrestrial carnivores.

Species:	**Reference sources:**
Ailuridae: panda, red panda	[10-12]
Canidae: dogs, foxes, wolves, dingo, coyote, jackal, bush dog, raccoon dog, Cape Hunting dog	[4, 11, 13-32]
Felidae: lion, tiger, leopard	[9, 20, 33-43]
Hyaenidae: hyenas	[37, 44, 45]
Mustelidae: weasel, ferrets, mink, badger, stoat, marten, otter, pole cat, skunk	[11, 13, 14, 20, 29, 32, 46-49]
Procyonidae: raccoon, bassariscus, coati, kinkajou	[11, 14, 20, 50]
Ursidae: polar bear, black bear, grizzly bear	[51-53]
Viverridae: binturong, mongoose, meerkat, masked palm civet	[14, 20, 54, 55]

The second outbreak occurred in the Serengeti National Park, Tanzania, in a large closely monitored lion population in early 1994. It was estimated that one-third of the lions died from CD encephalitis and pneumonia. By August 1994, 85% of the surviving Serengeti lion population had anti-CDV antibodies. The epizootic spread north to lions in the Masai Mara National reserve, Kenya. Hyenas, jackals, bat-eared foxes, and leopards were also affected [37, 42]. Fifty-five percent of the Masai Mara lions were later found to be CDV seropositive [41]. Virus isolations from the Serengeti outbreak were made from a lion, a bat-eared fox, a hyena and from a domestic dog with distemper in a nearby village [37].

Small differences in the H and P genes of CDV were found in the American and African outbreaks [35, 40]. Similar differences have been observed in field isolates from CDV infected dogs [56-60]. Although differences could be demonstrated between CDV isolates from Europe/Africa on one hand and North America on the other [35], the essential observation was that CDV isolates from raccoons and large cats in California and from domestic dogs, hyenas, bat-eared foxes and lions in Tanzania were identical. It appears that CDV was transmitted from infected raccoons to large cats in California and from infected domestic dogs to hyenas and from hyenas to lions in the Serengeti [43]. In contrast to phocine and dolphin distemper virus, which was shown to be different from CDV [59, 61, 62], the CDV involved in outbreaks in large cats were identical to the CDV causing distemper in raccoons and lions in California and in dogs and lions in the Serengeti [9, 35, 37, 40, 42, 44].

Interestingly, we found a significant difference in neutralizing antibody when sera from CDV infected large cats were tested against the Onderstepoort strain, the Rockborn strain of CDV, and against a Vero cell adapted lion isolate of CDV. Responses to the Rockborn strain and the lion isolate were similar while a response to the Onderstepoort strain was considerably delayed [9]. The Onderstepoort strain of CDV is an atypical strain of CDV. Unfortunately, it has frequently been used for comparison with field isolates.

Isolated cases of CD in large cats have been reported earlier [33, 34] and retrospectively CDV antigen was found in lion and tiger tissues in Switzerland [38]. However, the epizootic proportion of the recent CD outbreaks in large cats is difficult to explain. Domestic cats become subclinically infected with CDV and they do not shed virus [63]. Initially we speculated that a dual infection with FIV and CDV could cause fatal disease in large cats. Antibody to FIV was found in only one lion in California, but in all CDV infected lions in the Serengeti [9, 42, 64] regardless whether they recovered or succumbed to CDV infection. Another possibility is enhanced exposure of large cats to CDV infected carnivores. However, that is unlikely as well, because distemper outbreaks in zoos in canids earlier this century were common but large cats were not involved.

The CDV isolates both from California and from the Serengeti had characteristics of virulent CDV in tissue culture. They replicated readily in dog lymphocyte culture [65] but not in dog kidney or Vero cells. Canine distemper virus isolates from California caused subclinical infection in domestic cats. However, the virus was first adapted and passaged in Vero cells, which can attenuate virulent virus [36]. Both CDV isolates from California and from the Serengeti caused fatal infections in domestic ferrets [49]. There appeared to be a difference in the incubation time and in the pathogenicity. In laboratory studies using SPF beagle dogs "biotypes" of CDV isolates showed different incubation periods and a different pathology: acute encephalitis with predominantly grey matter involvement or with predominantly white matter involvement with demyelination and subacute disease [66]. The incubation time in ferrets differed as well: the Snyder Hill strain of CDV which induced "grey matter disease" in dogs, killed ferrets in 10-14 days while ferrets exposed to the A75-17 strain of CDV, which caused "white matter disease" in dogs became moribund between 20 and 28 days after inoculation [Appel, unpublished].

Another unexpected episode of canine distemper occurred in 1989 in javelinas (collared peccaries, *Tayassu tajacu*) in Arizona. Signs of encephalitis (blindness, myoclonus, reluctance to move, circling) were observed with significant mortality. Histologic lesions were confined to the CNS. The isolated virus was identical to CDV when tested with monoclonal antibodies [67]. In an earlier study, javelinas, which belong to the *Tayassuidae* showed clinical signs when inoculated with rinderpest virus [68]. In contrast, domestic pigs *(Suidae)* were previously found to be susceptible to infection with CDV [63] and rinderpest virus [68] without developing disease. Both viruses replicate in lymphatic tissues of pigs without causing clinical signs and virus shedding.

Diseases induced with modified live CDV vaccines

The introduction of ML-CDV vaccines in the 1960s reduced the incidence of distemper in dogs significantly. Both the chicken embryo adapted [69] and the canine cell culture adapted vaccines [70] have been successful. It appears that the chicken embryo adapted vaccine is safer but the efficacy of the cell culture adapted vaccine is superior. In exceptional cases, a post-vaccinal fatal encephalitis may occur in puppies seven to 14 days after vaccination with the tissue culture vaccine. Lesions are usually most severe in the pontomedullary grey matter [1, 71]. CD virus can be isolated from these cases in canine kidney cell culture without adaptation, consistent with a vaccinal strain.

While both types of ML-CDV vaccines in general are safe for the immunization of dogs, they can induce fatal disease in a variety of wildlife and zoo animals [72, 20]. There are several species that can be safely vaccinated with the egg adapted vaccine, as for example the gray fox [15], bush dogs, maned wolves, or fennec foxes [11, 73, 74]. Cell culture adapted CDV vaccines are fatal for these and other CD susceptible species.

The potential virulence of ML-CDV virus in different carnivores became apparent in the mid-1970s. Vaccine-induced distemper was reported in 1976 almost simultaneously in red pandas [10] and in black-footed ferrets [46]. Similar episodes were later reported in kinkajous [50], in African cape hunting dogs [16, 21, 75], and in European mink [76]. Clinical signs of post-vaccinal CD usually consist of anorexia, mucopurulent ocular and nasal discharge followed by seizures and death.

For the past 20 years, we, at the Baker Institute, have produced inactivated CDV vaccine for zoo animals and for the endangered black-footed ferrets in Wyoming because inactivated CDV vaccine was not available in North America. A recombinant CDV-canarypox virus is now on the market [77] that has been tested in black-footed ferret-polecat crosses and can replace the inactivated vaccine.

Diagnosis

Most of the information available for the diagnosis of CD comes from dogs. The course of the disease is similar in wildlife species. Most diagnostic tests, therefore, would apply to other carnivores as well.

Clinical signs of respiratory, gastro-intestinal and neurological disease are the first step for a diagnosis. Haematologic findings during the acute phase of the disease include lymphopenia caused by lymphoid depletion, which results in immunosuppression [78]. Inclusion bodies can be found by examination of stained peripheral blood films or by fluorescent antibody (FA) staining [79, 80]. Serum biochemistry changes are usually non-specific.

Cytologic smears prepared from conjunctival, tonsillar, or genital epithelium, from bronchial washings, or from urine sediment [81] can be used for direct FA staining, immunocytochemistry, or histochemical staining for inclusion bodies. Positive results are usually found during the first 2 or 3 weeks of the disease. Negative results are not sufficient to rule out distemper. During the subacute phase, and frequently in dogs with CD neurological disease, CDV specific antibody develops in the host and these tests usually become negative. In the presence of antibody, virus may persist in the CNS, skin, foot pads, and uvea [82] and can be demonstrated by direct FA or immunocytochemistry in biopsies [79, 83].

Dogs and other carnivores may die or recover before the virus reaches the CNS. However, in most cases, encephalitis is involved. Inflammatory changes in the CNS are indicators for CD [84, 85]. The CSF protein content is usually increased, primarily as CDV specific IgG [86-88]. Increased anti-CDV IgG in the CSF offers definitive evidence for distemper encephalitis, provided there is no leakage in the blood/brain barrier. The serum/CSF antibody ratio can be compared with antibody to canine adenovirus or canine parvovirus [89]. Leakage of albumin into the CSF in distemper encephalitis has been reported [88, 90]. Lymphocyte pleocytosis is a common finding [91, 92]. Cells in the CSF can be stained by FA or immunocytochemistry for CDV antigen [93]. As long as virus persists in the CNS, interferon can be found in the CSF [94]. However, few diagnostic laboratories are prepared to test for canine interferon.

Serology is of limited value for the diagnosis of CD unless paired serum samples are available. During the early phase of the disease antibody titers are usually negative. Non-neutralizing antibody can be detected by ELISA before neutralizing antibody with the appearance of H and F antibody can be detected [95]. High serum neutralizing titers [96] protect from infection but are often present in dogs with persistent infection. In the subacute phase of the disease, high serum neutralizing antibody titers can be found that cannot be differentiated from vaccine titers. A positive IgM titer would be an indication of CD provided the dog has not been vaccinated within the last three weeks [97]. An immunocapture ELISA test has been used to detect viral antigen in serum and CSF [98]. Such a test would be valuable for a rapid diagnosis.

Virus isolation can be attempted during the acute phase of CD from buffy coat cells, bronchial washings, urine sediment, or conjunctival or tonsillar swabs. Isolation of virulent CDV can best be accomplished in mitogen stimulated buffy coat cells from healthy dogs or ferrets [65], or in dog or ferret macrophage cultures [99]. Virulent CDV does not readily replicate in epithelial monolayers without adaptation. This observation is of value for the differentiation of virulent CDV *versus* vaccine induced distemper. Vaccine virus replicates readily in epithelial monolayers.

More recently, PCR and nucleic acid hybridization studies have been performed to detect virus nucleic acid in infected cells and tissues [100-103]. These tests will be used more commonly in the future, provided the tests are well controlled and specific.

Post mortem histopathology and the demonstration of characteristic lesions with cells harboring inclusion bodies and CDV antigen by FA and immunocytochemistry in tissue sections determine the diagnosis. CDV monoclonal antibody (kindly provided by Claes Örvell [104]), is superior to polyclonal antibody for the staining of tissue sections by FA or immunocytochemistry.

Public health aspects

Cook *et al.* [105] suggested that there might be an association between CD in dogs and multiple sclerosis (MS). This hypothesis has not been confirmed [106, 107]. It is very unlikely for the following reasons: before ML-CDV vaccines became available in the 1960s, CD in dogs was very common worldwide. There was a dramatic reduction of CD thereafter. If CDV is involved in MS with any frequency, a decline in MS cases should be noticed after more than 30 years. The incubation period of MS, if caused by an infectious agent, is shorter. Unfortunately, there is no reduction in MS cases worldwide.

Paget's disease, a focal destructive disease of bone common in elderly people in the United States and Europe, has been linked to a paramyxovirus including CDV. By *in situ* hybridization and PCR, CDV transcripts were found in osteoclasts, osteoblasts, and osteocytes of Paget's disease patients [108-110]. Similar findings were reported in bone cells from dogs with CD [111, 112]. Canine distemper associated metaphyseal bone lesions were found in young dogs after experimental infection [113]. However, other studies have failed to support the hypothesis of CDV involvement in Paget's disease [114, 115].

References

1. Greene CE, Appel M. Canine distemper. In: Greene CE, ed. *Infectious Diseases of the Dog and Cat*, 2nd edition. Philadelphia: W.B. Saunders, 1998: 9-22.
2. Baker JA, Robson DS, Gillespie JH, *et al.* A nomograph that predicts the age to vaccinate puppies against distemper. *Cornell Vet* 1959; 49: 158-67.
3. Krakowka S, Confer A, Koestner A. Evidence for transplacental transmission of canine distemper virus: two case reports. *Am J Vet Res* 1974; 35: 1251-3.
4. Murray DL, Kapke CA, Evermann JF, Fuller TK. Infectious disease and the conservation of free-ranging large carnivores. *Anim Conservat* 1999; 2: 241-54.
5. Ek-Kommonen C, Sihvonen L, Pekkanen K, *et al.* Outbreak of canine distemper in vaccinated dogs in Finland. *Vet Record* 1997; 141: 380-3.
6. Blixenkrone-Møller M, Svansson V, Have P, *et al.* Studies on manifestations of canine distemper virus infection in an urban dog population. *Vet Microbiol* 1993; 37: 163-73.

7. Bohm J, Blixenkrone-Møller M, Lund E. A serious outbreak of canine distemper among sled-dogs in northern Greenland. *Arctic Med Res* 1989; 48: 195-203.
8. Johnson R, Glickman LT, Emerick TJ, Patronek GJ. Canine distemper infection in pet dogs: I. Surveillance in Indiana during a suspected outbreak. *J Am Anim Hosp Assoc* 1995; 31: 223-9.
9. Appel MJG, Yates RA, Foley GL, *et al.* Canine distemper epizootic in lions, tigers, and leopards in North America. *J Vet Diagn Invest* 1994; 6: 277-88.
10. Bush M, Montali RJ, Brownstein D, *et al.* Vaccine-induced canine distemper in a lesser panda. *J Am Vet Med Assoc* 1976; 169: 959-60.
11. Montali RJ, Bartz CR, Bush M. Canine distemper virus. In: Appel M, ed. *Virus Infections of Carnivores.* Amsterdam: Elsevier Science Publishers, 1987: 437-43.
12. Mainka SA, Xianmeng Q, Tingmei H, Appel MJ. Serologic survey of giant pandas *(Ailuropoda melanoleuca)* and domestic dogs and cats in the Wolong Reserve, China. *J Wildl Dis* 1994; 30: 86-9.
13. Appel M, Gillespie JE. Canine distemper monograph. In: Gard S, Hallauer C, Meyer KF, eds. *Handbook of Virus Research.* New York: Springer-Verlag, 1972: 34-63.
14. Budd J. Distemper. In: Davis JW, Karstad LH, Trainer DO, eds. *Infectious Diseases of Wild Mammals.* Ames, IA: The Iowa State University Press, 1981: 31-44.
15. Halbrooks RD, Swango LJ, Schnurrenberger PR, *et al.* Response of gray foxes to modified live-virus canine distemper vaccine. *J Am Vet Med Assoc* 1981; 179: 1170-4.
16. McCormick AE. Canine distemper in African cape hunting dogs *(Lycaon pictus)* – possibly vaccine induced. *J Zoo Anim Med* 1983; 14: 66-71.
17. Nicholson WS, Hill EP. Mortality in grey foxes from east-central Alabama. *J Wildl Manag* 1984; 48: 1429-32.
18. Guo W, Evermann JF, Foreyt WJ, *et al.* Canine distemper virus in coyotes: a serologic survey. *J Am Vet Med Assoc* 1986; 189: 1099-1100.
19. Appel MJ. Canine distemper virus. In: Horzinek M, ed. *Virus Infections of Carnivores.* Vol. 1: Virus Infections of Vertebrates. Amsterdam: Elsevier Science Publishers, 1987: 133-59.
20. Appel MJG, Summers BA. Pathogenicity of morbilliviruses for terrestrial carnivores. *Vet Microbiol* 1995; 44: 187-91.
21. Durchfeld B, Baumgärtner W, Herbst W, Brahm R. Vaccine-associated canine distemper infection in a litter of African hunting dogs *(Lycaon pictus). Zentralbl Veterinarmed* [B] 1990; 37: 203-12.
22. Gese EM, Schultz RD, Rongstad OJ, Andersen DE. Prevalence of antibodies against canine parvovirus and canine distemper virus in wild coyotes in southeastern Colorado. *J Wildl Dis* 1991; 27: 320-3.
23. Holtzman S, Conroy MJ, Davidson WR. Diseases, parasites and survival of coyotes in south-central Georgia. *J Wildl Dis* 1992; 28: 572-80.
24. Machida N, Kiryu K, Oh-ishi K, *et al.* Pathology and epidemiology of canine distemper in raccoon dogs *(Nyctereutes procyonides). J Comp Pathol* 1993; 108: 383-92.
25. Alexander KA, Appel MJG. African wild dogs *(Lycaon pictus)* endangered by a canine distemper epizootic among domestic dogs near the Masai Mara National Reserve, Kenya. *J Wildl Dis* 1994; 30: 481-5.
26. Alexander KA, Kat PW, Wayne RK, Fuller TK. Serologic survey of selected canine pathogens among free-ranging jackals in Kenya. *J Wildl Dis* 1994; 30: 486-91.
27. Johnson MR, Boyd DK, Pletscher DH. Serologic investigations of canine parvovirus and canine distemper in relation to wolf *(Canis lupus)* pup mortalities. *J Wildl Dis* 1994; 30: 270-3.
28. Anderson EC. Morbillivirus infections in wildlife (in relation to their population biology and disease control in domestic animals). *Vet Microbiol* 1995; 44: 319-32.
29. van Moll P, Alldinger S, Baumgärtner W, Adami M. Distemper in wild carnivores: An epidemiological, histological and immunocytochemical study. *Vet Microbiol* 1995; 44: 193-9.
30. Creel S, Creel NM, Munson L, *et al.* Serosurvey for selected viral diseases and demography of African wild dogs in Tanzania. *J Wildlife Dis* 1997; 33: 823-32.
31. Laurenson K, Van Heerden J, Stander P, Van Vuuren MJ. Seroepidemiological survey of sympatric domestic and wild dogs *(Lycaon pictus)* in Tsumkwe District, northeastern Namibia. *Onderstepoort J Vet Res* 1997; 64: 313-6.
32. Frölich K, Czupalla O, Haas L, *et al.* Epizootiological investigations of canine distemper virus in free-ranging carnivores from Germany. *Vet Microbiol* 2000; 74: 283-92.
33. Blythe LL, Schmitz JA, Roelke M, Skinner S. Chronic encephalomyelitis caused by canine distemper virus in a Bengal tiger. *J Am Vet Med Assoc* 1983; 183: 1159-62.
34. Gould DH, Fenner WR. Paramyxovirus-like nucleocapsids associated with encephalitis in a captive Siberian tiger. *J Am Vet Med Assoc* 1983; 183: 1319-22.

35. Harder TC, Kenter M, Appel MJG, *et al.* Phylogenetic evidence of canine distemper virus in Serengeti's lions. *Vaccine* 1995; 13: 521-3.
36. Harder TC, Kenter M, Vos H, *et al.* Canine distemper virus from diseased large felids: biological properties and phylogenetic relationships. *J Gen Virol* 1996; 77: 397-405.
37. Roelke-Parker ME, Munson L, Packer C, *et al.* A canine distemper virus epidemic in Serengeti lions *(Panthera leo)*. *Nature* 1996; 379: 441-5.
38. Myers DL, Zurbriggen A, Lutz H, Pospischil A. Distemper: Not a new disease in lions and tigers. *Clin Diagn Lab Immunol* 1997; 4: 180-4.
39. Van Vuuren MJ, Stylianedes E, du Rand A. The precence of viral infections in lions and leopards in southern Africa. Proceedings of a symposium on lions and leopards as game ranch animals, Onderstepoort, South Africa, 1997: 168-73.
40. Carpenter MA, Appel MJG, Roelke-Parker ME, *et al.* Genetic characterization of canine distemper virus in Serengeti carnivores. *Vet Immunol Immunopathol* 1998; 65: 259-66.
41. Kock R, Chalmers WS, Mwanzia J, *et al.* Canine distemper antibodies in lions of the Masai Mara [published erratum appears in *Vet Record* 1998; 142 (26): 721]. *Vet Record* 1998; 142: 662-5.
42. Packer C, Altizer S, Appel M, *et al.* Viruses of the Serengeti: patterns of infection and mortality in African lions. *J Anim Ecol* 1999; 68: 1161-78.
43. Cleaveland S, Appel MGJ, Chalmers WSK, *et al.* Serological and demographic evidence for domestic dogs as a source of canine distemper virus infection for Serengeti wildlife. *Vet Microbiol* 2000; 72: 217-27.
44. Alexander KA, Kat PW, Frank LG, *et al.* Evidence of canine distemper virus infection among free-ranging spotted hyenas *(Crocuta crocuta)* in the Masai Mara, Kenya. *J Zoo Wildl Med* 1995; 26: 201-6.
45. Haas L, Hofer H, East M, *et al.* Canine distemper virus infection in Serengeti spotted hyaenas. *Vet Microbiol* 1996; 49: 147-52.
46. Carpenter JW, Appel MJG, Erickson RC, Novilla MN. Fatal vaccine-induced canine distemper virus infection in black-footed ferrets. *J Am Vet Med Assoc* 1976; 169: 961-4.
47. Woolf A, Gremillion-Smith C, Evans RH. Evidence of canine distemper virus infection in skunks negative for antibody against rabies virus. *J Am Vet Med Assoc* 1986; 198: 1086-8.
48. Williams ES, Thorne ET, Appel MJG, Belitsky DW. Canine distemper in black-footed ferrets *(Mustela Nigripes)* from Wyoming. *J Wildlife Dis* 1988; 24: 385-98.
49. Evermann JF, Leathers CW, Gorham JR, McKeirnan AJ, Appel MJG. Pathogenesis of two strains of lion *(Panthera leo)* morbillivirus in ferrets *(Mustela putorius furo)*. *Vet Pathol* 2001; 38: 311-6.
50. Kazacos KR, Thacker HL, Shivaprasad HL. Vaccination-induced distemper in kinkajous. *J Am Vet Med Assoc* 1981; 179: 1166-9.
51. Schönbauer M. Perinatal distemper infection of three polor bears *(Ursus maritimus)* and one spectacled bear *(Tremarctos ornatus)*. *Proc Intl Symp Dis Zoo An* 1984; 26: 131-6.
52. Follmann EH, Garner GW, Evermann JF, *et al.* Serologic evidence for the occurrence of morbillivirus infection in polar bears from Alaska and Russia. *Vet Rec* 1996; 138: 615-8.
53. Chomel BB, Kasten RW, Chappuis G, *et al.* Serological survey of selected canine viral pathogens and zoonoses in grizzly bears *(Ursus arctos horribilis)* and black bears *(Ursus americanus)* from Alaska. *Rev Sci Tech Off Int Epiz* 1998; 17: 756-66.
54. Machida N, Izumisawa N, Nakamura J, Kirgu K. Canine distemper virus infection in a masked palm civet *(Paguma larvata)*. *J Comp Pathol* 1992; 107: 439-43.
55. Hur K, Bae JS, Choi JH, *et al.* Canine distemper virus infection in binturongs *(Arctictis binturong)*. *J Comp Path* 1999; 121: 295-9.
56. Bolt G, Jensen TD, Gottschalck E, *et al.* Genetic diversity of the attachment (H) protein gene of current field isolates of canine distemper virus. *J Gen Virol* 1997; 78: 367-72.
57. Haas L, Martens W, Greiser-Wilke I, *et al.* Analysis of the haemagglutinin gene of current wild-type canine distemper virus isolates from Germany. *Virus Res* 1997; 48: 165-71.
58. Iwatsuki K, Miyashita N, Yoshida E, *et al.* Molecular and phylogenetic analyses of the hemagglutinin (H) proteins of field isolates of canine distemper virus from naturally infected dogs. *J Gen Virol* 1997; 78: 373-80.
59. Barrett T. Morbillivirus infections, with special emphasis on morbillivirus of carnivores. *Vet Microbiol* 1999; 69: 3-13.
60. Mochizuki M, Hashimoto M, Hagiwara S, *et al.* Genotypes of canine distemper virus determined by analysis of the hemagglutinin genes of recent isolates from dogs in Japan. *J Clin Microbiol* 1999; 37: 2936-42.
61. Kennedy S. Morbillivirus infections in aquatic animals. *J Comp Lab Immunol* 1997; 4: 180-4.

62. Barrett T, Visser IKG, Mamaev L, *et al.* Dolphin and porpoise morbilliviruses are genetically distinct from phocine distemper virus. *Virology* 1993; 193: 1010-2.
63. Appel M, Sheffy BE, Percy DH, Gaskin JM. Canine distemper virus in domesticated cats and pigs. *Am J Vet Res* 1974: 35: 803-6.
64. Olmsted RA, Langley R, Roelke ME, *et al.* Worldwide prevalence of lentivirus infection in wild feline species: epidemiologic and phylogenetic aspects. *J Virol* 1992; 66: 6008-18.
65. Appel MJG, Pearce-Kelling S, Summers BA. Dog lymphocyte cultures facilitate the isolation and growth of virulent canine distemper virus. *J Vet Diagn Invest* 1992; 4: 258-63.
66. Summers BA, Greisen HA, Appel MJG. Canine distemper encephalomyelitis: variation with virus strain. *J Comp Pathol* 1984; 94: 65-75.
67. Appel MJG, Reggiardo C, Summers BA, *et al.* Canine distemper virus infection and encephalitis in javelinas (collared peccaries). *Arch Virol* 1991; 119: 147-52.
68. Dardiri AH, Yedloutschnig RJ, Taylor WD. Clinical and serologic response of American white-collored peccaries to African swine fever, foot-and-mouth disease, vesicular stomatitis, vesicular exanthema of swine, hog cholera, and rinderpest viruses. In: *Proceedings 73rd Annual Meeting US Animal Health Assoc.*, 1969: 437-52.
69. Haig DA. Canine distemper-immunization with avianised virus. *Onderstepoort J Vet Res* 1956; 27: 19-53.
70. Rockborn G. An attenuated strain of canine distemper virus in tissue culture. *Nature (London)* 1959; 184: 822.
71. Hartley WJ. A post-vaccinal inclusion body encephalitis in dogs. *Vet Pathol* 1974; 11: 301-12.
72. Montali RJ, Cambre RC, Sutherland-Smith M, Appel MJG. Vaccination against canine distemper in exotic carnivores: successes and failures. In: Junge, ed. *Proc Am Assoc Zoo Vet*. Pittsburgh, PA, 1994: 340-4.
73. Thomas-Baker B. Vaccination-induced distemper in maned wolves, vaccination-induced corneal opacity in a maned wolf. *Proc Am Assoc Zoo Vet, Ann Rep*, Scottsdale, AZ, 1985, 53.
74. McInnes EF, Burroughs RE, Duncan NM. Possible vaccine-induced canine distemper in a South American bush dog *(Speothos venaticus)*. *J Wildlife Dis* 1992; 28: 614-7.
75. VanHeerden J, Bainbridge N, Burroughs REJ, Kriek NPJ. Distemper-like disease and encephalitozoonosis in wild dogs *(Lycaon pictus)*. *J Wildlife Dis* 1989; 25: 70-5.
76. Sutherland-Smith MR, Rideout BA, Mikolon AB, *et al.* Vaccine-induced canine distemper in european mink, *Mustela Lutreola*. *J Zoo Wildl Med* 1997; 28: 312-8.
77. Pardo MC, Bauman JE, Mackowiak M. Protection of dogs against canine distemper by vaccination with a canarypox virus recombinant expressing canine distemper virus fusion and hemagglutinin glycoproteins. *Am J Vet Res* 1997; 58: 833-6.
78. Krakowka S, Cockerell G, Koestner A. Effects of canine distemper virus infection on lymphoid function *in vitro* and *in vivo*. *Infect Immun* 1975; 11: 1069-78.
79. Appel M. Pathogenesis of canine distemper. *Am J Vet Res* 1969; 30: 1167-82.
80. Shen DT, Gorham JR, Pedersen V. Viruria in dogs infected with canine distemper. *Vet Med Sm Anim Clin* 1981; 76: 1175-7.
81. Brown RAL, Morrow A, Heron I, Chong SN. Immunocytological confirmation of a diagnosis of canine distemper using cells in urine. *J Sm Anim Prac* 1987; 28: 845-51.
82. Summers BA, Greisen HA, Appel MJG. Does virus persist in the uvea in multiple sclerosis, as in canine distemper encephalomyelitis? *Lancet* 1983; 2: 372-5.
83. Haines DM, Martin CL, Chelack BJ, *et al.* Immunohistochemical detection of canine distemper virus in haired skin, nasal mucosa, and footpad epithelium: a method for antimortem diagnosis of infection. *J Vet Diagn Invest* 1999; 11: 396-9.
84. Tipold A, Vandevelde M, Jaggy A. Neurological manifestations of canine distemper virus infection. *J Sm Anim Pract* 1992; 33: 466-70.
85. Tipold A. Diagnosis of inflammatory and infectious diseases of the central nervous system in dogs: a retrospective study. *J Vet Int Med* 1995; 9: 304-14.
86. Cutler RW, Averill DRJ. Cerebrospinal fluid gamma globulins in canine distemper encephalitis. An immunoelectrophoretic study. *Neurology* 1969; 19: 1111-4.
87. Johnson GC, Fenner WR, Krakowka S. Production of immunoglobulin G and increased antiviral antibody in cerebrospinal fluid of dogs with delayed-onset canine distemper viral encephalitis. *J Neuroimmunol* 1988; 17: 237-51.

88. Sorjonen DC, Cox NR, Swango CJ. Electrophoretic determination of albumin and gamma globulin concentration in the cerebrospinal fluid of dogs with encephalomyelitis attributable to canine distemper virus infection: 13 cases (1980-1087). *J Am Vet Med Assoc* 1989; 195: 977-80.
89. Tipold A, Pfister H, Vandevelde M. Determination of the IgG index for the detection of intrathecal immunoglubulin synthesis in dogs using an ELISA. *Res Vet Sci* 1993; 54: 40-4.
90. Johnson GC, Krakowka S, Axthelm MK. Albumin leakage into cerebrospinal fluid of dogs lethally infected with R252 canine distemper virus. *J Neuroimmunol* 1987; 14: 61-74.
91. Abate O, Bollo E, Lotti D, Bo S. Cytological, immunocytochemical and biochemical cerebrospinal fluid investigations in selected central nervous system disorders of dogs. *Zentralbl Veterinarmed* [B] 1998; 45: 73-85.
92. Vandevelde M, Spano JS. Cerebrospinal fluid cytology in canine neurologic disease. *Am J Vet Res* 1977; 38: 1827-32.
93. Alleman AR, Christopher MM, Steiner DA, Homer BL. Identification of intracytoplasmic inclusion bodies in mononuclear cells from the cerebrospinal fluid of a dog with canine distemper. *Vet Pathol* 1992; 29: 84-5.
94. Tsai SC, Summers BA, Appel MJ. Interferon in cerebrospinal fluid: A marker for viral persistence in canine distemper encephalomyelitis. *Arch Virol* 1982; 72: 257-65.
95. Rima BK, Duffy N, Mitchell WJ, *et al.* Correlation between humoral immune responses and presence of virus in the CNS in dogs experimentally infected with canine distemper virus. *Arch Virol* 1991; 121: 1-8.
96. Appel M, Robson DA. A microneutralization test for canine distemper virus. *Am J Vet Res* 1973; 34: 1459-63.
97. Blixenkrone-Møller M, Pedersen IR, Appel MJ, Griot C. Detection of IgM antibodies against canine distemper virus in dog and mink sera employing enzyme-linked immunosorbent assay (ELISA). *J Vet Diagn Invest* 1991; 3: 3-9.
98. Gemma T, Iwatsuki K, Shin YS, *et al.* Serological analysis of canine distemper virus using an immunocapture ELISA. *J Vet Med Sci* 1996; 58: 791-4.
99. Appel M, Jones OR. Use of alveolar macrophages for cultivation of canine distemper virus. *Proc Soc Exp Bio Med* 1967; 126: 571-4.
100. Zurbriggen A, Muller C, Vandevelde M. *In situ* hybridization of virulent canine distemper virus in brain tissue using digoxigenin-labeled probes. *Am J Vet Res* 1993; 54: 1457-61.
101. Shin Y, Mori T, Okita M, *et al.* Detection of canine distemper virus nucleocapsid protein gene in canine peripheral blood mononuclear cells by RT-PCR. *J Vet Med Sci* 1995; 57: 439-45.
102. Grone A, Frisk AL, Baumgärtner W. Cytokine mRNA expression in whole blood samples from dogs with natural canine distemper virus infection. *Vet Immunol Immunopathol* 1998; 65: 11-27.
103. Frisk AL, Konig M, Moritz A, Baumgärtner W. Detection of canine distemper virus nucleoprotein RNA by reverse transcription-PCR using serum, whole blood, and cerebrospinal fluid from dogs with distemper. *J Clin Microbiol* 1999; 37: 3634-43.
104. Örvell C, Sheshberadaran H, Norrby E. Preparation and characterization of monoclonal antibodies directed against four structural components of canine distemper virus. *J Gen Virol* 1985; 66: 443-56.
105. Cook SD, Rohowsky-Kochan C, Bansil S, Dowling PC. Evidence for multiple sclerosis as an infectious disease. *Acta Neurol Scand Suppl* 1995; 161: 34-42.
106. Kurtzke JF, Hyllested K, Arbuckle JD, *et al.* Multiple sclerosis in the Faroe Islands. IV. The lack of a relationship between canine distemper and the epidemics of MS. *Acta Neurol Scand* 1988; 78: 484-500.
107. Hodge MJ, Wolfson C. Canine distemper virus and multiple sclerosis. *Neurology* 1997; 49: S62-S6.
108. Gordon MT, Anderson DC, Sharpe PT. Canine distemper virus localised in bone cells of patients with Paget's Disease. *Bone* 1991; 12: 195-201.
109. Gordon MT, Mee AP, Anderson DC, Sharpe PT. Canine distemper virus transcripts sequenced from pagetic bone. *Bone Miner* 1992; 19: 159-74.
110. Mee AP, Dixon JA, Hoyland JA, *et al.* Detection of canine distemper virus in 100% of Paget's disease samples by *in situ*-reverse transcriptase-polymerase chain reaction. *Bone* 1998; 23: 171-5.
111. Mee AP, Webber DM, May C, *et al.* Detection of canine distemper virus in bone cells in the metaphyses of distemper-infected dogs. *J Bone Miner Res* 1992; 7: 829-34.
112. Mee AP, Gordon MT, May C, *et al.* Canine distemper virus transcripts detected in the bone cells of dogs with metaphyseal osteopathy. *Bone* 1993; 14: 59-67.

113. Baumgärtner W, Boyce RW, Weisbrode SE, *et al.* Histologic and immunocytochemical characterization of canine distemper-associated metaphyseal bone lesions in young dogs following experimental infection. *Vet Pathol* 32: 702-9.
114. Ralston SH, Digiovine FS, Gallacher SJ, *et al.* Failure to detect paramyxovirus sequences in Paget's disease of bone using the polymerase chain reaction. *J Bone Miner Res* 1991; 6: 1243-8.
115. Fraser WD. Paget's disease of bone. *Curr Opin Rheumatol* 1997; 9: 347-54.

Emergence and Control of Zoonotic Ortho- and Paramyxovirus Diseases
B. Dodet, M. Vicari, eds.

Morbillivirus outbreaks among aquatic mammals

Albert D.M.E. Osterhaus
Institute of Virology, Erasmus University, Rotterdam, The Netherlands

In 1988, the seal populations of northwestern Europe suffered heavy losses due to an apparent newly emerging infectious disease [1]. About 50% of the harbour seal *(Phoca vitulina)* population died, with symptoms that varied greatly depending on the geographical area. In some areas respiratory symptoms predominated, whereas in other areas gastrointestinal or neurological symptoms were most frequently seen. The combined symptoms found throughout the epidemic indicated that a generalised profound immune suppression was the basis of the observed pathogenesis. Although it was widely speculated that factors like environmental pollution and food shortage played a major role in this outbreak, based on the epidemiological data, our working hypothesis was that an infectious agent was the primary cause. Besides a plethora of bacteria, several viruses were isolated from the animals. Some of these had previously been identified, such as an alphaherpesvirus [2] and an ortho- as well as parapoxviruses [3], whereas others, such as a picornavirus [1], had not been found previously. Serological studies revealed that the primary cause of the outbreak was probably a morbillivirus: virtually all the animals that had suffered from the disease and recovered, developed serum antibodies that neutralised canine distemper virus (CDV) [4, 5]. Experimental infection of SPF dogs with a newly discovered morbillivirus (phocine distempervirus: PDV) that was isolated from seals that had died during the outbreak, resulted in a mild form of canine distemper. Final proof that PDV was indeed the primary cause of the outbreak, came from a vaccination experiment: harbour seals, seronegative for CDV antibodies were vaccinated with an inactivated morbillivirus vaccine or sham-vaccinated. Subsequently, the animals were challenged with organ material from affected seals. The vaccinated animals did not develop any symptoms, whereas the sham-vaccinated seals died [6]. The vaccine was subsequently successfully used in rehabilitation centres. Just before the PDV outbreak in northwestern Europe, a similar outbreak had taken place amongst Lake Baikal seals *(Phoca sibirica)*. A morbillivirus was also isolated from these animals, and serological as well as sequence analyses showed that the latter virus was a CDV strain that occurred locally in the dog population, whereas the PDV from northwestern Europe was indeed a newly discovered morbillivirus from seals [7]. The origin of the PDV that caused the disease outbreak among the seals of northwestern Europe has not been established. However, we showed that PDV has been present along the East-coast of the USA from the early eighties onward [8]. It seems likely that PDV was transmitted to the European seal population, when, due to intensive fishing in the seas around Greenland, harp seals *(Phoca groenlandica)* migrated eastward foraging in the Scandinavian coastal waters, thus introducing PDV into the European seal populations. In the early nineties several similar outbreaks of a disease with high mortality among dolphin and other cetacean species were observed in European and other coastal waters. Again, the combined symptoms suggested that an immunosuppressive agent was at the basis of the pathogenesis [9-11]. Also in these outbreaks several infectious agents were identified, some of which had not been found before, like a newly discovered dolphin rhabdovirus (DRV) [12]. The primary cause of these outbreaks proved to be yet another group of previously unidentified morbilliviruses, of which the dolphin morbillivirus (DMV) and the porpoise morbillivirus (PMV) were the prototype viruses [9-11]. They proved only distantly related to CDV and PDV, as appears in the phylogenetic tree presented in *Figure 1*. Subsequently, several outbreaks of morbillivirus infections have been noted in both pinniped and cetacean species inhabiting coastal waters all over the world.

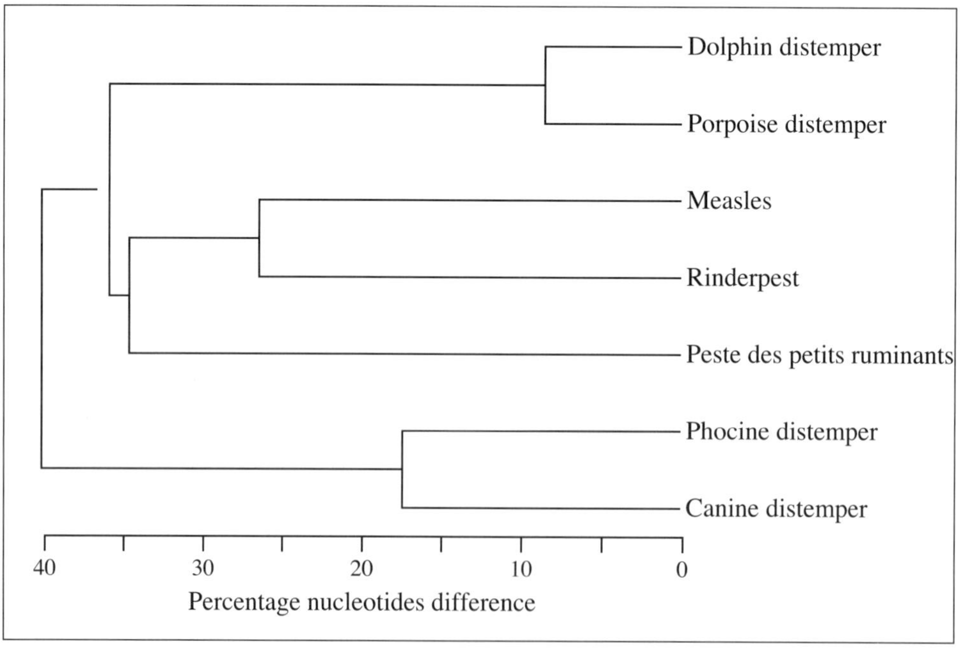

Figure 1. Phylogenetic tree of P gene fragment of different morbilliviruses, derived using the Phylip program DNA-dist. The percentage nucleotide difference between the viruses is indicated [11].

A serious outbreak of a mysterious disease killed more than two thirds of the about 350 – strong population of highly endangered Mediterranean monk seals *(Monachus monachus)* off the coast of Mauritania in West Africa in 1997. The disease outbreak was associated with a DMV-like virus that had probably spilled over from dolphins during a mass mortality among these animals that had just preceeded that in the Mediterranean monk seals [13]. Although there were also indications that an algal bloom had played a role during the outbreak [14], more recent data indicated the pathogenic nature of the DVM-like virus for the Mediterranean monk seals. Similarly, it was shown that a Mediterranean monk seal that had died in Greek waters during the same period was infected with a PMV-like virus [13].

Recent mass mortality that is currently still ongoing among Caspian seals *(Phoca caspica)* in the Caspian sea, proved to be caused by CDV infection, that probably spilled over from terrestrial carnivores [15]. This has probably also been the case for mass mortality among crab-eating seals *(Lobodon carcinophagus)* that took place in Antarctica in 1955, shortly after an expedition with sledge dogs of the USA army to the area [16]. Collectively, our data show that interspecies transmission of morbilliviruses from terrestrial and aquatic carnivores has been at the basis of many disease outbreaks with high mortality rates among aquatic mammals in the past decades. Similar interspecies transmissions of *e.g.* CDV have been noted by us and others in terrestrial mammals like lions in the Serengeti [17] and leopards in zoos in the USA [18].

It was clear that the primary cause of the above mentioned disease outbreaks among aquatic mammals was infection with CDV or one of the newly discovered morbilliviruses, which in most cases led to a profound immune suppression which predisposed the animals for many secondary bacterial or virus infections, thus causing mass mortalities. However, since most of the outbreaks had occurred in highly polluted coastal waters, we speculated that environmental pollution had contributed to the severity and extent of the outbreaks by having a negative influence on the functioning of the immune system of the aquatic mammals as top predators [19]. To test this hypothesis we conducted a semi-field feeding experiment with harbour seals.

To this end, two groups of 11 recently weaned harbour seal pups were caught off the western coast of Scotland, within a relatively clean area. The animals were kept in two groups under identical conditions. One group was fed herring from the highly polluted Baltic sea, the other herring from the relatively unpolluted Atlantic sea. Both herring batches were intended for human consumption, and had passed all quality tests for this purpose. Changes in immune function were monitored over a 2.5 year period. The seals fed contaminated Baltic herring developed significantly higher body burdens of potentially immunotoxic organochlorines, and displayed impaired immune responses as evidenced by suppression of natural killer cell activity and specific T cell responses *(Table I)*. These results clearly demonstrated that chronic exposure to environmental contaminants accumulated through the food chain affects immune function in harbour seals [20-26]. The seals of this study had not been exposed perinatally to the high levels of environmental chemicals, and body burdens of organochlorines measured towards the end of the study were lower than those generally observed in free-ranging seals inhabiting contaminated coastal areas. Therefore, it may be expected that environmental contaminants adversely affect immune functions of free-ranging seals at least as seriously as observed in these studies.

Therefore it seems likely that exposure to immunotoxic chemicals acted as a co-factor in the recently observed outbreaks of morbillivirus infections. It may well have facilitated the emergence of the recent epizootics by aggravating the severity and the extent of the infections, leading to increased numbers of affected animals and case fatality rates [20-26].

Table I. Summary of differences in immunological parameters between two groups of seals in a feeding experiment [20-26].

Parameter	Assay	Effect*
NK cell	^{51}Cr release assay	↓[1]
T lymphocyte	Mitogen-induced proliferation	↓
	Antigen-induced proliferation	↓
	Mixed lymphocyte reaction	↓
	Delayed type hypersensitivity skin test	↓
B lymphocyte	Mitogen-induced proliferation	→[2]
	Specific serum antibody response	→/↓
	Ex vivo/in vitro Ig production	→
Overall	Lymphocyte counts in peripheral blood	→
	Neutrophil counts in peripheral blood	↑[3]

1. Significantly lower responses in the seals fed Baltic herring, as compared to the seals fed Atlantic herring.
2. No significant differences over time between both groups of seals.
3. Significantly higher responses in the seals fed Baltic herring, as compared to the seals fed Atlantic herring.

References

1. Osterhaus ADME. Seal death. *Nature* 1988; 334: 301-2.
2. Osterhaus ADME, Yang H, Spijkers HEM, Groen J, Teppema JS, Steenis G van. The isolation and partial characterization of a highly pathogenic herpesvirus from the harbor seal *(Phoca vitulina)*. *Arch Virol* 1985; 86: 239-51.
3. Osterhaus ADME, Broeders WHJ, Visser IKG, Teppema JS, Vedder EJ. Isolation of an Orthopoxvirus from pox-like lesions of a grey seal *(Halichoerus grypus)*. *Vet Rec* 1990; 127: 91-2.
4. Osterhaus ADME, Vedder EJ. Identification of virus causing recent seal deaths. *Nature* 1988; 335: 20.
5. Osterhaus A, Groen J, De Vries P, UytdeHaag F, Klingeborn B, Zarnke R. Canine distemper virus in seals. *Nature* 1988; 335: 403.
6. Osterhaus ADME, UytdeHaag FGCM, Visser IKG, Vedder EJ, Reijnders PJM, Kuiper J, Brugge HN. Seal vaccination success. *Nature* 1989; 337: 21.
7. Osterhaus ADME, Groen J, UytdeHaag FGCM, Visser IKG, Van de Bildt MWG, Bergman A, Klingeborn B. Distemper virus in Baikal seals. *Nature* 1989; 338: 209-10.
8. Ross PS, Visser IKG, Broeders HWJ, Van de Bildt MWG, Bowen WD, Osterhaus ADME. Antibodies to phocine distemper virus in Canadian seals. *Vet Rec* 1992; 130: 514-6.
9. Van Bressem MF, Visser IKG, Van de Bildt MWG, Teppema JS, Raga JA, Osterhaus ADME. Morbillivirus infection in Mediterranean striped dolphins *(Stenella coeruleoalba)*. *Vet Rec* 1991; 129: 471-2.
10. Visser IKG, Van Bressem MF, De Swart RL, Van de Bildt MWG, Vos HW, Van der Heijden RWJ, Saliki JT, Örvell C, Kitching P, Kuiken T, Barrett T, Osterhaus ADME. Characterization of morbilliviruses isolated from dolphins and porpoises in Europe. *J Gen Virol* 1993; 74: 631-41.
11. Barrett T, Visser IKG, Mamaev L, Goatley L, Van Bressem MF, Osterhaus ADME. Dolphin and porpoise morbilliviruses are genetically distinct from phocine distemper viruses. *Virology* 1993; 193: 1010-2.
12. Osterhaus ADME, Broeders HWJ, Teppema KS, Kuiken T, House JA, Vos HW, Visser IKG. Isolation of a virus with rhabdovirus morphology from a white-beaked dolphin *(Lagenorhynchus albirostris)*. *Arch Virol* 1993; 133: 189-93.
13. Osterhaus A, Groen J, Niesters H, Van de Bildt M, Martina B, Vedder L, Vos J, Van Egmond H, Ba Abou Sidi, Mohamed Ely Ould Barham. Morbillivirus in monk seal mass mortality. *Nature* 1997; 388: 838-9.
14. Osterhaus A, Van de Bildt M, Vedder L, Martina B, Niesters H, Vos J, Van Egmond H, Liem D, Baumann R, Androukaki E, Kotomatas S, Komnenou A, Ba Abou Sidi, Azza Bent Jiddou, Mohamed Ely Ould Barham. Monk seal mortality: virus or toxin? *Vaccine* 1998; 16: 979-81.

15. Kennedy S, Kuiken T, Jepson PD, Deaville R, Forsyth M, Barret T, Van de Bildt MWG, Osterhaus ADME, Eybatov T, Duck C, Kydyrmanov A, Mitrofanov I, Wilson S. Mass die-off of Caspian seals caused by canine distemper virus. *Emerg Infect Dis* 2000; 6: 637-9.
16. Bengston JL, Boveng P, Franzen U, Have P, Heide-Jorgensen MP, Harkonen TL. Antibodies to canine distemper virus in Antarctic seals. *Marine Mammal Sci* 1991; 7: 85-7.
17. Harder TC, Kenter M, Appel MJG, Roelke-Parker ME, Barrett T, Osterhaus ADME. Phylogenetic evidence of canine distemper virus in Serengeti's lions. *Vaccine* 1995; 13: 521-3.
18. Harder TC, Harder M, Vos H, Kulonen K, Kennedy-Stoskopf S, Liess B, Appel MJG, Osterhaus ADME. Characterization of phocid herpesvirus-1 and -2 as putative alpha- and gamma-herpesviruses of North American and European pinnipeds. *J Gen Virol* 1996; 77: 27-35.
19. Osterhaus ADME, Vedder EJ. No simplification in the etiology of recent seal deaths. *Ambio* 1989; 18: 297-8.
20. De Swart RL, Ross PS, Vedder EJ, Timmerman HH, Heisterkamp SH, Van Loveren H, Vos JG, Reijders PJH, Osterhaus ADME. Impairment of immune function in harbour seals *(Phoca vitulina)* feeding on fish from polluted waters. *Ambio* 1994; 23: 155-9.
21. Ross PS, De Swart RL, Reijnders PJH, Van Loveren H, Vos JG, Osterhaus ADME. Contaminant-related suppression of delayed-type hypersensitivity (DTH) and antibody responses in harbor seals fed herring from the Baltic Sea. *Env Health Perspectives* 1995; 103: 162-7.
22. De Swart RL, Ross PS, Timmerman HH, Vos HW, Reijnders PJH, Vos JG, Osterhaus ADME. Impaired cellular immune response in harbour seals *(Phoca vitulina)* feeding on environmentally contaminated herring. *Clin Exp Immunol* 1995; 101: 480-6.
23. Ross PS, De Swart RL, Timmerman HH, Reijnders PJH, Vos JG, Van Loveren H, Osterhaus ADME. Suppression of natural killer cell activity in harbour seals *(Phoca vitulina)* fed Baltic Sea herring. *Aquatic Toxicology* 1996; 34: 71-84.
24. De Swart RL, Ross PS, Vos JG, Osterhaus ADME. Impaired immunity in harbour seals *(Phoca vitulina)* exposed to bioaccumulated environmental contaminants: review of a long-term feeding study. *Env Health Perspectives* 1996; 104 (Suppl. 4): 823-8.
25. Harvell CD, Kim K, Burkholder JM, Colwell RR, Epstein PR, Grimes J, Hofmann EE, Lipp E, Osterhaus ADME, Overstreet R, Porter JW, Smityh GW, Vasta G. Emerging marine diseases – Climate links and anthropogenic factors. *Science* 1999; 285: 1505-10.
26. Ross PS, Vos JG, Birnbaum LS, Osterhaus ADME. PCBs are a health risk for humans and wildlife. *Science (letter)* 2000; 289: 1878-9.

Emergence and Control of Zoonotic Ortho- and Paramyxovirus Diseases
B. Dodet, M. Vicari, eds.

Serological evidence of morbillivirus (canine distemper-like) in free-ranging North-American bears *(Ursus americanus, U. arctos,* and *U. maritimus)*: an update

Bruno B. Chomel[1], G. Chappuis[2], M. Soulier[2], E.H. Follmann[3], G.W. Garner[4], J.F. Evermann[5], A.J. McKeirnan[5], J.A. Mortenson[6], D.A. Immell[7]

[1] *Department of Population Health and Reproduction, School of Veterinary Medicine, University of California, Davis, CA, USA*
[2] *Mérial, Lyon, France*
[3] *Institute of Arctic Biology, University of Alaska, Fairbanks, AK, USA*
[4] *US National Biological Service, Alaska Science Center, Anchorage, AK, USA*
[5] *Washington Animal Disease Diagnostic Laboratory, College of Veterinary Medicine, Washington State University, Pullman, WA, USA*
[6] *Department of Fisheries and Wildlife, Oregon State University, Corvallis, OR, USA*
[7] *Oregon Department of Fish and Wildlife, Roseburg, OR, USA*

Abstract – Evidence of distemper-like infection in free-ranging North-American bears, including black bears *(Ursus americanus)*, grizzly bears *(Ursus arctos)* and polar bears *(Ursus maritimus)* is reported, based on serological testing of 351 black bears, 480 grizzly bears and 186 polar bears captured between 1984 and 1997. In black bears, overall canine distemper virus (CDV) antibody prevalence was 6% (21/351). Among these black bears, 5 (6.2%) of the 80 bears from Virginia had CDV antibodies. In Florida [1], 8% of 66 free-ranging bears captured between 1993 and 1995 had CDV antibodies. On the West Coast States, 1 (5%) of 21 bears from Northern California, 6 (6.4%) of 94 black bears from Oregon and 1 (2%) of 50 bears from Washington State were seropositive, whereas none of the 40 black bears from central Alaska had specific antibodies. CDV antibody prevalence was much higher in Alaskan grizzly bears (8.3%, 40/480) and polar bears (33.9%, 63/186) from Alaska and Russia. In grizzly bears, animals from Southern Alaska were 2.5 times more likely to be seropositive than grizzly bears from other areas. Prevalence was the highest (30%) for grizzly bears from Kodiak Island (30%, 23/77) and the Alaskan Peninsula (8%, 7/86). High titres were mainly observed in adult bears > 8 years of age. For polar bears, the highest prevalence of CDV antibodies also occurred in adults (43.9%). Polar bears with morbillivirus antibodies were present in all the areas sampled during each year, suggesting widespread exposure to the virus in the Bering, Chukchi and East Siberian seas. Recent data suggest that North American bears are infected by a morbillivirus closer to canine morbillivirus than to pinniped morbillivirus.

In North-America, the black bear *(Ursus americanus)* population is estimated to be between 400,000 and 750,000 individuals, whereas the world population of polar bears *(U. maritimus)* is estimated at 21,000 to 28,000 animals (www.beartrust.org). For Alaska only, there are an estimated 30,000 grizzly bears *(Ursus arctos horribilis)* and 140,000 black bears [2].

The emergence of severe epizootics of morbillivirus in many wildlife species, including terrestrial carnivores in North America, such as gray foxes *(Urocyon cinereoargenteus)* and raccoons *(Procyon lotor)* [3] or in lions in Africa [4], as well as in pinnipeds and cetaceans worldwide [5, 6] raised interest in investigating the presence of canine distemper virus (CDV) or distemper-like antibodies in free-ranging bear populations, especially in North America. Canine distemper has been reported as a cause of death in captive polar bears and one spectacled bear *(Tremarctos ornatus)* in Austria [7]. Antibodies to canine distemper virus have been reported from giant pandas *(Ailuropoda melanoleuca)* in China [8], and more recently from polar bears [9], free-ranging and captive Italian brown bears [10], grizzly bears [11] and black bears [1, 11, 12]. It will be important to determine if free-ranging bears are a natural reservoir for CDV or a related morbillivirus or are accidental victims during epidemics in wild or domestic canids. For instance, seroprevalence ranging from 2.3% to 12% has been reported in Alaskan wolf populations [13-15]. The infection is supposed to be enzootic in these free-ranging canid populations rather than being introduced sporadically from domestic dogs [15].

The present manuscript describes most of the recent seroepidemiological studies, including new data concerning the seroprevalence of CDV antibodies in various free-ranging bear populations from North America and Siberia.

Material and methods

Polar bears from Alaska and Russia [9]

One hundred and ninety-one serum samples collected from 186 polar bears were collected between 1984 and 1992. Females accounted for 75.8% (141/186) of the bears tested. Five females were bled twice during the study. Polar bears were captured by helicopter immobilization procedures and the remote injection of immobilizing drugs on the seasonal and permanent polar pack ice and on Arctic islands in the Bering, Chukchi and East Siberian seas, including both US and Russian regions. The bears were grouped into three age categories: cubs (one to two years of age), sub-adults (three to five years of age) and adults (six or more years of age).

The serum samples were stored at - 70 °C until they were tested by the microtitre virus neutralization test, with CDV as the challenge virus [16], as described previously [9].

Grizzly and black bears from Alaska [11]

Personnel of the Alaska Department of Fish and Game and the US Fish and Wildlife Service captured 480 grizzly bears and 40 black bears in the course of performing population ecology studies between 1988 and 1991. Sampling was opportunistic and some bears were captured more than once; 644 serum samples were available for testing. 76 blood samples were collected from 40 black bears in interior Alaska on the Tanana Flats, south of Fairbanks. The 568 grizzly bear blood samples were collected from 8 different areas: in Southern Alaska, 79 samples were collected on Kodiak Island, and 86 samples from the Alaska Peninsula (Katmai Coast: 38 samples and Black Lake: 48 samples). In interior Alaska, 53 samples were collected in the Tanana Flats, Denali Park, and Fairbanks areas. In Western Alaska, 40 samples came from the Seward Peninsula and 99 from the Noatak River drainage. In Northern Alaska, 133 samples came from the North-West, 6 from the North-Central (Prudhoe Bay), and 72 from the North-East. Blood samples were collected by femoral, saphenous or cephalic venipuncture. Serum was separated by centrifugation and stored at - 20 °C until tested. Blood was collected from 25 (63%) of the 40 black bears more than once: 4 bears had blood taken 4 times; 3 bears 3 times; and 18 bears twice. Among the grizzly bears, samples were obtained 3 times from 11 bears and twice from 67 bears.

Serologic tests for canine distemper virus were performed at the Virology Laboratory, Merial, Lyons, France. Sera were tested for evidence of antibodies to canine distemper virus by competitive ELISA. Briefly, 100 µl per well of capture monoclonal anti-H glycoprotein neutralizing antibodies at a 1:1,500 dilution in carbonate bicarbonate buffer, pH 9.6, were bound to 96-well flat bottom microtitration plates (ELISA Nunc Maxisorp, Nunc Inc., Rochester, NY, USA) by overnight incubation at room temperature. On cell culture plates, 50 µl of distemper virus and 50 µl of each serum dilution (0.9, 1.8 and 2.7), and respective controls, were incubated for 1 hr at 37 °C with continuous shaking. After 3 washes, 50 µl of the virus-serum mix was transferred onto the monoclonal antibody-sensitized plates and incubated with continous shaking for 1 hr at 37 °C. Then, 50 µl of the monoclonal anti-H glycoprotein neutralizing antibody labelled with peroxidase was added to each well and plates were incubated with continous shaking for 1 hr at 37 °C. The plates were washed 3 times, then 100 µl of substrate (orthophenylene diamine, Sigma Co.) was added. The reaction was stopped after 25 min with 50 µl of 2.5 M H_2SO_4. Microtitration plates were read at a wavelength of 490 nm. Results were expressed as percent OD compared to a control without serum (100%). Serum titers were given as log of the reciprocal dilution with a 50% OD.

In order to validate the ELISA test and define the cut-off point (COP) for seropositivity, 23 serum samples from bears with an ELISA titer $\geq$ 0.8 were also tested by the classical serum-neutralization (SN) test [16]. Titres by SN were usually lower than by ELISA, which led to defining the COP at $\geq$ 1.0. For further validation, ELISA positive samples and a random sample of ELISA negative serum samples were also tested using an immunoperoxidase antibody test, which is similar to a fluorescence test, using immunoperoxidase instead of fluorescein isothyocyanate. ELISA positive samples were also found to be immunoperoxidase positive and ELISA negative samples negative by the immunoperoxidase antibody test.

Ages were estimated by examining cementum annuli of premolar teeth for black bears and grizzly bears. Black bears were classified in 4 inclusive age groups: 0-2 year old, 2.5-4 year old, 4.5-8 year old and ≥ 9 year old. Grizzly bears were classified into 5 inclusive age groups: 0.5-2 year, 2.5-4 year, 4.5-8 year, 8.5-12 year, and ≥ 13 year. Grizzly bears from the Seward Peninsula and Denali Park were reported as being adults (*i.e.* ≥ 4.5 years). Sixty-two percent (297/480) of the grizzly bears and 55% (22/40) of the black bears were females. Among the grizzly bears, 12% were ≤ 2 years old, whereas 31.5% of the black bears were ≤ 2 years old. Demographic data (*i.e.* species, sex, age) were analyzed using Epi Info version 6.02. Frequency distributions were obtained and χ^2 statistics for 2×2 contingency tables were calculated to obtain measures of association, and the statistical significance of such associations.

Black bears from California, Oregon and Washington [12]

- **Northern California:** blood samples were collected by the California Department of Fish and Game personnel between 1993 and 1997 from Shasta National forest (10 samples) and Klamath National forest (37 samples).

- **Oregon:** blood samples were obtained from two different sites. At Willamette National Forest, 93 samples were collected by the Oregon Department of Fish and Wildlife between 1993 and 1997. Nine bear samples were obtained from the Coast Range from damage-causing bears killed by private trappers in 1997.

- **Washington:** blood samples from the two sites in Olympic National Park (23 samples) and Snoqualmie National Forest (27 samples) were obtained in 1996-1997 by the Washington Department of Fish and Wildlife.

Black bears from Florida and Virginia

- **Florida** [1]: bears were captured in three different sites: 21 bears (14 males, 7 females) from the Apalachicola region (Florida panhandle) between June and August 1995; 8 (6 males, 2 females) from Osceola National Forest/Pinhook Swamp region (North peninsular Florida) between July and August 1994 and 37 bears (21 males, 16 females) from the Wekiva River region (central Florida) between November 1993 and June 1995. Presence of CDV antibodies was determined by serum neutralization performed at Cornell University, College of Veterinary Medicine, Diagnostic laboratory, as previously described [16].

- **Virginia:** 84 blood samples were collected from 80 black bears (61 males and 19 females) from the Great Dismal Swamp area in Virginia between 1984 and 1986. Blood samples were collected in 1984 from 20 bears (19 males, 1 female), in 1985 from 41 bears (26 males and 15 females) and in 1986 from 23 bears (19 males and 4 females). Among these 80 bears, four were bled twice. Age of bears ranged from 1 year to 16 years (mode and mean: 4 years). Serum samples were tested by Mérial laboratories, as described above.

Results

Polar bears, Alaska and Russia [9]

Sixty-eight of the 191 samples had morbillivirus antibodies, including 5 females that were positive in samples collected in two different years. Overall, 33.9% (63/186) of the bears, including 53 females and 10 males, had CDV antibodies. A higher percentage of females (37.7%) were seropositive than males (27%). The highest prevalence of morbillivirus antibodies occurred in the adult bears (43.9%) followed by the cubs (37.9%) and the sub-adults (35.7%). Polar bears with morbillivirus antibodies were present in all the areas samples during each year.

Grizzly and black bears, Alaska [11]

Prevalence was not significantly different in females than in males ($p = 0.2$). It primarily varied with bears' origin *(Table I)*, grizzly bears from Southern Alaska being 2.5 times more likely to be seropositive than grizzly bears from other areas (95% confidence interval (CI) = 1.28, 4.96). Among the 41 positive samples (one bear tested positive twice), 73% (30/41) had titres $\geq$ 2.0, of which 77% (23/30) were from Southern Alaska *(Table II)*. Distemper seropositive grizzly bears were also more likely to be positive for CIH (odds ratio (OR) = 2.65, 95% CI = 1.18, 5.60). Age prevalences are presented in *Table III*. Mean age of seropositive grizzly bears was 12.5 years (standard error (SE) = 0.85), whereas mean age of seronegative bears was 8.4 ± 0.27 years ($p < 0.05$). High titers were mainly observed in grizzly bears > 8 years old. In Southwest and Western Alaska, all positive grizzly bears were > 7 years old, whereas, in Northern Alaska, 40% of the positive bears were $\leq$ 4 year-old. Annualized prevalence for Kodiak Island was stable (32% in1988 and 29% in 1989) and ranged from 2.6% to 7.6% in Northern Alaska.

Black bears from California, Oregon, Washington [Mortenson JA, Chomel BB, Immell DA, Wildlife Disease Association, Madison, WI, August 10-13, 1998]

Of the 165 bears tested, eight (4.8%) had CDV antibodies *(Table IV)*. In Northern California, only one bear was seropositive among the Klamath bears (1/11; 9.1%) whereas 6 bears from Oregon had CDV antibodies, 5 bears from the Willamette National Forest (5/85, 9%) and one bear from the Coast Range area (1/9, 11%). In Washington, one bear only from Olympic National Park (1/23, 4.4%) was seropositive. There was no significant prevalence difference by sex (males: 3.9%, 4/104; females: 6.6%, 4/61).

Black bears from Virginia and Florida

• **Florida** [1]: five (8%) of the 66 bears had CDV antibodies *(Table IV)*. Four bears were from Wekika River region (4/37, 10.8%) and one from Apachicola region (1/21, 4.8%). The positive bears were three females (5, 12 and 14 years old) and one 12 years old male.

Table I. Seroprevalence of canine distemper antibody in grizzly bears, Alaska.

Location	No. tested	No. positive (%)	Sex (%)
Kodiak Island	77	23 (30)	2M, 21F
Katmai coast/Black Lake	86	7 (8)	2M, 5F
Tanana Flats/Denali	40	1 (2.5)	1M
Seward Peninsula	40	1 (2.5)	1M
Noatak River Drainage	87	0 (0)	
Northwest Arctic	96	6 (6)	2M, 4F
North central/east Arctic	54	2 (4)	2M
Total	480	40 (8.3)	10M (5.4) 30F (10.2)

Table II. Canine distemper antibody titre distribution in grizzly bears, Alaska.

Location	Distemper OD			
	< 1	1-1.9	2-2.9	≥ 3
Kodiak Island	55	6	15	3
Katmai coast/Black Lake	79	1	5	1
Tanana Flats/Denali	52	0	1	0
Seward Peninsula	39	0	0	1
Noatak River Drainage	98	0	0	1
Northwest Arctic	127	4	1	1
North central/east Arctic	74	1	1	2

Table III. Canine distemper virus antibody prevalence by age groups, grizzly bears, Alaska.

Age	No. samples tested	No. positive (%)
0 to 2 years	70	1 (1.5)
2.5 to 4 years	97	3 (3)
4.5 to 8 years	89	4 (4.5)
8.5 to 12 years	101	14 (14)
> 12 years	167	20 (12)
Adult*	44	2 (4.5)
Total	568	44 (8)

* 40 bears from Seward Peninsula and 4 bears from Denali.

• **Virginia:** five bears (6.2%) were seropositive for canine distemper antibodies *(Table IV)*. One 6 year old male in 1984 (titer: 2.9), two females (4 and 3 years old, titres of 2.7 and 1.8, respectively) in 1985 and two young males (both 2 years old, titres of 3.6 and 1.8, respectively) in 1986. None of the four bears bled twice had specific antibodies.

Table IV. Seroprevalence of canine distemper virus antibodies in American black bears *(U. americanus)*.

State	Location	No. positive/No. tested (%)	
Washington	Olympic Natl. Park	1/23 (4.4)	
	Snoqualmie Natl. Forest	0/27 (0)	
Oregon	Willamette Natl. Forest	5/85 (9)	
	Coastal Range	1/9 (11)	
California	Klamath Natl. Forest	1/11 (9.1)	
	Shasta Natl. Forest	0/10 (0)	
Virginia	Great Dismal Swamp	5/80 (6.2)	
Florida	Osceola/Pinhook	0/8 (0)	(Dunbar *et al.*, *J Wildl Dis* 1998)
	Wekika River	4/37 (10.8)	
	Apalachicola	1/21 (4.8)	
Alaska	Tanana Flats	0/40 (0)	

Discussion

The present review indicates that most populations of free-ranging bears, including polar bears, grizzly bears and black bears from various part of North America and Siberia have experienced exposure to a morbillivirus, as diagnosed by the presence of canine distemper virus antibodies. Infection appears to be enzootic in these various bear populations with a seroprevalence ranging from 6% in average in black bears to up to 35.6% in polar bears. Regional variations in prevalence were observed within each bear species; however high prevalence was observed in all polar bear populations and specifically in grizzly bears from Southern Alaska. Positive bears were identified throughout the study period, and cases were not clustered in time. In most surveys, concurrent epidemics of distemper in other wild or domestic carnivores were not documented or reported. These data raise questions about the epidemiology of morbillivirus infection in free-ranging bear populations. For instance, as grizzly bears' potential exposure to wild canids is concerned, antibody prevalence was more evenly distributed among wolf packs in all geographic areas [15, 17]. Therefore, a source of infection from wolves seems less likely, despite the fact that distemper antibodies are more widespread and evenly distributed in Alaskan wolves, because of their sparse distribution. However, the much higher densities of foxes *(Vulpes vulpes)*, which are known to be susceptible to distemper, make them more likely to be spreading the infection to other wild species. The possibility of infection by a virus of canine origin also seems less likely, as domestic dogs are found throughout inhabited areas of Alaska, and none of the black bears and a very small percentage of grizzly bears from central Alaska had CDV antibodies.

For polar bears, feeding mainly on seals, it could be hypothesized that they acquire their infection from phocine morbilliviruses, as several major epidemics have been reported in these species in recent years [5, 6]. The recent work of Garner *et al.* [18] brings important information on the characteristics of the polar bear morbillivirus. Differential seroneutralization tests using four different morbilliviruses (CDV, phocine distemper virus (PDV), dolphin morbillivirus (DMV) and porpoise morbillivirus (PMV)) on 47 of 75 previously CDV positive samples showed higher titers for CDV than for PDV, DVM and PMV. These authors concluded that CDV or a virus more closely related to it than the three other morbilliviruses was most probably the homologous virus that induced the antibodies in these bears. The low (< 10%) prevalence of CDV antibodies in most black bear populations could also support the hypothesis of a morbillivirus endemic to bears. Definitive identification of this virus would require isolation of the virus from an infected bear. At present, blood plasma could also be screened for morbillivirus RNA by polymerase chain reaction and partial sequencing.

Acknowledgments

Serum samples from grizzly bears from Alaska and black bears from Alaska and Virginia were kindly provided by Dr. R.L. Zarnke, Alaska Department of Fish and Game. The authors thanks Gary Koehler, Tim Burton, Bob Gilman and Richard Green for their assistance in collecting the black bear samples from Washington, Oregon and California.

References

1. Dunbar MR, Cunningham MW, Roof JC. Seroprevalence of selected disease agents from free-ranging black bears in Florida. *J Wildl Dis* 1998; 34: 612-9.
2. Hummel M, Pettigrew S. *Wild hunters, predators in peril.* Niwot, Colorado: P Roberts Rinehart publ., 1991: 251 p.
3. Forrester DJ. *Parasites and diseases of wild mammals in Florida.* Gainesville, Florida: University Press of Florida, 1992: 459 p.
4. Harder TC, Kenter M, Appel MJ, Roelke-Parker ME, Barrett T, Osterhaus AD. Phylogenetic evidence of canine distemper virus in Serengeti's lions. *Vaccine* 1995; 13: 521-3.
5. Duignan PJ, Saliki JT, St. Aubin DJ, Early G, Sadove S, House JA, Kovacs K, Geraci JR. Epizootiology of morbillivirus infection in North American harbor seals *(Phoca vitulina)* and gray seals *(Halichoerus grypus). J Wildl Dis* 1995; 31: 491-501.
6. Kennedy S. Morbillivirus infections in aquatic mammals. *J Comp Pathol* 1998; 119: 201-25.
7. Schonbauer M. Perinatal distemper infection of three polar bears *(Ursus maritimus)* and one spectacled bear *(Tremarctos ornatus). Proc Intl Symp Diseases Zoo Animals* 1984; 26: 131-6.
8. Mainka SA, Xianmeng Q, Tingmei H, Appel MJ. Serologic survey of giant pandas *(Ailuropoda melanoleuca)*, and domestic dogs and cats in the Wolong reserve, China. *J Wildl Dis* 1994; 30: 86-9.
9. Follmann EH, Garner GW, Evermann JF, McKeirnan AJ. Serological evidence of morbillivirus infection in polar bears *(Ursus maritimus)* from Alaska and Russia. *Vet Rec* 1996; 138: 615-8.
10. Marsilio F, Tiscar PG, Gentile L, Roth HU, Boscagli G. Tempesta M, Gatti A. Serological survey for selected viral pathogens in brown bears from Italy. *J Wildl Dis* 1997; 33: 304-7.

11. Chomel BB, Kasten RW, Chappuis G, Soulier M, Kikuchi Y. Serological survey of selected canine viral pathogens and zoonoses in grizzly bears *(Ursus arctos horribilis)* and black bears *(Ursus americanus)* from Alaska. *Rev Sci Tech Off Int Epiz* 1998; 17: 756-66.
12. Mortenson JA. Serologic survey of infectious disease agents in black bears *(Ursus americanus)* of California, Oregon and Washington. Master of Science thesis, Oregon State University, November 1998, 57 p.
13. Choquette LPE, Kuyt E. Serological indication of canine distemper and of infectious canine hepatitis in wolves *(Canis lupus)* in northern Canada. *J Wildl Dis* 1974; 10: 321-4.
14. Stephenson RO, Ritter DG, Nielsen CA. Serologic survey for canine distemper and infectious canine hepatitis in wolves in Alaska. *J Wildl Dis* 1982; 18: 419-24.
15. Zarnke RL, Ballard WB. Serologic survey for selected microbial pathogens of wolves in Alaska, 1975-1982. *J Wildl Dis* 1987; 23: 77-85.
16. Appel M, Robson DS. A microneutralization test for canine distemper virus. *Am J Vet Res* 1973; 34: 1459-63.
17. Zarnke RL, Yuill TM. Serologic survey for selected microbioal agents in mammals from Alberta, 1976. *J Wildl Dis* 1981; 17: 453-61.
18. Garner GW, Evermann JF, Saliki JT, Follmann EH, McKeirnan AJ. Morbillivirus ecology in polar bears *(Ursus maritimus)*. *Polar Biol* 2000; 23: 474-8.

Emergence and Control of Zoonotic Ortho- and Paramyxovirus Diseases
B. Dodet, M. Vicari, eds.

Hendra virus: a new zoonotic paramyxovirus from flying foxes (fruit bats) in Australia

John S. Mackenzie[1], Hume E. Field[2]
[1] *Department of Microbiology and Parasitology, The University of Western Australia, Brisbane, Queensland, Australia*
[2] *Animal Research Institute, Department of Primary Industries, Queensland, Australia*

In September 1994, a sudden outbreak of an acute respiratory syndrome occurred among thoroughbred horses in a training complex in Brisbane, Australia, during which thirteen horses and their trainer died. Seven horses and a stablehand were also infected but recovered. This outbreak marked the first appearance of a novel virus, Hendra virus, formerly called equine morbillivirus, a member of a new genus within the family *Paramyxoviridae*. Two further incidences of disease due to Hendra virus have occurred; the first of these actually preceded the initial outbreak but was not recognised until thirteen months afterwards, and the second occurred in January 1999 but only involved a single horse. Hendra virus has subsequently been shown to be a virus associated with fruit bats, or flying foxes, of the genus *Pteropus*, family Pteropodidae, sub-order Megachiroptera, and was the first of three novel zoonotic viruses to be described from fruit bats in Australia; the other two being Australian bat lyssavirus in 1996, and Menangle virus, a member of the genus *Rubulavirus* in the family *Paramyxoviridae*, in 1997 [1]. The importance of the emergence of Hendra virus has been underscored by the subsequent emergence of a closely related virus, Nipah virus, in Malaysia in 1999. This brief review describes the events surrounding the emergence of Hendra virus in Australia.

The first incident: the Brisbane outbreak

The initial outbreak took place in the city of Brisbane in South-East Queensland in September 1994. The index case was a pregnant mare that fell sick in a spelling paddock in the Brisbane suburb of Cannon Hill. The mare was moved to the training stable approximately 6 km away in the suburb of Hendra on 7th September, 1994, where it died two days later of acute respiratory disease. Between eight and 11 days later, 12 further horses became ill and died. The stable hand fell ill five days after the death of the index case with an influenza-like illness, and the trainer became ill a day later with similar symptoms, and subsequently died from acute respiratory disease. A further seven horses were also infected, and they together with the stablehand, recovered.

When the outbreak was first recognised, the cause of the horses' illness was not clear, and poisoning, bacterial, viral, and exotic diseases were all investigated [2; Lee, personal communication]. The clinical features of the affected horses included anorexia, depression, fever, ataxia, tachycardia, tachypnoea, dyspnoea, and a copious frothy nasal discharge. At autopsy, a marked sub-pleural oedema was observed with congestion and ventral consolidation of the lungs. An interstitial pneumonia with focal necrotising alveolitis, oedema, and syncytial formation affecting the vascular endothelium was evident from histological investigation [2-4]. Several other horses had a subclinical infection as determined by seropositivity, and seven horses with mild or subclinical infections were subsequently euthanased. A virus was isolated from tissues of several of the horses, which caused syncytia in cell culture. On the basis of antigenicity and sequence homology, the virus was deduced to be a distant member of the morbillivirus genus of the family *Paramyxoviridae* [3, 5]. Epidemiologically, the most surprising aspect of the outbreak was the absence of further cases, particularly once the aetiological agent was recognised to be a respiratory virus. It is believed that the virus was introduced from the index case to the other horses by a parenteral route through human intervention, probably by the trainer.

The trainer and stablehand were infected following exposure to the index case. Both had close contact with the index case, particularly the trainer who was exposed to nasal discharge while trying to feed her, acquiring abrasions on his hands and arms. The symptoms of the stablehand were myalgia, headaches, lethargy and vertigo. He did not develop respiratory symptoms or require hospital admission. His lethargy persisted for six weeks [4]. The horse trainer became ill with similar symptoms, and four days after onset of symptoms he developed nausea and vomiting and became dehydrated. He was admitted to hospital on the fifth day, and transferred to the intensive care unit for ventilation. Chest radiographs showed a diffuse alveolar shadowing. The differential diagnosis considered included legionaire's disease, viral pneumonitis, melioidosis or glanders, and toxic pneumonitis. His renal function deteriorated and continuous dialysis was instituted. Although he showed some improvement, he developed cardiac irritability on the seventh day, which led to prolonged periods of asystole and death [4]. At autopsy, findings were consistent with viral infection. Both lungs were congested, haemorragic and filled with serous fluid. Lung histology revealed focal necrotising alveolitis with many giant cells, and viral inclusions. Pre-existing lung disease was also observed, including small adenocarcinoma in the terminal bronchiole, as well as areas of inflammation with necrosis scattered throughout the kidneys and pulmonary embolism. A virus was subsequently cultured from the kidney. Neutralising antibodies to the horse virus were found in the serum of the trainer taken six days prior to his death and at *postmortem*. Neutralising antibodies were also found in sera collected from the stablehand.

Two horses experimentally inoculated with lung and spleen tissue from the infected horses became ill at six and 10 days post-inoculation with high fever and severe respiratory signs, and were euthanased two days later. The signs and symptoms were similar to those observed during the outbreak, demonstrating that the disease was transmissible, and virus was re-isolated from various tissues at necroscopy. Two further horses were experimentally infected with tissue culture-grown virus, and after a short severe clinical episode, were destroyed four and five days after infection. The gross histopathological lesions were primarily respiratory, and consistent with the natural disease. Virus was re-isolated from lungs, liver, spleen, kidney, lymph nodes and blood [2, 3, 6]. Thus the virus isolated from horses in the Brisbane outbreak was unequivocally shown to be responsible for the disease.

The second incident: the Mackay outbreak

The second incident of Hendra virus infection came to light about 13 months after the Brisbane outbreak when a 35-year-old farmer from Mackay in central Queensland died from severe encephalitis in October 1995 [7]. He had been admitted to hospital after two weeks of irritable mood and low back pain, with a generalised tonic-clonic seizure. He had had three focal motor seizures involving the right arm two days previously. During the following week, recurrent focal motor seizures involving the right face, secondarily generalised seizures, and a low grade fever occurred despite antibiotic, antiviral, and anticonvulsant therapy. Seven days after admission, dense right hemiplegia, signs of brainstem involvement, and depressed consciousness had developed and he required intubation. He remained deeply unconscious with persisting fever, and died 25 days after admission. Serum samples showed high titres of neutralising antibodies to Hendra virus, and a primary PCR on cerebrospinal fluid and nested PCR on brain material identified Hendra viral matrix protein gene sequences.

However, subsequent investigation showed that he had been infected 14 months previously and a month prior to the Brisbane outbreak. This incident started with the deaths of two horses on his farm in August 1994 [8]. The first horse, a mare in late pregnancy, was reported to have had severe respiratory distress, ataxia, and marked swelling of the head, particularly of the infraorbital fossa and cheeks, and died 24 hr after clinical signs were noted on 1st August, 1994. The second horse, a stallion, was reported to exhibit aimless pacing, muscle trembling and a haemorrhagic nasal discharge. Death also occurred 24 hr after the clinical signs were noticed on 12th August. The second horse had had a brief contact with the carcase of the first horse; thus the incubation time was consistent with those observed during the Hendra outbreak. A definitive diagnosis was not reached for either horse, although avocado poisoning and brown snake bite were considered as differential diagnoses. However, tissue was available for one horse and it was subsequently shown to have been infected with Hendra virus by PCR, immunofluorescence and consistent lung pathology [8, 9].

The patient had cared for the two sick horses on his property and assisted in their necropsies. Shortly after he had presented with a 12 day history of sore throat, headache, drowsiness, vomiting and neck stiffness. A provisional diagnosis of partially treated meningitis was made and he had made a full recovery. Serum collected from the patient at the time of this first illness was available and neutralising antibodies to Hendra virus were detected, and a nested PCR on the serum amplified a 500 nucleotide sequence of the Hendra virus matrix gene, demonstrating that he had been infected with Hendra virus [7]. Furthermore, the rise in neutralising antibody titre and the antibody class profile during the second encephalitic illness suggested an anamnestic response to the virus [7]. Thus, the Mackay incident demonstrated that the patient had been infected with Hendra virus from the infected horses one month prior to the Brisbane outbreak, and after a short meningitic illness, the virus remained latent for a year before reactivating and causing the second fatal encephalitis.

The third incident: the Cairns case

The third incident occurred in January 1999 when a 9-year-old thoroughbred horse became infected with Hendra virus at Trinity Beach, 15 km North of Cairns in North Queensland [10, 11]. The horse became unwell with depression, inappetance, and oedema of the face, lips and neck. It was initially diagnosed as an allergic reaction, and treated accordingly. On the following morning it was found in sternal recumbency, but soon progressed to lateral recumbency, and was subsequently euthanased. As Hendra virus pneumonia was considered in the differential diagnosis, lung tissue was collected from a single small chest incision. Excess pleural fluid, a yellow frothy nasal discharge and jaundice of the ocular sclera were other findings [10]. Histopathology with immunohistochemistry, electron microscopy and PCR-amplified sequence analysis in the matrix gene region and flanking sequences, all confirmed that the mare had died of Hendra virus. Sequence analysis indicated 5 nucleotide substitutions had occurred in approximately 700 nucleotides sequenced, compared to the original sequence on Genbank from the Brisbane outbreak virus [11]. Thus this third incident only involved a single horse. The horse had been found to be pregnant two months prior to becoming ill, but although it should have been in mid-pregnancy at the time of death, it was found to be non-pregnant when the uterus was examined by small flank incision [10].

Hendra virus: source of infection and the role of pteropid bats

Following the isolation of a morbilli-like virus from autopsy tissues obtained from horses that died in the initial Brisbane outbreak, a major seroepidemiological investigation was undertaken to determine the incidence of the virus in horses in Queensland. Nearly 2,500 horses throughout Queensland were tested for the presence of antibody to equine morbillivirus, but all were negative [12], demonstrating that the virus was neither common nor widespread in the horse population, and suggesting that horses are not the normal host of the virus. Attention then focussed on possible wildlife and domestic animal sources, and over 5,000 sera from 46 species were tested, but no antibodies to Hendra virus were found [8, 13, 14]. In considering the characteristics of a potential reservoir host, it was suggested that: (a) any reservoir host should be present in both Brisbane and Mackay, the sites of the two outbreaks, either as a contiguous population and/or migratory; (b) the reservoir host should have the opportunity to come into contact with horses; and (c) the reservoir host would be unlikely to show any ill effects from infection with the virus [14, 15]. The two possible reservoir animals which would fit these requirements were fruit bats (flying foxes) and certain birds, especially nomadic waterfowl.

Flying foxes were chosen initially, and were quickly found to exhibit a significant incidence of seropositivity to Hendra virus [13, 14]. Indeed antibodies to Hendra virus were detected in all four species of pteropid fruit bats, or flying foxes, found in Australia. These are the spectacled flying fox *(Pteropus conspicillatus)*, which occurs in Northern and Eastern parts of Queensland; the black flying fox *(P. alecto)*, which has a wide distribution across Northern Australia; the little red flying fox *(P. scapulatus)*, which is found across Northern and Eastern Australia; and the grey-headed flying fox *(P. poliocephalus)*, which occurs in Eastern and South-Eastern Australia [16, 17].

Approximately 47% of flying foxes sampled over their full geographic range have been found to have antibodies to Hendra virus [16], although differences in seropositivity have been observed between different species [17]. Three virus isolates were obtained from uterine fluid and a pool of foetal lung and liver from one grey-headed flying fox and from foetal lung of a black flying fox [14-16, 18]. The virus was indistinguishable antigenically and genetically from Hendra virus. Clinical disease has not been observed in naturally infected [16] or experimentally infected [19, 20] flying foxes, but the virus does cause a subclinical disease as indicated by virus isolation, seroconversion, vascular lesions and positive immunostaining [19, 20]. Indeed immunostaining was also observed in the placental veins, but there was no immunostaining of foetal tissues [20].

Thus all results suggest that flying foxes are the probable reservoir host of Hendra virus, and that the virus is a relatively common among flying foxes throughout their geographic range in Australia. These results also indicate that the original name given to the virus, equine morbillivirus, was incorrect with respect to the host.

Hendra virus: characteristics and properties

The virus isolated from the horses during the Brisbane outbreak was morphologically similar to other morbilliviruses, being enveloped and pleomorphic, and containing herringbone nucleocapsids 18 mm wide with a 5 mm periodicity. However, it was unusual in that it had “double-fringed” surface projections [21]. The surface glycoproteins did not exhibit either haemagglutinin or neuraminidase activities. In addition, the virus displayed a wide *in vitro* host range [2, 3, 21]. The *in vivo* host range was also relatively broad compared to other morbilliviruses, causing disease in experimentally infected cats [19, 22-24] and guinea-pigs [20, 23, 24], but not in rats, rabbits, chickens, dogs or mice [24]. Experimentally infected cats became ill 4-8 days after being inoculated with virus by oral, intra-nasal, and sub-cutaneous routes. The disease and the lesions were similar to those observed in horses, and virus was isolated from various feline tissues [22]. The most important gross findings in all cats displaying clinical disease were hydrothorax and pulmonary oedema accompanied by various degrees of congestion and pulmonary haemorrhage [23], and histologically, lung lesions consistent with the gross findings and accompanied by intravascular thrombosis and vascular endothelial lesions with syncytia [23]. In guinea-pigs, subcutaneous inoculation also gave rise to severe respiratory disease [23], but neurological disease was also observed in some animals (Eaton, personal communication). At necropsy, all guinea pigs were cyanosed and had congestion and oedema in the gastrointestinal tract; however, there was no histological evidence of the severe pulmonary oedema seen in horses and cats [23]. In pregnant guinea-pigs, virus was isolated from the uterus (and placenta) with titres as high as, or greater than, titres in other tissues [20]. There was necrosis and strong positive immunostaining in the placenta in an indirect test for viral antigen. Virus could also be isolated from foetuses [20]. Virus was found in the urine of infected cats [19, 22], and horses [19]. Transmission studies with cats and horses have demonstrated that direct contact or exposure to infected urine is probably needed to initiate infection; there is no evidence to support aerosol transmission [19].

Sequence studies have shown that the genomic structure of Hendra virus is similar to other members of the *Paramyxovirinae* subfamily (that is, members of the

Respirovirus, *Morbillivirus*, and *Rubulavirus* genera) in having 6 genes in the order 3'-N-P/V/C-M-F-G-L-5' [25, 26]. Each of the genes has been sequenced and the deduced amino acid sequence determined [5, 25, 27-29]. A number of specific differences between the virion proteins of Hendra virus and those of other members of the family *Paramyxoviridae* were noted and discussed [5, 25-29]. The genome size is significantly larger (18,234 nucleotides) than other members of the subfamily *Paramyxovirinae* [25, 26] due to a larger P protein gene [27] and to longer non-coding intragenic sequences. This large genome size, unique complementary genome terminal sequences, and limited homology with other members of the subfamily have suggested that Hendra virus should be the first member of a new genus in the *Paramyxovirinae*, for which the name *Henipavirus* has been proposed [25, 26]. In addition to size, a number of unusual properties have been determined which have interesting implications for furthering our knowledge of the evolution of the non-segmented negative strand viruses comprising the order *Mononegavirales* [25, 26]. Thus these findings also indicate that the original name of the virus, equine morbillivirus, was incorrect as the virus is not a morbillivirus.

Some unanswered questions

A number of major questions about the transmission, pathogenicity, ecology and phylogeny of Hendra virus still remain unanswered. Of particular importance is its transmissibility, both to humans and to horses. In this regard, it is interesting to note that the three human infections have arisen from contact with infected horses and not from flying foxes. Indeed, no evidence of prior infection was found among bat carers, most of whom have a close relationship with many flying foxes each year and therefore ample opportunity for exposure [30], nor among people who had variable levels of exposure to infected horses (such as veterinarians with necropsy contact) and humans [31]. In addition, no cases of Hendra virus infection were detected in over 75 archival tissue specimens from patients who had died of pneumonia of unknown aetiology during the period 1989-1993 in Brisbane and elsewhere in Queensland (Allan, Selvey, Mackenzie, unpublished results). Thus these data suggest that the virus is not very contagious and transmission to humans is a very rare event.

The mechanism of transmission from flying foxes to horses has not been resolved. The lack of any evidence of previous infection among more than 5,000 horses in different geographic regions of Queensland [12] suggests that it is also a rare event, and indeed it has not been possible to demonstrate transmission from infected flying foxes to in-contact horses experimentally [19]. Various possible methods of transmission, such as ingestion of pasture contaminated by foetal tissues or fluids, or from masticated pellets of residual fruit pulp spat out by flying foxes, have been proposed [16]. Horses excrete virus in urine and saliva, but transmission between horses has not been observed experimentally [20], although it probably occurred in the field during the second incident at Mackay. However, transmission has been observed between cats [22] and from infected cats to a horse [19], probably through infected urine.

There has been a strong link between incidence of disease and pregnancy that may be important in understanding the ecology of the virus and its transmission. Thus, the index cases in the first and second incidents, in Brisbane and Mackay respectively, were pregnant mares, and both incidents occurred during the birthing season of the grey-headed and black flying foxes. The single case in the third incident at Cairns was a mare which had been pregnant shortly before her illness, and this occurred during the birthing season of the spectacled flying fox. Isolation of Hendra virus was first achieved from uterine fluid after an injured flying fox had aborted twin foetuses, from which virus was also isolated [18]. In experimentally infected grey-headed flying foxes, subclinical infection resulted in transplacental transmission as indicated by positive immunostaining in two placentas and virus isolation from one of the associated foetuses [20]. Thus, although pregnancy appears to be associated with possible transmission periods, the importance of these observations to our understanding of the ecology of the virus remains to be determined.

The geographic range of Hendra virus has not been resolved. Although the virus is widespread among pteropid bats in Australia, there are differences in the seroprevalence in different species of flying foxes [17]. Three of the pteropid bat species found in Australia are also found in Papua New Guinea and at least one, the black flying fox, is also found in some islands of the Indonesian archipelago. Antibodies to a Hendra-like virus have been found in the sera of fruit bats in Papua New Guinea, and it seems likely that other related viruses are endemic to fruit bat species elsewhere, such as Nipah virus. This concept is extended further in a companion paper [17].

Finally, evidence described above indicates that Hendra virus is the first member of a new genus in the family *Paramyxoviridae*, with a suggested name of *Henipavirus* [25]. The various properties of Hendra virus and its proteins to support this contention, and the evolutionary relationship of Hendra virus to other members of the nonsegmented negative strand RNA viruses are discussed in a companion paper [26].

Acknowledgements

The authors would like to thank the Fondation Mérieux for the opportunity to present this work. We would like to acknowledge our many colleagues whose work has been included in this brief review, especially Kim Halpin, Linda Selvey, Cathy Allan, Peter Young, and our colleagues at the Australian Animal Health laboratory. We would also like to acknowledge the financial support from the National Health and Medical Research Council for some of the unpublished work described in this report.

References

1. Mackenzie JS. Emerging viral diseases: an Australian perspective. *Emerg Infect Dis* 1999; 5: 1-8.
2. Murray K, Rogers R, Selvey L, Selleck P, Hyatt A, Gould A, *et al.* A novel morbillivirus pneumonia of horses and its transmission to humans. *Emerg Infect Dis* 1995; 1: 31-3.
3. Murray K, Selleck P, Hooper P, Hyatt A, Gould A, Gleeson L, *et al.* A morbillivirus that caused fatal disease in horses and humans. *Science* 1995; 268: 94-7.
4. Selvey LA, Wells RM, McCormack JG, Ansford AJ, Murray K, Rogers RJ, *et al.* Infection of humans and horses by a newly described morbillivirus. *Med J Aust* 1995; 162: 642-5.
5. Gould A. Comparison of the deduced matrix and fusion protein sequences of equine morbillivirus with cognate genes of the Paramyxoviridae. *Virus Res* 1996; 43: 17-31.
6. Hooper PT, Ketterer PJ, Hyatt AD, Russell GM. Lesions of experimental equine morbillivirus pneumonia in horses. *Vet Pathol* 1997; 34: 312-22.

7. O'Sullivan JD, Allworth AM, Paterson DL, Snow TM, Boots R, Gleeson LJ, *et al.* Fatal encephalitis due to novel paramyxovirus transmitted from horses. *Lancet* 1997; 349: 93-5.
8. Rogers RJ, Douglas IC, Baldock FC, Glanville RJ, Seppanen KT, Gleeson LJ, *et al.* Investigation of a second focus of equine morbillivirus infection in coastal Queensland. *Aust Vet J* 1996; 74: 243-4.
9. Hooper PT, Gould AR, Russell GM, Kattenbelt JA, Mitchell G. The retrospective diagnosis of a second outbreak of equine morbillivirus infection. *Aust Vet J* 1996; 74:244-5.
10. Field HE, Barratt PC, Hughes RJ, Shield J, Sullivan ND. A fatal case of Hendra virus infection in a horse in north Queensland: clinical and epidemiological features. *Aust Vet J* 2000; 78: 279-80.
11. Hooper PT, Gould AR, Hyatt AD, Braun MA, Kattenbelt JA, Hengstberger SG, *et al.* Identification and molecular characterisation of Hendra virus in a horse in Queensland. *Aust Vet J* 2000; 78: 281-2.
12. Ward MP, Black PF, Childs AJ, Baldock FC, Webster WR, Rodwell BJ, *et al.* Negative findings from serological studies of equine morbillivirus in the Queensland horse population. *Aust Vet J* 1996; 74: 241-2.
13. Young PL. Halpin K, Selleck PW, Field H, Gravel JL, Kelly MA, *et al.* Serologic evidence for the presence in pteropus bats of a paramyxovirus related to equine morbillivirus. *Emerg Infect Dis* 1996; 2: 239-40.
14. Young P, Halpin K, Field H, Mackenzie J. Finding the wildlife reservoir of equine morbillivirus. In: Asche V, ed. *Recent advances in microbiology*, Vol 5. Melbourne: Australian Society for Microbiology Inc, 1997: 1-12.
15. Halpin H, Young PL, Field H, Mackenzie JS. Newly discovered viruses of flying foxes. *Vet Microbiol* 1999; 68: 83-7.
16. Field H, Young P, Yob JMd, Mills J, Hall L, Mackenzie J. The natural history of Hendra and Nipah viruses. *Microb Infect* 2001; 3: 307-14.
17. Field HE, Mackenzie JS, Hall LS. Emerging zoonotic paramyxoviruses – the role of pteropid bats. In: Dodet B, Vicari M, eds. *Emergence and control of zoonotic ortho- and paramyxoviruses.* Paris: John Libbey, 2001: 205-9.
18. Halpin K, Young PL, Field HE, Mackenzie JS. Isolation of Hendra virus from pteropid bats: a natural reservoir of Hendra virus. *J Gen Virol* 2000; 81: 1927-32.
19. Williamson MM, Hooper, PT, Selleck PW, Gleeson LJ, Daniels PW, Westbury HA, *et al.* Transmission studies of Hendra virus (equine morbillivirus) in fruit bats, horses and cats. *Aust Vet J* 1998; 76: 813-8.
20. Williamson MM, Hooper PT, Selleck PW, Westbury HA, Slocombe RF. Experimental Hendra virus infection in pregnant guinea-pigs and fruit bats *(Pteropus poliocephalus). J Comp Pathol* 2000; 122: 201-7.
21. Hyatt AD, Selleck PW. Ultrastructure of equine morbillivirus. *Virus Res* 1996; 43: 1-15.
22. Westbury HA, Hooper PT, Brouwer S, Selleck PW. Susceptibility of cats to equine morbillivirus. *Aust Vet J* 1996; 74: 132-4.
23. Hooper PT, Westbury HA, Russell GM The lesions of experimental equine morbillivirus disease in cats and guinea pigs. *Vet Pathol* 1997; 34: 323-9.
24. Westbury HA, Hooper PT, Selleck PW, Murray PK. Equine morbillivirus pneumonia: susceptibility of laboratory animals to the virus. *Aust Vet J* 1995; 72: 278-9.
25. Wang LF, Yu M, Hansson E, Pritchard LI, Shiell B, Michalski WP, Eaton BT. The exceptionally large genome of Hendra virus: support for creation of a new genus within the family *Paramyxoviridae. J Virol* 2000; 74: 9972-9.
26. Wang LF, Yu M, Eaton BT. Molecular biology of Hendra virus. In: Dodet B, Vicari M, eds. *Emergence and control of zoonotic ortho- and paramyxoviruses.* Paris: John Libbey Eurotext, 2001; 185-97.
27. Wang LF, Michalski WP, Yu M, Pritchard LI, Crameri G, Shiell B, *et al.* A novel P/V/C gene in a new member of the Paramyxoviridae family, which causes lethal infection in humans, horses and other animals. *J Virol* 1998; 72: 1482-90.
28. Yu M, Hansson E, Langedijk JP, Eaton BT, Wang LF. The attachment protein of Hendra virus has high structural similarity but limited primary sequence homology compared with viruses in the genus Paramyxovirus. *Virology* 1998; 251: 227-33.
29. Yu M, Hansson E, Shiell B, Michalski W, Eaton BT, Wang LF. Sequence analysis of the Hendra virus nucleoprotein gene: comparison with other members of the subfamily Paramyxovirinae. *J Gen Virol* 1998; 79: 1775-80.
30. Selvey L, Taylor R, Arklay A, Gerrard J. Screening of bat carers for antibodies to equine morbillivirus. *Comm Dis Intell* 1996; 477-8.
31. McCormack JG, Allworth AM, Selvey LA, Selleck PW. Transmissibility from horses to humans of a novel paramyxovirus, equine morbillivirus (EMV). *J Infect* 1999; 38: 22-3.

Emergence and Control of Zoonotic Ortho- and Paramyxovirus Diseases
B. Dodet, M. Vicari, eds.

Molecular biology of Hendra virus

Lin-Fa Wang, Meng Yu, Bryan T. Eaton
CSIRO Livestock Industries, Australian Animal Health Laboratory, Geelong, Victoria, Australia

Abstract – An outbreak of acute respiratory disease in Hendra, a suburb of Brisbane, Australia, in September 1994 resulted in the deaths of 14 racing horses and a horse trainer. The causative agent was a new member of the family *Paramyxoviridae*. The virus was originally called equine morbillivirus, but was renamed Hendra virus (HeV) when molecular characterization highlighted differences between it and members of the genus *Morbillivirus*. Further characterization of the entire virus genome has revealed several important features for this novel zoonotic paramyxovirus. Some of the highlights include: 1) a much larger genome whose size (18.2 kb) is actually closer to filoviruses (18.9-19.1 kb) than to other paramyxoviruses (15.2-15.9 kb); 2) much longer untranslated regions, especially at the 3' ends of mRNAs; 3) a larger and complex P/V/C gene; 4) an unusual cleavage site for the fusion protein; 5) an unusual attachment protein lacking both neuraminidase and hemagglutination activities; 6) an RNA polymerase with changes in the catalytic site; and 7) a unique genome terminal sequence not seen in other paramyxoviruses. Less than five years later, the closely related Nipah virus (NiV) emerged in Malaysia, spread rapidly through the pig population and caused the death of over one hundred people. It is now evident that HeV and NiV share a high degree (70-90%) of sequence homology and have almost identical genomic features, and that antisera against the two viruses could cross neutralize each other. Based on these findings and the lack of significant sequence homology and antibody cross reactivity with other members of the *Paramyxoviridae*, it has been proposed that HeV, together with NiV, should be classified in a new genus in this family. The large genome of HeV also fills a gap in the spectrum of genome sizes observed in non-segmented negative-strand (NNS) RNA virus genomes. As such it provides a further piece in the puzzle of NNS RNA virus evolution.

Viruses in the families *Filoviridae*, *Paramyxoviridae*, *Rhabdoviridae* and *Bornaviridae* contain a non-segmented, negative stranded (NNS) RNA genome and share similar genome organization, replication strategy, and domain structure and amino acid sequence in the polymerase proteins. These four families are grouped taxonomically in the order *Mononegavirales*, the first taxon above family level to be recognized in virus taxonomy [1-3]. The genome size of viruses in the order varies significantly, ranging from 8.9 kb in the *Bornaviridae* to 19.1 kb in the *Filoviridae*. Members of *Paramyxoviridae* have intermediate genome sizes from 15.1 to 15.9 kb, and have traditionally been described as having a "uniform genome size" [1, 4]. The universality of this family feature is now challenged with the discovery of a much larger genome of Hendra virus (HeV). Classification within the family has undergone major changes in recent years and the current taxonomy [3-5] divides the family into two subfamilies, *Paramyxovirinae* and *Pneumovirinae*. The *Paramyxovirinae* include three genera, *Respirovirus* (formerly known as *Paramyxovirus*), *Morbillivirus* and *Rubulavirus*, whereas the *Pneumovirinae* contains two genera, *Pneumovirus* and *Metapneumovirus.*

HeV has received a great deal of publicity because of its ability to cause lethal infection of humans and a variety of animals [6-9]. Its profile was further boosted with the discovery of the closely related Nipah virus (NiV) in Malaysia some five years later [10-13]. These viruses have also significantly expanded our perception of the extent of viral diversity in the *Paramyxoviridae* and raised questions about the nature of virus evolution within the order *Mononegavirales*. Here, important molecular features of HeV will be summarized to demonstrate that HeV, together with NiV, represents a group of new viruses within the subfamily *Paramyxovirinae*. In addition, the potential correlation of the genetic characteristics of these new viruses with their novel biological properties will be discussed.

Biological features of Hendra virus

HeV grows to high titre in a range of cultured cells from diverse species and has been purified by rate zonal centrifugation in sucrose gradients. Virus structural proteins have been characterised by polyacrylamide gel electrophoresis and individual proteins identified using monospecific rabbit antisera generated against bacterially expressed HeV proteins. The protein profile resembles that of a typical member of the subfamily *Paramyxovirinae* although the P protein is significantly larger than cognate proteins in the subfamily [14]. Both cleaved (F_1) and uncleaved (F_0) forms of the fusion protein are present in approximately equivalent amounts in HeV produced by Vero cells and a range of other cultured cells and from the allantoic fluid of infected chicken embryos [15]. In contrast, the fusion protein in Vero cell-derived NiV appears to be completely cleaved.

HeV displays a number of interesting biological properties. In addition to infecting a wide range of cells *in vitro*, the virus causes systemic infections *in vivo* in species as diverse as flying foxes, humans, cats and horses, displaying a predilection for endothelial cells. HeV does not agglutinate erythrocytes from a variety of sources, nor does it display neuraminidase activity when tested on fetuin, activities that characterize members of the *Respirovirus* and *Rubulavirus* genera. Antigenically, HeV was not related to any known paramyxovirus at the time of discovery [6].

Overall genome features of Hendra virus

The complete genome sequence of HeV has been determined [14, 16-19]. As with other viruses in the subfamily *Paramyxovirinae*, there is a total of six transcription units encoding six major structural proteins. They are nucleocapsid protein (N), phosphoprotein (P), matrix protein (M), fusion protein (F), glycoprotein (G) or attachment (A) protein, and large protein (L) or RNA polymerase, in the order 3’-N-P-M-F-G-L-5’. Overall, the arrangement of genes of the HeV genome is most closely related to that of the *Respirovirus* and *Morbillivirus* genera. However, several features make HeV unique in the subfamily *Paramyxovirinae*. HeV has a genome size of 18.2 kb, which is approximately 15% larger than the relatively uniform genome size of all other known members of the *Paramyxovirinae*. This makes the size of HeV genome closer to those of members of the family *Filoviridae* (18.9-19.1 kb). HeV has longer untranslated regions than other members of the *Paramyxovirinae*, mostly at the 3' end, with the exception of the last transcription unit coding for the L gene [18]. This feature has also been observed for filoviruses, including Ebola and Marburg viruses [20]. On the other hand and with the exception of the P protein, the size of the six major structural proteins is similar to those of other paramyxoviruses *(see Table I)*. In other words, the increase in genome size is largely due to the expansion of non-translated regions.

Table I. Size comparison of major structural proteins from selected *Paramyxovirinae* members*.

Genus	Virus	N	P	M	F	A	L
	HeV	532	707	352	546	604	2,244
Respirovirus	SeV	524	568	348	565	575	2,228
	HPIV3	515	603		539	572	2,233
Morbillivirus	MeV	525	507	335	550	614	2,183
	CDV	523	507	335	662	604	2,161
Rubulavirus	NDV	489	395	364	553	577	2,204
	MuV	549	391	375	538	583	2,261
	SV41	543	394	382	561	568	2,269

* Numbers given in the table are amino acid residue numbers. Abbreviations: SeV, Sendai virus; HPIV3, human parainfluenza virus-3; MeV, measles virus; CDV, canine distemper virus; NDV, Newcastle disease virus; MuV, mumps virus; SV41, simian virus 41.

The genomes of paramyxoviruses have a 3' leader sequence that contains the promoter for transcription of positive-sense mRNA and a 5' trailer that contains the promoter responsible for the synthesis of the negative strand RNA during virus replication. The first 12 nt of the 3' and 5' genomic termini are highly conserved and complementary. For HeV the termini of the genome and anti-genome are identical for the first 12 nt positions and for 19 of the first 23 nt positions. A comparison of the first 12 nt of the HeV anti-genome with other members of the *Paramyxovirinae* indicated that HeV is more closely related to respiroviruses and morbilliviruses than to rubulaviruses [18]. It is interesting to note that HeV is unique in having a G residue at the 4th nt position whereas all other members of the subfamily have an A residue in that location [18].

The gene start, gene stop and intergenic sequences (IGS) are usually conserved among different members of the same genus in the *Paramyxovirinae*. The gene start regions are more GC-rich than the gene stop regions which are AT-rich and always end with a series of Us (or As in the anti-genome sequence). The size of the IGS varies from genus to genus, but is uniform in length for members of the *Respirovirus* and *Morbillivirus* genera. For these two genera, the IGS is a highly conserved trinucleotide sequence of 3'-GAA-5'. The gene start and stop signals of HeV are highly conserved and show much greater homology to the gene start and stop sequences found in respiroviruses and morbilliviruses than in rubulaviruses. Moreover, the 3-nt IGS is absolutely conserved for all seven positions in HeV. To our knowledge, this is the first paramyxovirus to be characterized with a completely conserved IGS for all of the possible positions [18].

The template for paramyxovirus RNA synthesis is not naked RNA but the helical ribonucleoprotein core of the virus, a structure in which nucleotide hexamers are believed to be associated with individual nucleocapsid (N) protein molecules [21]. As a consequence, many *Paramyxovirinae* members have a genome length that is a multiple of 6. Moreover, it has been shown that these genomes are effectively replicated only when they are a multiple of 6 nt [21]. In addition, it is found that within a genus, the transcription start site for each gene tends to be conserved in relation to the hexamer phasing position as shown in *Table II*. It is interesting to note that HeV genes have a unique hexamer phasing pattern "2, 3, 4, 4, 4, 3" that is significantly different from other viruses in the subfamily. The hexamer phasing positions for the HeV P, A (G) and L genes are unique and not used by cognate genes in the subfamily. HeV is also unique in that it uses hexamer phasing position 5 for the P editing site. This position is not used by any other virus for either a P editing site or transcription start site [21].

Table II. Comparison of hexamer phasing patterns of selected *Paramyxovirinae* members*.

Genus/Virus	Genone length	Rule of Six (length/6)	Hexamer phasing position					
			N	P(e)	M	F	A	L
HeV	18,234	3,039	2	3(5)	4	4	4	3
Morbillivirus								
MeV	15,894	2,649	2	2(6)	4	3	3	2
CDV	15,690	2,616	2	2(2)	4	2	3	2
Respirovirus								
SeV	15,384	2,564	2	1(1)	1	1	1	2
hPIV3	15,462	2,577	2	1(2)	1	1	1	2
Rubulavirus								
MuV	15,384	2,564	2	1(3)	1	6	1	6
SV5	15,246	2,541	2	1(3)	1	6	1	6
NDV	15,186	2,531	2	4(1)	4	4	3	6

* Number given is the hexamer phasing position at each of the six gene start sites and, for the P gene, the editing site (in parenthesis).

Structural genes and their encoded products

The nucleocapsid protein (N) gene

The N protein of HeV is the most abundant protein in the purified virion, and has an apparent molecular weight of 58 kDa, which is in good agreement with the calculated molecular weight of 58,481 Da. The deduced N protein sequence of 532 amino acids (aa) was confirmed by direct amino acid sequencing of peptides obtained by proteolytic digestion of purified viral N protein [17]. The size of the N protein is very similar to those of other members *(Table I)*. Overall, the N protein of HeV has only 20 to 30% sequence homology with the N proteins of other viruses in the subfamily *Paramyxo-*

virinae and this may explain the lack of antigenic cross-reactivity observed during the initial characterization of HeV [6].

The amino-acid (aa) sequence homology between the N proteins of HeV and other paramyxoviruses is mostly located in the central domain (aa 171-383). This is the domain believed to be important for N-N, N-P and N-L interactions. Most, if not all, paramyxovirus N proteins carry the so-called "invariant" sequence F-X_4-Y-P-X_3-S-Y-A-M-G [22]. This sequence is also present in the HeV N protein except that the second Y residue is replaced by an F residue, a relatively conserved change, yet unique for NiV and HeV [17].

The phosphoprotein (P) gene

As shown in *Figure 1*, the P gene of HeV is highly complex and has a coding capacity for five potential proteins encoded in three possible reading frames. The P gene in the *Paramyxovirinae* represents an example of a virus encoding as much information as possible in a single gene. The P gene can give rise to a number of different polypeptide products by means of internal translation initiation sites, overlapping reading frames and an unusual transcription process whereby one or several non-templated nucleotides are inserted, resulting in a shift of reading frame during translation [22, 23]. All of these mechanisms were found in the HeV P gene.

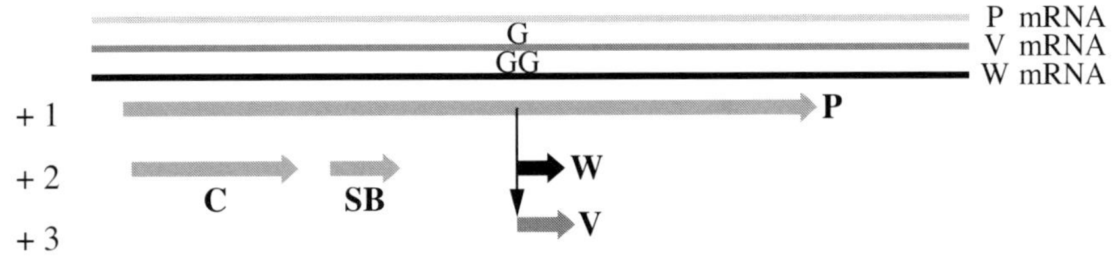

	P	V	W	C	SB
Size (aa)	707	457	448	166	65
MW (kDa)	78.3	50.6	49.4	19.6	7.6
pI	4.5	4.5	4.7	8.8	12.2

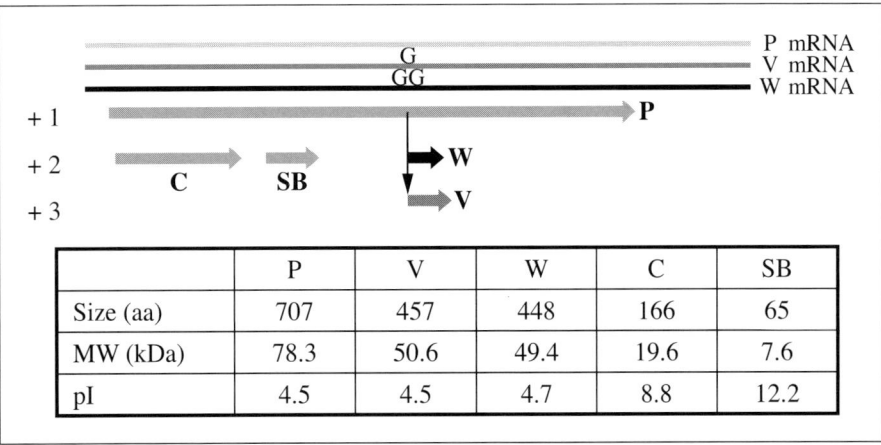

Figure 1. The coding capacity of HeV P gene. The top part of the diagram shows the three potential mRNA species that could be made by RNA editing *via* addition of non-templated G residue(s). The translation reading frames are shown at left as +1, +2 and +3. The P protein is translated from the +1 reading frame whereas the C, and SB proteins are derived from internal translation initiation sites in the +2 reading frame. The W- and V-specific domains are encoded in the +2 and +3 reading frames, respectively, and are only accessible in the edited mRNA as shown above. The fusion junction between P protein and W- or V-domain is shown by the down pointing arrow corresponding to the G-insertion site in the W- and V-mRNA. The table at the bottom summarizes the five gene products that could be made from the P gene.

The P protein is the largest protein encoded by the P gene of HeV. It is transcribed from an unedited mRNA that is co-linear with genomic RNA. The HeV P protein (707 aa) is more than 100 aa longer than any other known paramyxovirus P protein *(Table I)*. The calculated molecular weight of the HeV P protein is 78,305 Da, but the protein migrated with an apparent molecular weight of 98 kDa [14]. The identity of the 98 kDa band as the HeV P protein has been confirmed by direct sequencing of peptides after proteolytic digestions [14] and by Western blot analyses using monospecific rabbit sera raised against recombinant polypeptides corresponding to three different regions of the P protein (Wang, unpublished results). *In vivo* phosphorylation of the HeV P protein has been confirmed by radioactive labeling and by mass spectrometry (Michalski and Eaton, unpublished results).

As for morbilliviruses and respiroviruses, the addition of a single, non-templated G at the RNA editing site produces a V-mRNA which allows access to a cysteine-rich reading frame, producing the non-structural V protein that contains the amino terminal part of P and a unique V domain at the C-terminus *(Figure 1)*. The predicted HeV V protein is 457 aa long with a calculated molecular weight of 50,647 Da. On SDS-PAGE the HeV V protein migrates as a 70-kDa band, which is significantly larger than predicted, as observed for the P protein. The functional expression of HeV V protein has been confirmed by Western blot analysis using a rabbit anti-V antibody generated using a recombinant fusion protein containing the Cys-rich V-specific region (Wang, unpublished results).

The addition of two non-templated G residues to the P mRNA of HeV produces yet another mRNA (the W-mRNA) that allows access to a 47-amino-acid ORF and potentially encodes a protein that would be analogous to the W protein described for Newcastle disease virus and Sendai virus [24, 25]. It is not known whether this W protein is expressed *in vivo*.

Members of the *Respirovirus* and *Morbillivirus* genera synthesize a third P gene-derived protein. The C protein is encoded at the 5' end of the gene by a reading frame different from that used by the P and V proteins (reading frame +2, *see Figure 1*). An independent translation initiation site is used for expression of this relatively small protein (varying between approximately 160-210 aa). Although not required for replication *in vitro*, recent studies using reverse genetics suggest that the C protein is required for *in vivo* functions, such as virulence and efficient replication in certain cell types [26-28]. In HeV, the C protein is 166 aa in length with a calculated molecular weight of 19,647 Da. It has a pI of 8.8, and migrates as an 18-kDa band in SDS-PAGE. Although once considered a non-structural protein, C protein can be detected in purified HeV virions by Western blot analysis using antibodies raised against recombinant C protein (Wang, unpublished results).

In addition to coding for the P, V, W and C proteins, the HeV P gene also has a small open reading frame (ORF) located between the coding regions of the C and V proteins. This small ORF has the coding capacity for an extremely basic protein with a pI of 12.2. Although the functional expression of the SB protein in virus-infected cells has not been proven, it is interesting to note that the coding region for a similar small basic protein (SB) has been identified in the P gene equivalents of members of two related virus families within the order *Mononegavirales*. These are vesicular stomatitis virus (VSV) in the family *Rhabdoviridae* [29] and Marburg virus in the family *Filoviridae* [20]. Although the function of SB is not known, the expression of SB protein in VSV-infected cells has been unequivocally demonstrated [29, 30]. This ORF is not found in NiV [31].

The matrix protein (M) gene

The deduced M protein of HeV is 352 aa long with a calculated molecular weight of 39,827 Da. It is a basic protein with a pI of 9.44 and a net charge of +14 at neutral pH. These properties are very similar to other paramyxovirus M proteins, which range in size from approximately 341 to 375 aa residues and have net charges of +14 to +17 [19, 29]. Interestingly, the alignment of HeV M gene indicated that the translation initiation codon (AUG) normally utilized by morbilliviruses had been changed to AUA, and an upstream initiation codon was used instead. This resulted in the size difference between HeV M protein (352 aa) and the morbillivirus M proteins (335 aa) [19].

The fusion protein (F) gene

Paramyxovirus fusion proteins are type I membrane glycoproteins with a signal peptide at the N-terminus and a transmembrane anchor at the C-terminus. The fusion proteins are synthesized in an inactive precursor form (F_0) that is cleaved by a host cell protease into a biologically active form consisting of two disulfide-linked polypeptides (F_1 and F_2). The N-terminus of the F_1 protein is hydrophobic and responsible for membrane fusion activity of paramyxoviruses [22, 32].

The F protein of HeV is predicted to be a type I glycoprotein that is 546 aa in size. All cysteine residues outside of the signal sequence are conserved between HeV and other *Paramyxovirinae*. This suggests that the HeV F protein has structural features that are similar to those of the F proteins of other *Paramyxovirinae* [19].

There are six potential N-linked glycosylation sites in the extracellular domains of the HeV F protein, and these are equally distributed between F_2 and F_1 [15, 19]. The difference between the calculated molecular weight (12 kDa) and the observed molecular weight (19-23 kDa) of the F_2 protein of HeV suggests that at least one, and probably more, of these sites is utilized. This suggestion is consistent with the observation that whereas HeV F_2 can be radiolabelled with glucosamine and can bind glucosamine-specific lectins, HeV F_1 does not appear to contain carbohydrate moieties [15]. In this respect, although the HeV F1 protein resembles cognate proteins in the *Respirovirus* and *Rubulavirus* genera in having potential glycosylation sites, phenotypically HeV resembles members of the *Morbillivirus* genus in having an unglycosylated F_1 protein *(see Figure 2)*.

The most distinctive feature of the F protein of HeV is the unique cleavage site that has been shown experimentally to contain a single basic residue, lysine (K) in the sequence DVKLAG [15]. This cleavage site differs from the majority of the F protein cleavage sites that are found in the *Paramyxovirinae* which contain multiple basic residues, are arginine-rich, and are thought to be cleaved by furin, an ubiquitous serine protease localised in the *trans*-Golgi network of many eucaryotic cells [22, 33]. The minimum sequence requirement for efficient processing by furin *in vitro* is R-X-X-R [34], a sequence that is highly conserved in paramyxovirus F proteins [22, 32]. Although the enzyme responsible for the cleavage of HeV F protein is not known, it has been demonstrated that HeV replicates and the F protein is cleaved in LoVo cells [15], which lack furin, suggesting that HeV and possibly NiV utilize other host cell proteases.

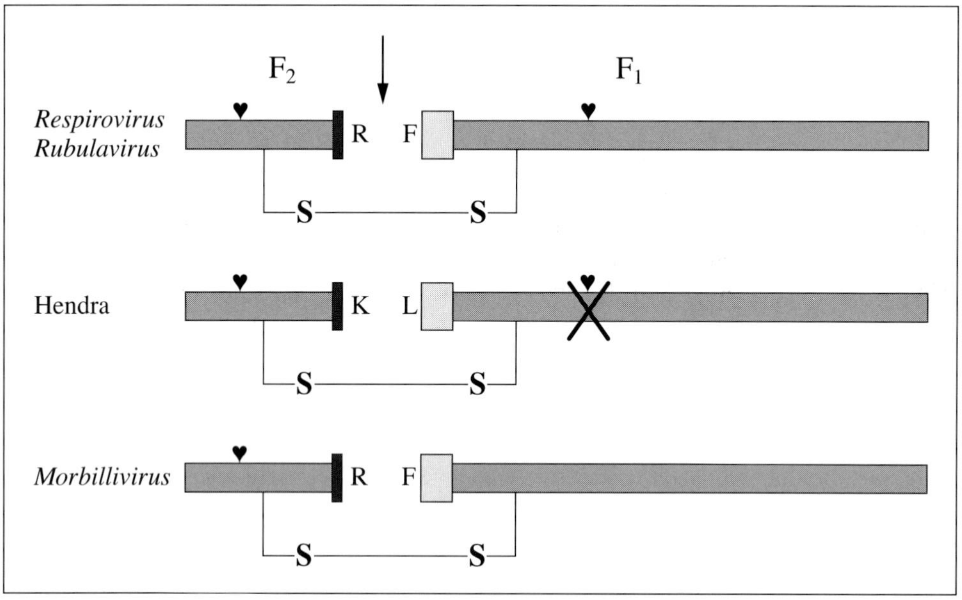

Figure 2. Comparison of important features of the HeV F gene with those of other members within the subfamily *Paramyxovirinae*. The disulfide-bonded F_2 and F_1 proteins are shown at the left and right of the cleavage site (down-pointing arrow), respectively. The solid box at the end of the F_2 protein represents the cleavage site sequence whereas the dotted box at the beginning of the F_1 protein represents the highly conserved fusion peptide domain. The amino acid residues immediately before and after the cleavage site are shown. The heart sign indicates the presence of N-glycosylation site(s). The cross sign indicates that the N-glycosylation site on the HeV F_1 protein is present, but not used.

Another interesting feature of the HeV F protein is that the F_1 protein begins with a leucine residue (L) whereas all other paramyxoviruses, except for some avirulent strains of NDV, have a phenylalanine [19, 22, 32] *(see Figure 2)*. The biological consequence of this amino acid change is unclear.

The attachment protein (G) gene

The cell attachment proteins of members of the family *Paramyxoviridae* can display haemagglutination (H) and neuraminidase (N) activities. Members of the *Respirovirus* and *Rubulavirus* genera have HN proteins, while those in the *Morbillivirus* genus have H proteins. However, the cognate protein in HeV is similar to the attachment proteins in the *Pneumovirus* genus in that they lack both haemagglutination and neuraminidase activities and are designated as G proteins [6, 16]. Sequence analysis of the HeV G gene predicted a type II membrane glycoprotein with structure similar to that of other paramyxovirus attachment proteins [16]. These proteins contain a cytoplasmic tail at the N-terminus followed by a hydrophobic transmembrane domain, a short extracellular stem region and a large globular extracellular "head" at the C-terminus. The G protein contains eight, potential N-linked glycosylation sites and glycosylation of HeV G protein *in vivo* has been confirmed by lectin binding analysis [15], but the exact location of glycosylation site(s) has not been determined.

Three-dimensional modeling studies of the globular head domain of the HeV G protein resulted in several interesting findings [16]. The HeV G protein shares structural features characteristic of viruses in the genus *Respirovirus*. The locations of all seven proposed disulfide bonds are absolutely conserved between HeV and the respiroviruses. A large number of structurally important aa residues (Gly, Pro, and aromatic aa residues) are conserved in the HeV G protein. The overall canonical folding pattern of six parallel sheets, which is conserved in viral, bacterial and eukaryotic neuraminidases, is also retained in the HeV G protein [16]. Among the seven active site residues known to be important for neuraminidase activity [35], only one is present in the HeV G protein whereas all are conserved in the neuraminidase-positive respiroviruses and rubulaviruses and four in morbilliviruses which are predominantly neuraminidase-negative *(see Table III)*.

It has been proposed that the conserved hexapeptide NRKSCS in HN proteins is close to the sialic acid binding site [36-38]. The failure of HeV to display hemagglutination is consistent with the presence of the hexapeptide TIHHCS in the cognate region of the G protein [16]. In addition, removal of sialic acid from susceptible cells by neuraminidase treatment did not abrogate infection by HeV (Eaton, unpublished results).

Table III. Comparison of conserved residues important for neuramidinase activity among *Paramyxovirinae* attachment proteins*.

Genus/Virus	Catalytic site residues							Sialic acid binding site
	R(1)	D(2)	E(3)	R(4)	R(5)	Y(6)	E(7)	NRKSCS
Respirovirus	✓	✓	✓	✓	✓	✓	✓	✓
Rubulavirus	✓	✓	✓	✓	✓	✓	✓	✓
Morbillivirus	✓	X	X	X	✓	✓	✓	XXXXCX
Hendra & Nipah	X	X	X	X	X	X	✓	XXXXCS

* Conserved residues are represented by ✓ whereas non-conserved residues are indicated by X.

The RNA polymerase (L) gene

The L protein of paramyxoviruses is the least abundant of viral structural proteins. Its gene is located at the most 5' promoter-distal region of the genome and is thus the last to be transcribed. The HeV L gene codes for a protein of 2,244 aa with a calculated molecular weight of 257,280 Da. The identity of the 200+ kDa band in purified virions as the L protein was confirmed by two different approaches. First by Western blot using rabbit mono-specific antibodies raised against a recombinant polypeptide located in the middle of the L gene, and second by mass spectrometric analysis of proteolytic peptides derived from the putative L protein band [18].

Like other paramyxoviruses, the HeV L protein is rich in leucine and isoleucine (19.3%). The linear domain structure of L proteins suggested by Poch *et al.* [39] is also identified in the HeV L protein, with the sequence of domain III being the most conserved in comparison to other L proteins. In a region predicted to contain the catalytic site of L proteins, all non-segmented negative sense RNA viruses characterized to date have the tetra-peptide sequence GDNQ. However, the HeV L protein has the sequence of GDNE *(see Figure 3)*. This Q to E change has also been found in NiV and the recently described Tupaia paramyxovirus (TPMV) [40] (and GenBank Accession Number AF079780). This change introduces a second negative charge in this functionally important region. In this regard, it is interesting to note that RNA polymerases from positive sense RNA viruses do carry a double negative charged consensus sequence GDD in the cognate catalytic site [39]. Whether this suggests a more ancient form of the catalytic domain for the HeV, NiV and TPMV RNA polymerases is difficult to predict at this time.

Hendra	IVQ	GDNE	SIA
		*	
Morbillivirus	LVQ	GDNQ	TIA
Respirovirus	MVQ	GDNQ	AIA
Rubulavirus	MVQ	GDNQ	AIA
RSV	LIN	GDNQ	SID
Rabies	LAQ	GDNQ	VLC
VSV	LAQ	GDNQ	VIC
Marburg	SVM	GDNQ	CIT
Ebola	AVM	GDNQ	CIT
BDV	LGQ	GDNQ	TII

Figure 3. Sequence alignment of the putative RNA polymerase (L) catalytic site from all four family members of the order *Mononegavirales*. The highly conserved GDNQ motif is boxed and the unique E residue in the HeV L protein sequence is indicated by a * sign beneath. Abbreviations: RSV, respiratory syncytial virus; VSV, vesicular stomatitis virus; BDV, borna disease virus.

Evolutionary relationships and virus classification

While there is no significant nucleotide sequence homology detected between the HeV genome and other members of the *Paramyxovirinae*, a clear, albeit limited, sequence homology can be found at the protein level. In general, the proteins encoded by HeV are similar in size, sequence and/or predicted functional domain structure to those of the respiroviruses and morbilliviruses. However, several unique features found in HeV proteins as described above point to a different evolutionary lineage for HeV.

Phylogenetic analysis of the deduced amino acid sequences of the N, P, M, F, G and L from representatives of the subfamily *Paramyxovirinae* showed that HeV consistently formed a unique cluster which was more closely related to the morbilliviruses and the respiroviruses than to the rubulaviruses. This is also true for NiV [31]. A representative phylogenetic tree based on the N proteins of selected *Paramyxovirinae* members is shown in *Figure 4*. All of the four new viruses characterized in the last few years (boxed in *Figure 4*) seem to be positioned between morbilliviruses and respiroviruses.

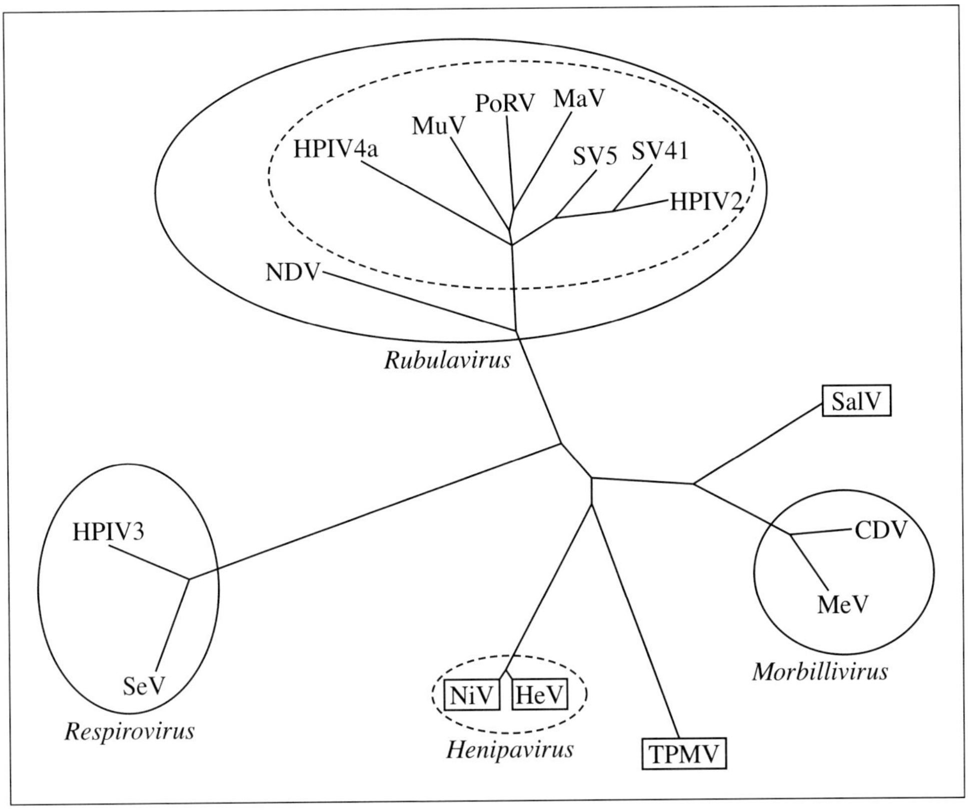

Figure 4. Phylogenetic analyses based on the N protein sequences from selected members of the subfamily *Paramyxovirinae*. Unclassified members are boxed. Members in an officially recognized genus classification are grouped inside a solid-line circle whereas the dotted-line circles indicated the proposed new genera for HeV and NiV [18, 42] and for rubulaviruses excluding NDV [43]. Abbreviations not in text: HPIV2, human parainfluenza virus-2; HPIV4a, human parainfluenza virus-4a; MaV, Mapuera virus; PoRV, porcine rubulavirus.

While strong serological cross reactivity has been demonstrated between HeV and NiV, that is not the case for the other two novel viruses, *i.e.* the tree shrew virus (TPMV) [40] and Salem virus (SalV) [41]. TPMV is more closely related to the HeV-NiV cluster while SalV is more related to morbilliviruses.

Many genomic features suggest that HeV and NiV are significantly different from members of the three existing genera within the subfamily. The genomes of HeV and NiV are more than 15% larger, due predominantly to the presence of long untranslated regions in the six transcription units. In addition, the HeV genome has unique terminal sequences and highly conserved gene start, stop and inter-genic sequences. Also significant in this context is the different tetra peptide sequence in the proposed catalytic site of the HeV and NiV L protein. It is interesting to note that TPMV also has a large genome (17,904 nt, GenBank Accession Number AF079780) and a GDNE tetra-peptide sequence at the putative catalytic site of its L protein.

In summary, all these data confirm that although HeV and NiV clearly belong to the subfamily *Paramyxovirinae*, they may not be confidently classified as members of the three existing genera. Instead, all the data gathered so far suggest that HeV and NiV should be considered as members of a fourth new genus within the *Paramyxovirinae*. It has therefore been proposed that a new genus, named *Henipavirus*, should be created within the subfamily *Paramyxovirinae* to accommodate the classification of these newly discovered paramyxoviruses [18, 42].

References

1. Pringle CR. The order Mononegavirales. *Arch Virol* 1991; 117: 137-40.
2. Pringle CR, Easton AJ. Monopartite negative strand RNA genomes. *Semin Virol* 1997; 8: 49-57.
3. Pringle CR. Virus taxonomy – San Diego 1998. *Arch Virol* 1998; 143: 1449-59.
4. Rima B, Alexander DJ, Billeter MA, Collins PL, Kingsbury DW, Lipkind MA, Nagai Y, Orvell C, Pringle CR, ter Meulen V. Family *Paramyxoviridae*. In: Murphy FA, Fauquet CM, Bishop DHL, Ghabrial SA, Jarvis AW, Martelli GP, Mayo MA, Summers MD, eds. *Virus taxonomy. Sixth report of the international committee on taxonomy of viruses*. Vienna-New York: Springer-Verlag, 1995: 268-74.
5. Mayo MA, Pringle CR. Virus taxonomy-1997. *J Gen Virol* 1998; 79: 649-57.
6. Murray K, Selleck P, Hooper P, Hyatt A, Gould A, Gleeson L, Westbury H, Hiley L, Selvey L, Rodwell B. A morbillivirus that caused fatal disease in horses and humans. *Science* 1995; 268: 94-7.
7. O'Sullivan JD, Allworth AM, Paterson DJ, Snow TM, Boots R, Gleeson LJ, Gould AR, Hyatt AD, Bradfield J. Fatal encephalitis due to novel paramyxovirus transmitted from horses. *Lancet* 1997; 349: 93-5.
8. Westbury HA, Hooper PT, Selleck PW, Murray PK. Equine morbillivirus pneumonia: susceptibility of laboratory animals to the virus. *Aust Vet J* 1996; 72: 278-9.
9. Williamson MM, Hooper PT, Selleck PW, Westbury HA, Slocombe RF. Experimental Hendra virus infection in pregnant guinea-pigs and fruit bats *(Pteropus poliocephalus)*. *J Comp Pathol* 2000; 122: 201-7.
10. Anonymous. Outbreak of Hendra-like virus – Malaysia and Singapore, 1998-1999. *MMWR* 1999; 48: 265-9.
11. Anonymous. Update: outbreak of Nipah virus – Malaysia and Singapore, 1999. *MMWR* 1999; 48: 335-7.
12. Chua KB, Bellini WJ, Rota PA, Harcourt BH, Tamin A, Lam SK, Ksiazek TG, Rollin PE, Zaki SR, Shieh WJ, Goldsmith CS, Gubler DJ, Roehrig JT, Eaton B, Gould AR, Olson J, Field H, Daniels P, Ling AE, Peters CJ, Anderson LJ, Mahy BWJ. Nipah virus: A recently emergent deadly paramyxovirus. *Science* 2000; 288: 1432-5.
13. Goh KJ, Tan CT, Chew NK, Tan PSK, Kamarulzaman A, Sarji SA, Wong KT, Abdullah BJJ, Chua KB, Lam SK. Clinical features of Nipah virus encephalitis among pig farmers in Malaysia. *N Engl J Med* 2000; 342: 1229-35.
14. Wang LF, Michalski WP, Yu M, Pritchard LI, Crameri G, Shiell B, Eaton BT. A novel P/V/C gene in a new member of the Paramyxoviridae family, which causes lethal infection in humans, horses, and other animals. *J Virol* 1998; 72: 1482-90.
15. Michalski WP, Crameri G, Wang LF, Shiell BJ, Eaton BT. The cleavage activation and sites of glycosylation in the fusion protein of Hendra virus. *Virus Res* 2000; 69: 73-83.
16. Yu M, Hansson E, Langedijk JP, Eaton BT, Wang LF. The attachment protein of Hendra virus has high structural similarity but limited primary sequence homology compared with viruses in the genus Paramyxovirus. *Virology* 1999; 251: 227-33.
17. Yu M, Hansson E, Shiell B, Michalski W, Eaton BT, Wang LF. Sequence analysis of the Hendra virus nucleoprotein gene: comparison with other members of the subfamily Paramyxovirinae. *J Gen Virol* 1998; 79: 1775-80.
18. Wang LF, Yu M, Hansson E, Pritchard LI, Michalski WP, Eaton BT. The exceptionally large genome of Hendra virus: support for the creation of a new genus within the family Paramyxoviridae. *J Virol* 2000; 74: 9972-9.

19. Gould AR. Comparison of the deduced matrix and fusion protein sequences of equine morbillivirus with cognate genes of the Paramyxoviridae. *Virus Res* 1996; 43: 17-31.
20. Feldmann H, Klenk HD. Marburg and Ebola viruses. *Adv Virus Res* 1996; 47: 1-53.
21. Kolakofsky D, Pelet T, Garcin D, Hausmann S, Curran J, Roux L. Paramyxovirus RNA synthesis and the requirement for hexamer genome length: the rule of six revisited. *J Virol* 1998; 72: 891-9.
22. Lamb RA, Kolakofsky D. *Paramyxoviridae*: the viruses and their replication. In: Fields BN, Knipe DM, Howley PM, Chanock RM, Melnick JL, Monath TP, Roizman B, Straus SE, eds. *Fields Virology*, 3rd ed. Philadelphia: Lippincott-Raven, 1996, 1177-204.
23. Thomas SM, Lamb RA, Paterson RG. Two mRNAs that differ by two nontemplated nucleotides encode the amino coterminal proteins P and V of the pramyxovirus SV 5. *Cell* 1988; 54: 891-902.
24. Steward M, Vipond BI, Millar NS, Emmerson PT. RNA editing in Newcastle disease virus. *J Gen Virol* 1993; 74: 2539-47.
25. Curran J, Boeck R, Kolakofsky D. The Sendai virus P gene expresses both an essential protein and an inhibitor of RNA synthesis by shuffling modules *via* RNA editing. *EMBO J* 1991; 10: 3079-985.
26. Escoffier C, Manie S, Vincent S, Muller CP, Billeter M, Gerlier D. Nonstructural C protein is required for efficient measles virus replication in human peripheral blood cells. *J Virol* 1999; 73: 1695-8.
27. Patterson JB, Thomas D, Lewicki H, Billeter MA, Oldstone MBA. V and C proteins of measles virus function as virulence factors *in vivo*. *Virology* 2000; 267: 80-9.
28. Baron MD, Barrett T. Rinderpest viruses lacking the C and V proteins show specific defects in growth and transcription of viral RNAs. *J Virol* 2000; 74: 2603-11.
29. Spiropoulou CF, Nichol ST. A small highly basic protein is encoded in overlapping frame within the P gene of vesicular stomatitis virus. *J Virol* 1993; 67: 3103-10.
30. Kretzschmar E, Peluso R, Schnell MJ, Whitt MA, Rose JK. Normal replication of vesicular stomatitis virus without C proteins. *Virology* 1996; 216: 309-16.
31. Harcourt BH, Tamin A, Ksiazek TG, Rollin PE, Anderson LJ, Bellini WJ, Rota PA. Molecular characterization of Nipah virus, a newly emergent paramyxovirus. *Virology* 2000; 271: 334-49.
32. Bellini WJ, Rota PA, Anderson LJ. Paramyxoviruses. In: Collier L, Balows A, Sussman M, eds. *Microbiology and microbial infections*, Vol. 1. London: Arnold, 1998: 435-61.
33. Hatsuzawa K, Hosaka M, Nakagawa T, Nagase M, Shoda A, Murakami K, Nakayama K. Structure and expression of mouse furin, a yeast Kex2-related protease. Lack of processing of coexpressed prorenin in GH4C1 cells. *J Biol Chem* 1990; 265: 22075-8.
34. Molloy SS, Bresnahan PA, Leppla SH, Klimpel KR, Thomas G. Human furin is a calcium-dependent serine endoprotease that recognizes the sequence Arg-X-X-Arg and efficiently cleaves anthrax toxin protective antigen. *J Biol Chem* 1992; 267: 16396-402.
35. Langedijk JP, Daus FJ, van Oirschot JT. Sequence and structure alignment of Paramyxoviridae attachment proteins and discovery of enzymatic activity for a morbillivirus hemagglutinin. *J Virol* 1997; 71: 6155-67.
36. Jorgensen ED, Collins PL, Lomedico PT. Cloning and nucleotide sequence of Newcastle disease virus hemagglutinin-neuraminidase mRNA: identification of a putative sialic acid binding site. *Virology* 1987; 156: 12-24.
37. Morrison TPA. Structure, function, and intracellular processing of the glycoproteins of Paramyxoviridae. In: Kingsbury DW, ed. *The Paramyxoviruses*. New York: Plenum, 1991: 347-82.
38. Mirza AM, Deng R, Iorio RM. Site-directed mutagenesis of a conserved hexapeptide in the paramyxovirus hemagglutinin-neuraminidase glycoprotein: effects on antigenic structure and function. *J Virol* 1994; 68: 5093-9.
39. Poch O, Blumberg BM, Bougueleret L, Tordo N. Sequence comparison of five polymerases (L proteins) of unsegmented negative-strand RNA viruses: theoretical assignment of functional domains. *J Gen Virol* 1990; 71: 1153-62.
40. Tidona CA, Kurz HW, Gelderblom HR, Darai G. Isolation and molecular characterization of a novel cytopathogenic paramyxovirus from tree shrews. *Virology* 1999; 258: 425-34.
41. Renshaw RW, Glaser AL, Van Campen H, Weiland F, Dubvi EJ. Identification and phylogenetic comparison of Salem virus, a novel paramyxovirus of horses. *Virology* 2000; 270: 417-29.
42. Wang LF, Eaton BT. Henipavirus (Paramyxoviridae). In: Tidona CA, Darai G, eds. *The Springer index of viruses*. Berlin, Heidelberg, New York, Toyko: Springer-Verlag, 2001 (in press).
43. De Leeuw O, Peeters B. Complete nucleotide sequence of Newcastle disease virus: evidence for the existence of a new genus within the subfamily Paramyxovirinae. *J Gen Virol* 1999; 80: 131-6.

Emergence and Control of Zoonotic Ortho- and Paramyxovirus Diseases
B. Dodet, M. Vicari, eds.

The Nipah outbreak and control response in Malaysia

Lam Sai Kit, Chua Kaw Bing
Department of Medical Microbiology, Faculty of Medicine, University of Malaya, Kuala Lumpur, Malaysia

An outbreak of severe febrile encephalitis associated with the deaths of pig farmers was reported in the state of Perak, Malaysia in September 1998 [1, 2]. The outbreak was associated with respiratory illness in pigs and was initially attributed to Japanese encephalitis (JE). JE is a mosquito-borne viral disease that is enzootic in the region, and pigs are among the amplifying vertebrate hosts. Despite efforts to control this mosquito-borne virus, by February 1999, similar diseases in pigs and humans were recognized in other states of Malaysia. This was associated with the illegal movement of infected pigs into the new outbreak areas. In March 1999, a cluster of 11 cases of respiratory and encephalitis illnesses was noted in Singapore in abattoir workers who had handled pigs from the outbreak areas in Malaysia [3]. The Singapore outbreak ended when the importation of pigs from Malaysia was prohibited, and the outbreak in Malaysia ceased when over 1 million pigs were culled from the outbreak and immediate surrounding areas [4, 5]. A total of 265 cases of encephalitis, including 105 deaths, were associated with the outbreak in Malaysia.

Although JE is endemic and occurs sporadically in Malaysia, the epidemiological characteristics of the present outbreak were distinct from those associated with JE. Most of the cases occurred in adult males who worked with pigs, with very few case patients among young children. Mosquito control and JE vaccination programmes did not affect the course of the outbreak. Illnesses and deaths among infected pigs discounted the possibility of JE.

Virology

In early March 1999, Vero cells inoculated with cerebrospinal fluid specimens from three fatal cases of encephalitis developed syncytia after 5 days [6]. The infected cells did not react with antibodies to known paramyxoviruses or other encephalitic viruses, including JE. However, the isolate stained positively with antibodies against Hendra virus by indirect immunofluorescence. Cross-neutralization studies resulted in an 8 to16-fold difference in neutralizing antibodies between the isolate and Hendra virus, indicating that the two viruses, though related, were not identical.

Electron microscopic (EM) studies of the virus, named Nipah virus, demonstrated features characteristic of a virus belonging to the family *Paramyxoviridae* [7]. This family of viruses typically possesses a single-stranded nonsegmental RNA genome of negative polarity that is fully encapsidated by protein. Virus particles vary in size from 120 to 500 nm. Thin-section EM studies of infected cells revealed filamentous nucleocapsids within cytoplasmic inclusions and incorporated into virions budding from the plasma membrane. Typical "herringbone" nucleocapsid structures were observed by means of negative stain preparations.

Initial RT-PCR experiments allowed the entire nucleoprotein (N) gene and 700 nucleotides from the 3' terminus of the phosphoprotein (P) gene to be amplified [8]. Nipah virus differed from Hendra by 21-25% at the nucleotide level in N and P, respectively. The predicted N protein of Nipah virus differed from that of Hendra at 42 amino acid positions (8.0%). Based on these findings, Hendra virus and Nipah virus represent a unique genus within the *Paramyxoviridae* family.

Clinical features

The clinical features of ninety-four patients seen in the University Hospital of Kuala Lumpur have been published [9]. The mean age of the patients was 37 years with a ratio of male to female patients of 4.5:1. Ninety-three percent had been in direct contact with pigs, usually within two weeks before the onset of illness. The main presenting features were fever, headache, dizziness and vomiting. Fifty-two patients had a reduced level of consciousness and prominent brainstem dysfunction. Distinctive clinical signs included segmental myoclonus, areflexia and hypotonia, hypertension and tachycardia, suggesting the involvement of the brainstem and the upper cervical spinal cord. Thirty patients died following rapid deterioration of their condition. An abnormal doll's eye reflex and tachycardia were factors associated with a poor prognosis. Fifty patients recovered fully, and fourteen had persistent neurologic deficits.

After one year of study and follow up, 12 patients developed relapses of encephalitic illness. These patients had either neurological symptoms after an initial illness without re-exposure to the pigs, or long latency from the initial exposure to the virus till the development of neurological symptoms. The onset of symptoms during relapses was acute. The symptoms and signs were fever, headache, focal neurological signs, seizure, dizziness, reduced consciousness and myoclonus. It was noted that 2 of the patients died, 3 patients developed cognitive impairment, 2 developed cerebellar signs, dyphasia and opthalmoplegia.

Histopathology

Post-mortem samples from virus cultured positive patients showed histological findings of endothelial damage and vasculitis, mainly in arterioles, capillaries and venules. The brain was the most severely affected organ, but other organs including the lungs, heart, and kidney were also affected. Vasculitic vessels were characterized by vessel-wall necrosis, thrombosis and inflammatory-cell infiltration of neutrophils and mononuclear cells. Syncytial cell formation was seen in the endothelium of affected blood vessels in the brain and lung, and in the Bowman's capsule of the glomerulus. Zones of microinfarction and ischaemia were commonly found around or adjacent to vasculitic blood vessels. In the brain, many neurons had eosinophilic cytoplasmic and nuclear viral inclusions such as seen with other paramyxovirus infections.

Imaging features [10]

The brains of Nipah patients were imaged by computed tomography (CT) or magnetic resonance imaging (MRI). There were no abnormalities found by CT but MRI of the brain performed on 31 patients with Nipah encephalitis demonstrated the presence of discrete high-signal-intensity lesions, measuring 2-7 mm, disseminated throughout the brain, mainly in the subcortical and deep white matter of the cerebral hemispheres. There was no correlation with the focal neurologic signs, depth of coma, and outcome of the patients. The lesions were attributed to widespread microinfarctions from underlying vasculitis of cerebral small vessels. Features found on MRI in relapsed and late-onset encephalitis differed from the features in acute encephalitis in that confluent cortical involvement was the prominent finding in the former, as opposed to discrete focal lesions in the subcortical and deep white matter in the latter.

Control measures and responses

As with most emerging infectious diseases, there was considerable panic and fear among the local population during the Nipah virus outbreak. When it was thought to be due to JE, the government response was to control the mosquito vectors in the pig farms by fogging and larviciding and at the same time to offer JE immunization to those at risk. Thousands of pigs in the outbreak areas were also immunized at substantial cost to the government.

With the discovery of Nipah virus as the causative agent, JE control measures were replaced by more appropriate measures. Health Education and advice to people working in porcine related activities was given through the distribution of health education materials and through the electronic media such as the national radio and TV channels.

Personal protection was issued to ensure that those involved in these areas were protected. The message focused on the proper use of goggles, gloves, gowns, boots and overalls when a worker had to deal with live and dead pigs. Since the virus is quite labile, advice was given on the use of soap and detergents to destroy the virus. Special instructions were given to high-risk groups through health officers and veterinary officers in the state and districts.

As with other zoonotic diseases involving humans and farm animals, culling of the animals in infected farms was conducted. These operations were carried out by the Health Department, the Armed Forces, Police, Veterinary Services Department, Local Authority, Public Works Department, Fire and Rescue Department, Welfare Services Department and many others. Altogether, over a million pigs were culled and this resulted in the decline of cases.

As far as the control response in clinical cases is concerned, active case control detection was initiated among farm workers and their families. Protocols and guidelines for patient management were developed and ribavirin was offered to anyone from the outbreak areas with early symptoms. Special wards were set up to cater to the increasing number of patients and universal precautions were practiced at all times to prevent nosocomial infections.

One of the control responses in the handling of emerging infectious diseases is the use of the appropriate approach in laboratory investigations. Instead of using serology and polymerase chain reaction to confirm that the outbreak was due to JE, the laboratory investigation after it had spread outside of Perak involved the "catch-all" method of virus isolation. The identification of the isolate included exclusion of all agents known to cause viral encephalitis in Malaysia. International assistance was sought from the Centers for Disease Control and Prevention, Atlanta, and the isolate was shown to be antigenically related but distinct from the Australian Hendra virus.

Twelve experts from the CDC, Atlanta, two from the Commonwealth Scientific and Industrial Research Organization (CSIRO), Geelong, and one from the Animal Research Institute, Queensland were invited to Malaysia to assist in the control and investigation of the outbreak. A Task Force Laboratory was promptly set up by the CDC to conduct serological diagnosis in human cases and a veterinary laboratory conducted the testing of animal sera under the supervision of the Australian scientists. The role played by these international experts was much appreciated in helping to bring the outbreak under control.

Conclusion

Emerging infectious diseases involving zoonosis are estimated to be three times more likely than non-zoonotic diseases and are likely to reappear. There were many lessons learned during the Nipah virus outbreak and many issues related to the control measures taken by Malaysia. It is felt that by analyzing the control responses taken in Malaysia, we should be placed in a better position to handle future outbreaks of a similar nature.

References

1. Outbreak of Hendra-like virus – Malaysia and Singapore, 1998-1999. *MMWR* 1999; 48: 265-9.
2. Update: outbreak of Nipah virus – Malaysia and Singapore, 1999. *MMWR* 1999; 48: 335-7.
3. Paton NI, Leo YS, Zaki SR, *et al.* Outbreak of Nipah-virus infection among abattoir workers in Singapore. *Lancet* 1999; 354: 1253-6.
4. Sering M. New virus fingered in Malaysian epidemic. *Science* 1999; 284: 407-10.
5. Parashar UD, Lye MS, Ong F, *et al.* Case-control study of risk factors for human infection with a new zoonotic paramyxovirus, Nipah virus, during a 1998-1999 outbreak of severe encephalitis in Malaysia. *J Infect Dis* 2000; 181: 1755-9.
6. Chua KB, Goh KJ, Wong KT, *et al.* Fatal encephalitis due to Nipah virus among pig farmers in Malaysia. *Lancet* 1999; 354: 1257-9.
7. Chua KB, Bellini WJ, Rota PA, *et al.* Nipah virus: A recently emergent deadly paramyxovirus. *Science* 2000; 288: 1432-5.

8. Harcourt BH, Tamin A, Ksiazek TG, *et al.* Molecular characterization of Nipah virus, a newly emergent paramyxovirus. *Virology* 2000; 271: 334-49.
9. Goh KJ, Tan CT, Chew NK, *et al.* Clinical features of Nipah virus encephalitis among pig farmers in Malaysia. *N Engl J Med* 2000; 342: 1229-35.
10. Sazilah Ahmad Sarji, *et al.* MR Imaging of Nipah encephalitis. *Am J Roentgenology* 2000; 175: 437-42.

Emergence and Control of Zoonotic Ortho- and Paramyxovirus Diseases
B. Dodet, M. Vicari, eds.

Emerging zoonotic paramyxoviruses: the role of pteropid bats

Hume E. Field[1], John S. Mackenzie[2], Leslie S. Hall[3]
[1] *Department of Primary Industries, Animal Research Institute, Moorooka, Australia*
[2] *Department of Microbiology and Parasitology, University of Queensland, Brisbane, Australia*
[3] *School of Veterinary Science, University of Queensland, Brisbane, Australia*

The behavioural ecology of many bat species identifies them as potentially efficient vertebrate disseminator hosts of mammalian viruses. Further, it has been suggested that bats are unique in their response to viral infections, in that they are able to sustain viral infections in the absence of overt disease [1]. Certainly a wide range of viral infections (including flaviviruses, alphaviruses, rhabdoviruses, arenaviruses, reoviruses, and paramyxoviruses) has been identified in bats [1], but their epidemiological significance has often been unclear. The recent emergence of Hendra and Nipah viruses represents a quantum leap in the significance of bat-associated viruses to human and animal health [2].

Novel paramyxo-viruses identified

Hendra virus, a novel zoonotic paramyxovirus (initially called equine morbillivirus), was first described in September 1994 in an outbreak of disease in horses in Australia. Twenty one horses[1] and two humans were infected, with the resultant deaths of 14 horses and one human [3-5]. In two foci further (the most recent in January 1999), three horses and one human were infected, all fatally [6-9]. Human cases have been attributed to exposure to infected horses [10, 11]. Extensive wildlife surveillance has identified pteropid bats (flying foxes) as a natural host of Hendra virus, with infection endemic in the four mainland Australian species *(Pteropus alecto*, *P. poliocephalus*, *P. scapulatus* and *P. conspicillatus)* [12, 13, Field: in preparation]. The related Nipah virus was first identified in 1999 as the primary aetiological agent in a major outbreak of disease in pigs and humans in Peninsular Malaysia [14, 15]. Approximately 1.1 million pigs were culled to contain the outbreak. Of 265 reported human cases, 105 were fatal. Direct contact with infected pigs was identified as the predominant mode of human infection [16, 17]. Preliminary wildlife surveillance found serological evidence of infection in two species of flying foxes, *Pteropus vampyrus* and *P. hypomelanus* [18]. The recent isolation of virus from *P. hypomelanus* (Chua *et al.*: manuscripted submitted) strengthens the contention that flying foxes are a natural host of Nipah virus.

1. The revised figures of 20 equine cases and 13 fatal equine cases are presented in some literature.

Another two novel paramyxoviruses (both members of the genus *Rubulavirus*) have also been recently associated with flying foxes. In Australia, Menangle virus was described in 1997 when it caused an outbreak of reproductive disease in pigs, and was the probable cause of a severe febrile illness in two piggery workers [19, 20]. In Malaysia, Tioman virus, closely related to Menangle virus, was isolated from *P. hypomelanus* during efforts to isolate Nipah virus from flying foxes [21].

Distribution and movement of pteropid bats

There are about 60 species of bats in the genus *Pteropus* which are commonly referred to as flying foxes. The world distribution of flying foxes extends from the West Indian Ocean islands of Mauritius, Madagascar and Comoro, along the sub-Himalayan region of Pakistan and India, through South-East Asia, the Philippines, Indonesia, New Guinea, the South-West Pacific Islands as far East as the Cook Islands, and Australia excluding Tasmania. They are not found on mainland Africa, Europe, Asia or North and South America. Thus they are often called Old World fruit bats, and based on their greatest diversity, originate from Sulawesi and Eastern New Guinea, where up to six species are found. Many species are restricted to islands, but a number are widespread. Flying foxes range in body weight from 300 g to over 1 kg, and in wingspan from 600 mm to 1.7 m. They are the largest bats in the world, do not echolocate and navigate at night by eyesight and their keen sense of smell. Females usually have only one young a year after a six month pregnancy. The young grow rapidly but are dependent on their mother for up to three months. All species eat plant products (most commonly fruits, flowers and pollen) and roost communally in trees [22-25].

Of the four species of flying foxes found on the Australian mainland, only the Grey-headed flying fox *(P. poliocephalus)* is restricted to Australia, and is found from Melbourne along coastal Eastern Australia to Bundaberg in Southern Queensland. Black flying foxes *(P. alecto)* are found from Kempsey in New South Wales, North around the coastal areas of Queensland, Northern Territory and Northern Western Australia down to about Carnarvon. Spectacled flying foxes *(P. conspicillatus)* are restricted to the wet tropics of Queensland, while Little Red flying foxes *(P. scapulatus)* have been recorded over a large part of the Eastern, Northern and Western parts of the Australian continent. All three are known to occur in New Guinea. The regional distribution of the Black flying fox extends across to the Indonesian islands of Sulawesi, Lombok, Kangean and Baeween. The Spectacled flying fox is found over coastal New Guinea and on the Indonesian island of Halmahera [22, 23].

Where species distributions overlap, roosting camps are commonly shared. For example, in Northern Australia, Black and Spectacled flying foxes share camps with each other, and in New Guinea and Indonesia, with other species of flying foxes found there [22, 26]. Observations of flying fox movements to the immediate North of Australia have shown a yearly movement cycle which involved flying foxes moving from New Guinea to the islands of Torres Strait, down to Cape York in Northern Australia, and back into New Guinea [27]. The possibility of movements of flying foxes between New Guinea, Indonesian islands and South-East Asia has never been studied; however, there is anecdotal evidence that flying foxes can cross large distances over water [25, 28]. Within Australia, flying foxes are known to travel over considerable distances. Radio-tagged Grey-headed flying foxes in Eastern Australia have been shown to undertake regular long distance movements covering up to 600 km. The species is also known to move from one camp to another following good flowering of native trees. These movements cause fluctuating numbers in roosting camps and indicate a state of population flux over the whole range [29, 30]. These host features led us to suggest the possibility of Hendra-related viruses in other pteropid species, and the potential for interspecies transmission of infectious agents. The subsequent discovery of anti-Hendra antibodies in *Pteropus* and *Dobsonia* bat species in New Guinea (Field *et al.*: in preparation), and of Nipah virus and Tioman virus in Malaysian flying foxes has added weight to this hypothesis. It is noteworthy that the overlapping distributions of only three species of flying foxes are needed to form a continuous link between the East coast of Australia and Pakistan. Black and Spectacled flying foxes overlap with the Island flying fox *(P. hypomelanus)* and the Malayan flying fox *(P. vampyrus)* in New Guinea and Indonesia, and these species, at the Northern extent of their range, overlap with the Indian flying fox *(P. giganteus)*, whose distribution extends Eastward (from Thailand and Burma) across to India and Pakistan [23, 31]. This link can be demonstrated with two separate groups of flying foxes.

Factors precipitating emergence?

The available evidence suggests that Hendra and Nipah are ancient viruses [2, 32], well adapted to their natural flying fox hosts, and in whose populations they have long circulated. The close phylogenetic relationship between Hendra and Nipah and between Mcnangle and Tioman suggests a common progenitor virus for each related pair. However, it also appears that flying fox populations in Australia and Malaysia have been separate for a length of time sufficient for the respective viruses of each pair to evolve further in geographic isolation. So why are we seeing these diseases emerge now? In answering this question, it is appropriate to distinguish between emergence and detection. The identification of flying foxes as a probable natural host of these viruses can largely be attributed to increased surveillance of bats after the initial discovery of antibodies to Hendra virus in Australian bats. However, improved surveillance efforts or diagnostic capabilities cannot adequately explain the emergence *per se* of the viruses. Disease emergence requires, in addition to the presence of an agent, an effective bridge from the natural host to a susceptible spillover host. Such bridges result from anthropogenic or natural changes to the agent, the host, or the environment. Available data on many fruit bat species suggests that populations in Australia and South-East Asia are in decline and disruption throughout their range. In South-East Asia, anthropogenic activities (primarily habitat loss and hunting) have been identified as constituting the major threats. Deforestation, whether for agricultural land, commercial logging, or urban development, is widespread and results in loss or abandonment of roosting sites, and the loss of feeding habitats. Secondarily, habitat loss due to clearing is commonly exacerbated by tropical storms, the remnant forest being particularly prone to high wind damage. Hunting, whether for consumption or crop protection, and at both a local and at a commercial level, results in the abandonment of roost and feeding sites [23]. A scenario emerges of fruit bat populations under stress, of altered foraging and behavioural patterns, of niche expansion, and of closer proximity to man. In Australia, the geographic redistribution of roosting sites has been increasingly into urban areas in recent decades (Hall: personal communication).

The emergence of Nipah virus disease provides a case study illustration of anthropogenic factors contributing to the process of disease emergence [33]. The establishment of pig farms in areas of high natural host activity facilitated the introduction of infection into the pig population; the maintenance of high densities of pigs led to the rapid dissemination of the infection within local pig populations, and the transport of pigs to other geographic areas for commerce led to the rapid spread of disease in pigs in Southern Malaysia and Singapore. The presence of a high-density, amplifying host population facilitated transmission of the virus to humans. Had horizontal transmission occurred in humans, the worst-case emergence scenario would have been realised.

If the necessary and sufficient precipitating factors exist across the distribution of all pteropid species, the emergence of further novel agents may be expected unless these factors can be addressed.

References

1. Sulkin S, Allen R. Virus infections in bats. In: Melnick J, ed. *Monographs in Virology*. Vol. 8. New York, 1974: 170-5.
2. Field H, Young P, Johara Mohd Yob, Mills J, Hall L, Mackenzie J. The natural history of Hendra and Nipah viruses. *Microb Infect* 2001; 3: 315-22.
3. Murray K, Selleck P, Hooper P, *et al.* A morbillivirus that caused fatal disease in horses and humans. *Science* 1995; 268: 94-7.
4. Douglas IC, Baldock FC, Black P. Outbreak investigation of an emerging disease (equine morbillivirus). In: *Epidemiol Sante Anim* – Proc of 8th ISVEE conference. Paris, 1997: 04.08.1-04.08.3.
5. Baldock FC, Douglas IC, Halpin K, Field H, Young PL, Black PF. Epidemiological investigations into the 1994 equine morbillivirus outbreaks in Queensland, Australia. *Sing Vet J* 1996; 20: 57-61.
6. Rogers RJ, Douglas IC, Baldock FC, *et al.* Investigation of a second focus of equine morbillivirus infection in coastal Queensland. *Aust Vet J* 1996; 74: 243-4.
7. Hooper PT, Gould AR, Russell GM, Kattenbelt JA, Mitchell G. The retrospective diagnosis of a second outbreak of equine morbillivirus infection. *Aust Vet J* 1996; 74: 244-5.
8. Field H, Barratt P, Hughes R, Shield J, Sullivan N. A fatal case of Hendra virus infection in a horse in north Queensland: clinical and epidemiological features. *Aust Vet J* 2000; 78: 279-80.
9. Hooper P, Gould A, Hyatt A, *et al.* Identification and molecular characterisation of Hendra virus in a horse in Queensland. *Aust Vet J* 2000; 78: 281-2.
10. Selvey L, Wells RM, McCormack JG, *et al.* Infection of humans and horses by a newly described morbillivirus. *Med J Aust* 1995; 162: 642-5.
11. O'Sullivan JD, Allworth AM, Paterson DL, *et al.* Fatal encephalitis due to novel paramyxovirus transmitted from horses. *Lancet* 1997; 349: 93-5.
12. Young PL, Halpin K, Selleck PW, *et al.* Serologic evidence for the presence in Pteropus bats of a paramyxovirus related to equine morbillivirus. *Emerg Infect Dis* 1996; 2: 239-40.
13. Halpin K, Young P, Field H, Mackenzie J. Isolation of Hendra virus from pteropid bats: a natural reservoir of Hendra virus. *J Gen Virol* 2000; 81: 1927-32.
14. CDC. Outbreak of Hendra-like virus – Malaysia and Singapore, 1998-1999. *MMWR* 1999; 48: 265-9.
15. CDC. Update: Outbreak of Nipah Virus – Malaysia and Singapore, 1999. *MMWR* 1999; 48.
16. Chua K, Bellini W, Rota P, *et al.* Nipah virus: A recently emergent deadly paramyxovirus. *Science* 2000; 288: 1432-5.
17. Goh KJ, Tan TC, Chew NK, *et al.* Clinical features of Nipah virus encephalitis among pig farmers in Malaysia. *N Engl J Med* 2000; 342 (17).
18. Mohd Yob J, Field H, Mohd Rashdi A, *et al.* Serological evidence of infection with Nipah virus in bats (order Chiroptera) in Peninsular Malaysia. *Emerg Infect Dis* (Accepted November 2000).

19. Philbey A, Kirkland P, Ross A, *et al.* An Apparently New Virus (Family *Paramyxoviridae*) Infectious for Pigs, Humans and Fruit bats. *Emerg Infect Dis* 1998; 4: 269-71.
20. Chant K, Chan R, Smith M, Dwyer D, Kirkland P. Probable Human Infection with a newly Described Virus in the Family *Paramyxoviridae*. *Emerg Infect Dis* 1998; 4: 273-5.
21. Chua K, Wang LF, Lam SK, Crameri G, Yu M, Wise T, Boyle D, Hyatt AD, Eaton BT. Tioman virus, a novel.
22. Hall L. Identification, distribution and taxonomy of Australian flying-foxes (Chiroptera: Pteropodidae). *Aust Mammol* 1987; 10: 75-9.
23. Mickleburg S, Hutson A, Racey P. *Old World Fruit Bats: an action plan for their conservation.* Gland, Switzerland: Internation Union for the Conservation of Nature and Natural Resources (IUCN), 1992.
24. Corbett G, Hill J. *A world list of mammalian species.* London: British Museum (Natural History), 1986.
25. Nowak R. *Walker's bats of the world.* Baltimore: The Johns Hopkins University Press, 1994.
26. Waithman J. A report on a collection of mammals from southwest Papua 1992-1993. *Aust Zool* 1979; 20: 313-26.
27. Hall L, Richards G. Flying-foxes, fruit and blossom bats of Australia. Sydney: University of New South Wales Press Ltd, 2000.
28. Daniel M. First report of an Australian fruit bat (Megachiroptera: Pteropodidae) reaching New Zealand. *NZ J Zool* 1975; 2: 227-31.
29. Eby P. Seasonal movements of Grey-headed flying-foxes, Pteropus poliocephalus (Chiroptera: Pteropodidae), from two maternity camps in northern New South Wales. *Wildlife Res* 1991; 18: 547-59.
30. Eby P. *The biology and management of flying-foxes in New South Wales.* Hurstville, Sydney: New South Wales National Parks and Wildlife Service, 1995: 72 p.
31. Corbet G, Hill J. *The mammals of the IndoMalayan region.* Oxford, UK: Natural History Museum Publications, Oxford University Press, 1992.
32. Gould AR. Comparison of the deduced matrix and fusion protein sequences of equine morbillivirus with cognate genes of the Paramyxoviridae. *Virus Res* 1996; 43: 17-31.
33. Morse SS. Factors in the emergence of infectious diseases. *Emerg Infect Dis* 1995; 1: 7-15.

List of contributors

Dennis J. ALEXANDER
Central Veterinary Laboratory Agency
Wooden Lane
New Haw
Addelstone/Weybridge Surrey KT15-3NB
United Kingdom
Tel. : 441 932 357 466
Fax : 441 932 357 856
Email : dalexander.vla@gtnet.gov.uk

Max J.G. APPEL
James A. Baker Institute for Animal Health
College of Veterinary Medicine
Cornell University
Box 53
Ithaca NY 14853 USA
Tel. : 1 607 256 56 03
Fax : 1 607 256 56 08
Email : mja13@cornell.edu

Michèle AYMARD
Laboratoire de Virologie
CHU de Lyon
Université Claude-Bernard Lyon 1
8, avenue Rockefeller
69373 Lyon Cedex 08, France
Tel. : 04 78 77 70 29
Fax : 04 78 01 48 87
Email : aymard@rockefeller univ-lyon1.fr

Ian H. BROWN
Central Veterinary Laboratory Agency
Weybridge
New Haw
Addlestone Surrey KT15-3NB
United Kingdom
Tel. : 44 1932 35 73 39
Fax : 44 1932 35 72 39
Email : Ian.I.H.Brown@vla.maff.gsi.gov.uk

Thomas M. CHAMBERS
Department of Veterinary Science
108 GROG Center
Kentucky University
Lexington Kentucky 405-099
Tel. : 1 606 257 34 07
Fax : 1 606 257 85 42
Email : tmcham1@pop.uky.edu

Thierry CHILLAUD
Office National des Épizooties
12, rue Prony
75017 Paris, Cedex 15 France
Tel. : 33 (0)1 44 15 18 88
Fax : 33 (0)1 42 67 09 87
Email : t.chillaud@oie.int

Bruno B. CHOMEL
University of California
Department of Population Health and Reproduction
School of Veterinary Medicine
Davis CA 95616, USA
Tel. : 1 530 752 81 12
Fax : 1 530 752 23 77
Email : bbchomel@ucdavis.edu

Peter DASZAK
Consortium for Conservation Medicine
LDEO, 61 Route 9W
Palisades
New York 10964-8000, USA
Tel. : +1 845 365 8337
Fax : +1 845 365 8177
Email : daszak@aol.com

Betty DODET
Fondation Mérieux
17, rue Bourgelat
BP 2021
69227 Lyon Cedex 02, France
Tel. : 33 (0)4 72 40 79 72
Fax : 33 (0)4 72 40 79 50
Email : betty.dodet@fond-merieux.org

Hume E. FIELD
DPI Animal Research Institute
Queensland Department of Primary Industries
LMB 4
Moorooka 4105
Brisbane, Australia
Tel. : 61 7 336 295 53
Fax : 61 7 336 294 57
Email : FieldH@prose.dpi.qld.gov.au

Lionel GÉRENTES
Laboratoire de Virologie
CHU de Lyon
Université Claude-Bernard Lyon 1
8, avenue Rockeffeler
69733 Lyon Cedex 03, France

Larisa V. GUBAREVA
University of Virginia
Department of internal medicine
PO Box 800473 Jeffersson Park Ave
Hospital West Multistory Blg Room 2153
Charlottesville Virginia 22 908, USA
Tel. : 1 804 243 27 05
Fax : 1 804 924 90 65
Email : LVG9B@virginia.edu

Nicole KESSLER
Laboratoire de Virologie
CHU de Lyon
Université Claude-Bernard Lyon 1
8, avenue Rockeffeler
69733 Lyon Cedex 03, France

Yoshihiro KAWAOKA
Department of Pathobiological Sciences
2015 Llndian Drive West
Madison Wiscounsin 53706, USA
Tel. : 1 608 265 49 25
Fax : 1 608 265 56 22
Email : kawaokay@svm.vetmed.wisc.edu

Lam Sai KIT
Department of Medical Microbiology
Faculty of Medicine
University of Malaya
50603 Kuala Lumpur, Malaysia
Tel. : 603 750 23 24
Fax : 603 758 28 01
Email : lamsk@medicine.med.um.edu.my

John S. MACKENZIE
Department of Microbiology and Parasitology
University of Queensland
Brisbane QLD 4072, Australia
Tel. : 1 61 7 3365 4648
Fax : 1 61 7 3365 6225
Email : jmac@biosci.uq.edu.au

François MOUTOU
AFSSA
BP 67
94703 Maisons-Alfort Cedex, France
Tel. : 01 49 77 13 33
Fax : 01 43 68 97 62
Email : f.moutou@afssa.fr

Jenny A. MUMFORD
Animal Health Trust
Lanwades Park
Kentford
New Market Suffolk CB8 7UU Grande-Bretagne
Tel. : 44 16 38 75 06 59
Fax : 44 16 38 75 07 94
Email : j.mumford@aht.org.uk

Albert D.M.E. OSTERHAUS
Erasmus University Rotterdam
Institute of Virology
National Influenza Center
PO Box 1738
3000DR Rotterdam, Pays-Bas
Tel. : 31 10 408 80 66
Fax : 31 10 408 94 85
Email : osterhaus@viro.fgg.eur.nl

Kennedy F. SHORTRIGE
The University of Hong Kong
Department of Microbiology
Pathology Building
Queen Mary Hospital Compound
Hong Kong, Hong Kong
Tel. : 852 28 55 43 45
Fax : 852 28 55 12 41
Email : microgen@hkuco.hku.hk

David E. SWAYNE
USDA
Agriculture Research Service
Southeast Poultry Research Laboratory
934 College Station Road
Athens GA 30605, USA
Tel. : 706 546 34 33
Fax : 1 706 546 31 61
Email : dswayne@seprl.usda.gov

Sylvie VAN DER WERF
Institut Pasteur
Génétique Moléculaire des Virus Respiratoires
28, rue du Dr-Roux
75724 Paris Cedex 15, France
Tel. : 01 45 68 87 22/25
Fax : 01 40 61 32 41
Email : swdwerf@pasteur.fr

Lin-Fa WANG
CSIRO Livesstock Industries
Australian Animal Health Laboratory
PO Bag 24
Geelong Victoria 3220, Australia
Tel. : 61 3 5227 5121
Fax : 61 3 5227 5555
Email : Linfa.Wang@li.csiro.au

Kristien VAN REETH
Faculty of Veterinary Medicine
Laboratory of Veterinary Virology
University of Gent
Salisburylaan 133
B-9820 Merelbeke, Belgium
Tel. : 32 9 264 73 69
Fax : 32 9 264 74 95
Email : kristien.VanReeth@rug.ac.be

John M. WOOD
National Institute for Biological Standards
and Control
Blanche Lane
South Mimms
Potters Bar Herts EN6 3QG
United Kingdom
Tel. : 44 1 707 654 753
Fax : 44 1 707 646 730
Email : jwood@nibsc.ac.uk

Achevé d'imprimer par Corlet, Imprimeur, S.A.
14110 Condé-sur-Noireau (France)
N° d'Imprimeur : 54048 - Dépôt légal : septembre 2001
Imprimé en U.E.